High Angle Rescue Techniques

HIGH ANGLE RESCUE TECHNIQUES

SECOND EDITION

TOM VINES
Training Officer
Carbon County Sheriff's Search and Rescue
Red Lodge, Montana

STEVE HUDSON
President, Pigeon Mountain Industries, Inc.
Deputy Director, Walker County Emergency
Management
Lafayette, Georgia

with 491 illustrations

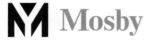 Mosby

St. Louis Baltimore Boston Carlsbad Chicago Minneapolis New York Philadelphia Portland
London Milan Sydney Tokyo Toronto

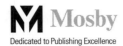
Mosby
Dedicated to Publishing Excellence

Vice President and Publisher: Don E. Ladig
Editor: Jennifer Roche
Developmental Editor: Tamara Myers
Project Manager: Mark Spann
Senior Production Editor: Julie Eddy
Senior Composition Specialist: Wendy Bellm
Book Design Manager: Judi Lang
Cover Designer: Teresa Breckwoldt
Manufacturing Supervisor: Don Carlisle
Illustrations by: Stella Carpenter Twilley
Photography by: David Scott Smith, William L. Renaker, Steve Hudson

SECOND EDITION

Copyright © 1999 by Mosby, Inc.

Previous Editions copyrighted 1989, 1992

Printed in the United States of America
Composition by Mosby Electronic Production
Illustration preparation by TOP Graphics
Printing/binding by R.R. Donnelley & Sons Company

Mosby, Inc.
11830 Westline Industrial Drive
St. Louis, MO 63146

Library of Congress Cataloging-in-Publication Data
Vines, Tom
    High angle rescue techniques/Tom Vines, Steve Hudson. —2nd ed.
        p.   cm.
    Includes bibliographical references (p. 245) and index.
    1. Rappelling.   2. Rope.   3. Knots and splices.
    4. Mountaineering—Search and rescue operations—United States.
    5. Rescue work—United States.   I. Hudson, Steve, 1950– .
    II. Title.
    GV200. 19.R34V56   1999
    363.14—dc21

                                                    98–31692
                                                    CIP

98 99 00 01 / 9 8 7 6 5 4 3 2 1

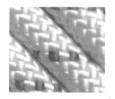

Surely the greatest test of friendship is writing a book together. Publishing has its rewards but by its very nature it involves constant pressures along with periods of frustration and disappointment. Working with others to publish a complex text such as this one, with the tension of deadlines, pressures to create, and the necessity to compromise, can easily stress the healthiest ego. The history of publishing is littered with former coauthors who now no longer speak to one another and even with authors' significant others who no longer speak to one another.

There are many who contributed to this book and who, over the years, enhanced our knowledge. But we hope that those many people who deserve mention will understand as we make an unconventional book dedication. Despite having created two editions of the book, both very difficult and challenging experiences, we still remain friends. Consequently, we dedicate this second edition of *High Angle Rescue Techniques* to one another. We both realize that without the other's contribution and perhaps more importantly, the tolerance, understanding, and encouragement from one another, this book would never have been possible.

Tom Vines
Steve Hudson

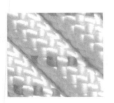

Introduction

About a decade has passed since the first publication of *High Angle Rescue Techniques,* and it seems like light years in rescue history. The past several years have seen a great revolution in all aspects of the high angle environment, particularly in rope rescue. There have been great changes in equipment (rope and hardware) and in techniques (how equipment is used). Much of the equipment and many of the techniques, formerly accepted, have been questioned. Only truly sound practices have survived.

Another important change has been the increased number of disciplines involved in rope rescue. Some time ago, it was primarily country and mountain rescuers who were involved in rope rescue. Now, those rescuers have been joined by the fire fighting community. The increasing number of National Fire Protection Agency standards that are related to rope rescue reflects this involvement. More recently, industry has become increasingly involved in rescue. The United States Federal Occupational Safety and Health Administration (OSHA) has become involved, issuing rules regulating industrial rescue, particularly confined space rescue.

Rope rescue concepts have leapt borders. During the past decade, the cross border union in North America has contributed greatly to the advances in rope rescue. The tandem Prusik belay system and load releasing hitch were both refined by British Columbia rescuers in collaborative efforts such as the Penticton Rescue Workshops during the 1970s and 1980s. These techniques found their way into the United States through forums such as the North American Technical Rescue Symposium and the Wildlands Rescue Workshop.

Perhaps most importantly, rope rescue has developed a sense of community. Knowledge is being developed and shared among the many professionals who practice in the field. No one ever stops learning. Each time we work with someone new, teach a class, work a rescue, or just discuss ropework with others, we learn more about the high angle environment. The greatest benefit for all of us in the rescue community is our working together to share this common knowledge. This sense of community and teamwork are vital to the advancement in rescue technology.

The world of rope rescue is too complex and changing to be dominated by any one authority or expert. Neither one of the authors considers himself to be *the* expert in the field. We do feel, however, that we have been in the fortunate position of having access to a great deal of information from many different sources in North America and Europe. Our feeling is that the best service we can make to the people in this field is to provide them with the best possible information available, collected from many reliable resources; this is what *High Angle Rescue Techniques* is all about.

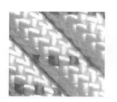

How To Use This Book

High Angle Rescue Techniques has evolved over many years. Many people have commented and made suggestions on the first edition. Where possible, we have implemented that feedback into this edition. We realize that this book's usefulness and popularity have been due to its simplicity. Consequently, this text will remain a manual for basic and team rope rescue. Remember that this book is designed as a training manual to be used under the guidance of a qualified instructor. High angle ropework is a dangerous activity. To be both safe and effective, you must have tools specifically designed for rope rescue and the knowledge to use them. For these reasons, this is not intended to be a self-instructional text.

High Angle Rescue Techniques is divided into two sections. The first nine chapters are concerned with personal rope skills basic to becoming a high angle rope technician. The second half of the book focuses on rescue skills that every rescue team must have.

High Angle Rescue Techniques is also a step-by-step manual, creating a series of building blocks in high angle training. In this manner, the most critical skills, such as knowledge of rope and equipment, are covered initially. These are followed by skills such as belaying and rappelling. Finally, everything is put together in the last chapters, which focus on team rescue skills.

Here is a list of some of the special features used in each chapter of this book:

WARNING BOXES
Warning boxes warn of an operational procedure, practice, or condition that may result in injury or death if not carefully observed. They are one of the most important features of this manual. Always remember that the high angle environment is a dangerous one; when you find one of these warnings in the text, *stop* and carefully *read* the warning. Make certain you understand it before proceeding.

CAUTION BOXES
Caution boxes warn of an operational procedure, practice, or condition that may result in damage to the equipment if not carefully observed. Although the Caution boxes are not as vital as the warning boxes, paying attention to these boxes will help you preserve equipment and prevent certain dangerous situations.

SUGGESTION BOXES
In many aspects of the high angle environment, there are small hints, often learned through years of experience, which may make the job easier. Throughout this text, these are listed in the Suggestion boxes.

OBJECTIVES
Each chapter lists a number of objectives that relate to knowledge or skills you should be able to display after completing that chapter. Mastery of this information or these skills indicates you have taken steps toward competency as a high angle rope technician. Proper instruction is critical in mastering the objectives. You cannot assume you have mastered a concept or skill without a qualified evaluation.

KEY TERMS

A command of the language of the high angle environment is essential for good communication in that environment. Terminology for high angle rope work comes from several different languages and from diverse activities such as mountaineering, caving, sailing, fire fighting, and textile manufacturing. It is important to know that some of these terms may have a unique or expanded meaning in high angle rescue terminology.

At the beginning of each chapter you will find lists of new words introduced in that particular chapter. All these words, in addition to some other terms of interest, are reproduced together in the Glossary at the end of the text. And all of the key terms and glossary terms are bold faced and italicized throughout the text.

EVALUATION EXERCISES

To help you in the learning process, the end of each chapter has Cognitive and Affective Exercises that focus on the major elements in that chapter. Use these questions to see if you have grasped the important concepts in the chapter and check to see if your answers are correct in the Answer Key at the end of the book.

In most chapters, there are also Psychomotor Exercises that are designed to help you review specific physical skills related to the high angle environment.

ADVANTAGES AND DISADVANTAGES

High angle rescue is a discipline in which some inflexible rules are necessary for safety. However, in some cases there are safe choices for both equipment and technique. In this manual, we have tried to provide all viable options. Our philosophy is that the ideal high angle rope technician is one who is well trained and has the ability to adapt to any kind of situation. A better-informed rescuer can make intelligent decisions, whatever the situation.

PREREQUISITES

Beginning with Chapter 9, Rappelling, Prerequisites are listed before each chapter. It is very important that you not move on to more advanced skills without first thoroughly mastering the prerequisite skills. If this progression is not followed, you will have problems executing the skills, which could result in unsafe conditions for yourself and others. This list of Prerequisites can also serve as ready guidelines for reviewing important basics.

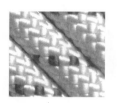

Acknowledgments

As with most projects the size of *High Angle Rescue Techniques,* this text, in both editions, represents the work of many more people than just the two authors. We would like to thank all those individuals and organizations who helped with the evolution of this project. It is impossible to list all of the individuals who have taught us techniques, made suggestions, listened to ideas, told us of mistakes (ours and theirs), introduced us to others with special skills, and all the other things that have helped shape our own knowledge. Many of these people were providing such help years before we started working on the new edition of this book. We are taking this opportunity to say, "Thank you!"

We would particularly like to acknowledge the contributors to the second edition: Mike Christie for emergency medical review and instructional materials, Loui Clem for technical review and standards information, Jon Heshka for technical review and Canadian perspective, and Ken Phillips for material on helicopter safety and operations.

Several individuals and organizations also deserve special acknowledgment for their direct contributions to our efforts over the years. Photographic resources, equipment and models, and other critical assistance were provided by: Billings Fire Department, Carbon County Montana Sheriff's Search and Rescue, Chattanooga-Hamilton County Rescue Service, Chattanooga Fire Department, Walker County Georgia Rescue, Pigeon Mountain Industries, Inc., Ken Fagen, Bill Renaker, Allen Padgett, Karen Padgett, Kenneth Huffines, Lisa Smith, Diane Cousineau, John Reid, Beth Elliott, Reggie Ferguson, Mark Wolinsky, Don Black, Sammy Manning, Bill Lord, Melinda Lord, Randolph Lane, Hank Moon, Buddy Lane, and Doranne Lane.

We also acknowledge Robert Canan, Linda Wilske, Michael J. Casey, Robin Pinkstaff, Steve Dewell, Joy Eden, Merle E. Froslie, Rob Spears, Russ Salo, Luke Furber, Tim Stavnes, Robert Golubski, David Gilbert, Sam Maness, and Sherry Cox. All of these people could not have donated their time unless their spouses, families, and employers were also willing to spare a little of their time. Once again, thank you all.

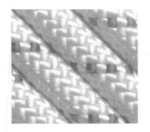

Contents

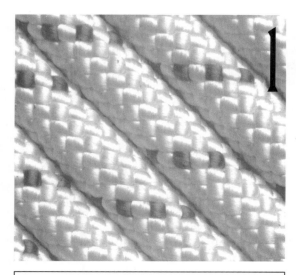

1 The High Angle Environment

Objectives ▼

At the completion of this chapter, you should be able to:

1. Define the primary difference between climbing and single rope technique (SRT).
2. Describe a situation that has potential for self-rescue.
3. State examples of equipment necessary for self-rescue situations.
4. Discuss the importance of practicing skills correctly every time and the use of evaluation tools.
5. State the universal warning call for falling or rolling objects.

Key Terms ▼

Belayer The person who controls a safety rope connected to another person or persons to keep them from falling.

Carabiner Metal snap links used to connect elements of a high angle system.

High Angle Very steep environment in which one must be secured with rope and other equipment to keep from falling.

Mountaineering The use of combined skills such as climbing and snow and ice travel to ascend a mountain.

Rappelling Using the friction of rope against one's body or through a descender to descend a rope under control.

Rock Climbing Ascending while making direct contact with the rock. Rope and other equipment may be used for safety in the event of a fall.

Rope Rescue The performing of rescue in high angle and steep slope environments where the use of rope and related equipment is necessary.

Single Rope Technique (SRT) Ascending and descending directly on the rope without direct aid by contact with the rock, walls, or structures.

System The combination of various components used in the high angle environment to construct a functioning unit; for example, a lowering or anchor system.

Vertical Caving Traveling through caves that have vertical, or near vertical, sections, which require the use of rope and ascending and descending equipment.

THE HIGH ANGLE ENVIRONMENT

Throughout history, humans have been able to conquer much of the world around them by devising means to operate comfortably in environments, such as the ocean, which nature had originally created hostile to them. One of the last environments conquered by humans is the high angle environment. Here, gravity is the great adversary. Although humans have not vanquished gravity, they have been able to create ways to temporarily overcome it and in some cases to use it to their advantage.

There are actually a number of different ways of operating in the high angle environment, depending on your needs.

Mountaineering

People have been engaged in the vertical sport of *mountaineering* for hundreds of years. Mountaineering combines a number of skills including climbing, camping, snow and ice travel, and often the test of will to survive against the very worst of natural forces. The most obvious goal may be reaching the top of a mountain, but there are often less obvious goals that include surviving the worst conditions in nature: cold, high wind, and high altitude illness.

Since World War II, there have been tremendous strides in mountaineering. Among the more significant is development of ropes using synthetic fibers.

Climbing

Climbing is a more specialized activity than mountaineering and is sometimes further defined as *rock climbing.* It may not involve much change in altitude or a walk much farther away than the parking lot. Furthermore it often may involve the ascent of a short piece of rock that is so difficult that the climber may spend weeks working out the right "moves" so that he or she can make the climb efficiently. Climbing can also involve "big walls" that take several days to ascend and can include ice, snow, or mixed terrain.

Climbing practice is often done by top roping. In top roping, one end of the rope is dropped to the beginning of the climb and is tied to the climber. A safety person or *belayer* controls the other end of the rope. It can be threaded through a carabiner at the top and given to the belayer either on the ground or at the top.

In lead climbing the first climber starts at the bottom of a climb with the rope attached to his or her harness and running back to a belayer. As the climb is ascended, the climber attaches the rope to intermediate anchors created by placing special pieces of climbing hardware known as *protection* into the rock. Such protection can be permanent bolts set into the rock or items such as cams, chocks, and pitons temporarily placed. *Carabiners* are clipped into the protection, and the rope is run through them. These intermediate pieces of protection reduce the potential falling distance of the "lead" climber as he or she makes progress up the route to the next belay station. Often the belayer follows the lead climber once the next belay station is reached. The former lead climber acts as belayer in a top-rope type climb for the former belayer.

Although "free solo climbing," which is ascent alone and without safety gear such as rope, is in vogue among a very few climbers, most climbing is still done while roped ("free climbing"). The essential elements of free climbing include: (1) a rope that has a great deal of stretch so that it will not only catch the falling climber but also absorb the shock created by the fall and (2) protection or anchoring hardware so that the rope can be attached to the rock and "protect" the climber.

In recent years, climbing has separated into several specialties. A more recent development has been climbing on artificial climbing walls located in indoor "climbing gyms." This is often done by top roping, but some of the more sophisticated gyms have walls with prebolted protection and lead routes on which individuals can place their own protection for lead climbing.

Vertical Caving

Vertical caving is one of the youngest of the vertical sports, beginning only in the 1950s. It also differs significantly from climbing. Instead of the vertical caver climbing the rock itself, he or she descends and ascends on the rope and usually does not intend to use the rope for protection in case of a fall from the rock. This method of climbing is known as *single rope technique* or *SRT* (see Chapter 3). Vertical caving uses two primary ropework skills.

One vertical caving technique is *rappelling,* which is the controlled descent on a rope. Vertical caving puts greater emphasis on the skill of rappelling than does climbing. This is because vertical cavers often have to rappel long distances, sometimes several hundred feet, and in adverse conditions such as darkness and wetness.

The other vertical caving skill is *ascending* directly on the rope using mechanical cams or specialized knots.

Vertical caving is not generally a widespread sport but it has had significant influence on the equipment and techniques used in other vertical activities, particularly high angle rescue. One of the most significant of these has been the development of a rope that is very durable and stretches very little (*static rope*).

HIGH ANGLE RESCUES
Rope Rescue

Rope rescue, depending on who is involved in it and the conditions, may also be called *vertical rescue* or sometimes, *technical rescue.* In these situations, a rope and other associated gear are necessary so the subject of the rescue can be moved from hazard, is kept stabilized and safe, and protected from falling.

Originally, most of the equipment and techniques used in rope rescue were the same as those used in mountaineering. But during the past generation, there has been a tremendous shift from these types of equipment and techniques to ones that are more specialized for rescue. One significant example is rescue rope, which has shifted from a stretchy line, as used in mountaineering, to a line with very little stretch and a more durable construction, similar to that used in vertical caving.

Fire Service Rescue

The use of life support rope and associated equipment in the fire service has undergone tremendous changes during the past decade. Part of this has been due to well-publicized tragic occurrences, such as the incident in New York City in June of 1980 when a rope broke during a rescue attempt and two firefighters fell to their deaths. Further impetus for these changes have come from fire service organizations such as the National Fire Protection Association (NFPA), the International Association of Fire Fighters (IAFF), and the International Society of Fire Service Instructors (ISFSI).

Perhaps the most significant of these changes has been the realization that the continued use of natural fiber rope for life safety is a dangerous and irresponsible practice, with the resulting massive changeover by most fire departments to synthetic fiber ropes.

Tactical Operations

The increase in the number of terrorist incidents and other forms of violence has lead to the greater preparation by law enforcement and the military to employ high angle operations. Many of these innovations have been in operational procedures, such as with helicopters. But the tactical practitioners have contributed to the high angle technology that is used by many other disciplines. One significant example of this is the *figure 8 with ears descender* (also called *rescue 8*). An early form of the device was developed by the Special Air Services (SAS) in England, but was then later adapted initially in North America through the joint effort of California Law Enforcement personnel and mountaineer and inventor, Russ Anderson. (See page 49 for a discussion of the advantages of the figure 8 with ears over the conventional figure 8).

Industrial Rescue

Industrial rescue incidents occur in high angle and confined areas where there is the potential for falls, entrapment, medical emergencies, and exposure to dangerous materials. Some examples would be re-fineries, chemical plants, and both open pit and underground mining. The principles for high angle rescue are the same in industrial environments as in natural environments, but environmental circumstances may either help or hinder industrial rescuers. In industrial rescue situations, there is usually an abundance of structural anchors available, and the response time is generally short. The rescue teams may either be on site or predesignated response units such as fire departments.

A very specialized type of industrial operation is called *confined space rescue*. Confined spaces often contain hazardous materials and dangerous machinery. Most significant are the hazardous atmospheres that mean the rescuers must protect themselves with protective clothing and breathing apparatus. In addition, the presence of hazardous materials can mean that the rescuers have to use specialized equipment, such as different rope materials, to protect the equipment from damage.

Because of the high death rate among persons attempting rescues in confined spaces, the U.S. Federal Occupational Safety and Health Administration (OSHA) has created laws specific to rescuers in confined spaces.

Other industrial situations may require rope access procedures to perform work. Such examples would be a worker climbing up a structural tower.

OTHER ROPEWORK USERS

The highly sophisticated entertainment environments require that lighting technicians, stagehands, and special effects workers climb in rigging high above the stage. They are increasingly using ropework techniques to access the rigging.

Other work situations where workers use ropework include workers on dams and bridges, arborists, and window cleaners.

THE HIGH ANGLE ROPE TECHNICIAN

There has been a tradition in the high angle environment of specializing in a particular discipline, such as rock climbing. But many people are taking those techniques and equipment from all disciplines in the high angle environment and putting them to use for their own particular needs. There are those who might be described as *high angle rope technicians,* who are competent in a number of high angle skills and who can use them for particular needs, such as rope rescue.

There are some basic principles that high angle rope technicians use to be both safe and successful in their work.

The Technology

Although most people associate the word *technology* with computers or space travel, the dictionary definition of the word is "the application of knowledge."

Thus high angle rope technicians are trained and experienced in the skills needed in the high angle environment. They use the technology of the high angle environment to conquer gravity and move about with ease in any direction needed to take their bodies. Or they use the technology of rope rescue to safely retrieve subjects from dangerous situations to those that are safe and where any injuries can be cared for.

The High Angle System

In this chapter the necessary elements of the high angle *system* and how their strengths and weaknesses determine the effectiveness of the system and, ultimately, the outcome of the operation will be examined.

One ideal that should be kept in mind by anyone working in the high angle environment is *think systems*. Although some elements are essential and important, it is the rare activity in the high angle environment that is completed with only a rope, only one piece of hardware, or only one person.

The high angle environment system consists of many elements such as rope, hardware, anchors, and other elements, which cannot be viewed in isolation. In order for the elements to operate safely and properly, they must be viewed together as a system.

Just as a chain is only as strong as its weakest link, the high angle system is only as effective as its weakest element. If, for example, your equipment system uses a rope that has a tensile test strength of 9,000 lb, but it is attached to an anchor that pulls out at 500 lb, then the strength of the entire system is only 500 lb.

The same idea applies to people systems in the high angle environment. It is human nature for a few motivated and aggressive individuals to be the ones who participate in every activity and attend every training session. It is also human nature for some persons to stand back and let others do the work.

But inevitably the well-trained individual is not available during the unexpected emergency, and the burden is shifted to the poorly trained and badly motivated person. In such an instance, the human chain can fail and disaster may result. And if a group has only a few well-trained members and the majority are inadequately trained and poorly motivated, then the team will probably be only as effective as this majority.

COMFORT IN THE HIGH ANGLE ENVIRONMENT

The fear of heights is natural to human beings and a degree of it is necessary for survival. A person without any fear or respect for the hazards involved in high angle work is a danger to himself or herself and others. But until a person feels at ease in operating in the high angle environment, his or her discomfort will prevent him or her from being effective in these activities. As with any unaccustomed environment,

there is a whole new approach to movement, to using equipment, and to working alongside other people. The only way to become accustomed to working in the high angle environment, and to become effective in it, is to spend time there. In other words, *practice*.

On the other hand, there is danger in being *too* comfortable in the high angle environment. Often, experienced climbers or high angle workers are too accustomed to being at heights with minimal protection. This familiarity often causes hazards in the adrenaline-charged and confused situation at a rescue site.

Attention to Detail

Attention to detail is necessary in the high angle environment not only to be effective but also to prevent injury to yourself and others. This environment is unforgiving, and the kind of lapse that might go unnoticed on level ground could result in severe injury or death in the high angle environment.

There is, of course, a need for balance. You must not be so obsessed that you are unable to complete a task. But it takes a focused mind to quickly examine a system and instantly know if all the necessary details are in place and this only comes with practice.

Although attention to detail is an essential trait to the high angle rope technician, the nature of high angle operations requires that a person have the ability to improvise.

Every high angle situation is different, with varying circumstances in terms of weather and terrain. Therefore a well-trained individual with good judgment is preferable to one who is well trained to perform only one way.

Prepare for Self-Rescue

Whatever the activity, a person who works in the high angle environment must always keep in mind that anything can go wrong and someday it probably will. Therefore you should be ready for something to go wrong and be ready to extricate yourself from it. This means that you should be mentally prepared and trained for an emergency. It also means always having the gear on your person that is necessary to perform self-rescue, including a small assortment of carabiners, a couple of slings made from webbing or rope, and either a set of Prusik loops or a pair of ascenders (see Chapter 10 for an explanation of the specific purpose of this gear).

Back up Others

In the same way, every person should be ready to extricate a partner or any other coworker who gets into a difficult situation. Whenever a team member is not performing a specific task in the high angle environment, he or she should be directing attention to the activities of others. Everyone, no matter how intelligent and experienced, has an occasional lapse. All team members should be ready to deal with any unsafe condition that may develop.

Care of Equipment

One sign of good mechanics and carpenters is their care of tools. The same is true of a high angle rope technician, who must care for rope and hardware. However, in the case of high angle gear, good care is even more critical because lives will depend upon these tools. Considerations for avoiding loss and damage to rescue gear include the following:

♦ Do not lay unsecured equipment at the edge of a drop. It has a good chance of being kicked or knocked over the edge, resulting in damage or loss or, even worse, causing injury to those below.

♦ Do not lay equipment on the ground or on the floor. High angle hardware, such as carabiners, is easily lost in leaves, dirt, or debris. Also, dirt and grit cause it to malfunction and wear out. When first arriving on site, hang a sling from a beam, a tree, or other convenient spot and clip all hardware to it when not in use.

♦ When working on a vertical face, keep all of your equipment attached to something. A convenient place is the equipment sling that many harnesses have.

♦ Inspect all gear after each operation. The time to discover that gear is damaged is during this inspection, not when it is being used.

♦ Ropes need special care (see Chapter 4). A traditional rule is *never step on a rope*. Many experienced vertical people have almost a fanaticism about never stepping on a rope, and there are good reasons for this rule. Stepping on a rope grinds grit into the core where it can damage the load-supporting fibers. But more than that, to many people, a person who steps on a rope displays a contempt for the well being of the person who uses the rope.

Attention to Skills

The difference between a competent high angle rope technician and one who can only talk about doing it, is that the competent technician really has the skills for the job. It is essential that the person has not just an understanding of the skills, but that use of the skills is instinctive. When there is a sudden and unexpected emergency, people react with actions that are instinctive. The only way to make high angle skills instinctive is practice.

An evaluation sheet should be used to assist in demonstrating that every student has indeed performed the skills satisfactorily. An example of an evaluation sheet is shown in Appendix B. Note that this checklist has a space for the instructor to indicate that the student has performed the skills satisfactorily and

a space for the student to confirm that he or she has performed the skills.

This method helps to double check the training system and may protect the instructor at a later date should the student fail to perform the skill correctly and claim the failure was due to a training lapse.

Continued Skills Maintenance

A student being instructed in high angle techniques is only the first step. The reality of the situation is that it is difficult for an individual to maintain his or her skills without constant and regular training. A training schedule should be an indispensable part of every high angle technician's routine.

Safety

There can be no doubt that the primary objective of high angle activity is *do it safely*. This primary objective is achieved through mental and physical concepts and through team organization.

Mental Concepts

♦ If you feel "spaced out" due to fatigue, heat, or cold, stand back from potentially dangerous activity.
♦ If you become overexcited, back off for a bit. (One technique is to feel your pulse. If it is racing well beyond your normal rate, sit down and cool off.)
♦ If you feel you are getting in over your head, ask for help (a belay, if appropriate) or back off.
♦ Everyone makes mistakes therefore everyone checks everyone else, even the most experienced, for possible lapses.
♦ No one goes into the high angle environment when alcohol or drugs diminish his or her capacities.
♦ Practicing technique helps people to perform safely in the high angle environment.

Physical Concepts

♦ Establish safety lines; everyone at the edge must be tied in.
♦ Use redundant systems, for example, more than one anchor.
♦ Everyone wears a helmet and other appropriate personal protection equipment.
♦ Check equipment constantly to make certain it is in safe condition.

Team Concepts

Many accidents or near misses occur because of organizational and management failures. One way to avoid this is to train together often so that individual skills are combined into one working unit. Another form of insurance is the use of a *safety officer*. The safety officer is an individual who makes certain that safe procedures are followed during training and real rescues. The safety officer should be someone other than the team leader because the leader is often too busy to check all safety systems. (See Chapter 11, The Rope Rescuer, for more about the safety officer.)

Warning Call

One of the most common dangers in the high angle environment is from falling objects, either hardware dropped by others or dislodged rocks. Whenever a hard object begins to fall, even if no one is thought to be below, the universal warning is to yell, "rock!" *very loudly.* Do not say, "look out," "heads up," or anything else other than "rock."

Evaluation Exercises

◆ COGNITIVE AND AFFECTIVE EXERCISES ◆

1. **Single rope technique implies which of the following:**
   A. The climber is using the rope to ascend or descend.
   B. The climber is using the rope to "safety" himself or herself.
   C. The climber is without a belay.
   D. The climber is climbing one rope length.

2. **Free climbing implies that:**
   A. The climber is climbing the rope to go upward.
   B. The climber is ascending, making direct contact with the surface he or she is on, while using rope and other equipment to provide safety in the event of a fall.
   C. The climber is rock or ice climbing.
   D. The climber is using a rope to make forward progress during a difficult vertical event.

3. **Which of the following might be considered a self-rescue situation?**
   A. While traversing a glacier, one of the rescue party falls into a crevasse.
   B. While rappelling the climber's shirt gets caught in the figure 8 device.
   C. The rescuer slips while climbing but is caught by the rope and is hanging upside down below an overhang.
   D. All of the above.

4. **Of the following, what would be considered minimal equipment for self-rescue preparedness?**
   A. In your pack: several locking carabiners, a figure 8 descender, several slings, and some Prusik loops.
   B. In your pack: several pieces of protection, ascenders, and Prusik loops or slings.
   C. On your person: a small assortment of carabiners, a couple of slings made from webbing or rope, and either a set of Prusik loops or a pair of ascenders.
   D. On your person: extra carabiners, a sling, and a rappel device.

5. **While performing a rescue operation, you notice something falling down from above your position. You should:**
   A. Yell, "rock!"
   B. Yell, "falling!"
   C. Shout in a loud voice, "something is falling toward you!"
   D. Shout, "look out!"

6. **It is important that personnel learn the correct way from the beginning because:**
   A. Under stressful situations in real incidents, people will revert to the way they did it the first time.
   B. People frequently cannot understand things until the fourth time.
   C. Participants must make mistakes before they can learn.
   D. It is not important; people can be remediated at any time.

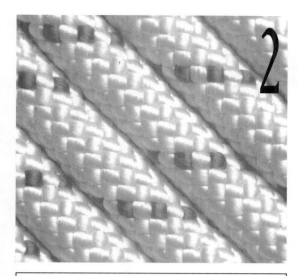

2 Personal Equipment and Protection

Objectives

At the completion of this chapter, you should be able to:

1. List four points to consider when selecting a helmet for use in the vertical environment.
2. List several considerations for the "shell" and "insulated" layers of clothing for rope rescue personnel.
3. List several considerations for hand and foot protection in rope rescue.
4. List several considerations for a secure and comfortable seat harness.
5. Demonstrate how to tie a ring bend ("water knot").
6. Demonstrate how to tie an emergency seat harness.
7. Demonstrate how to tie a figure 8 on a bight.
8. Cite an example of the safety standards that apply to safety equipment in the vertical environment.
9. Describe the considerations for selection of personal equipment for use in the high angle environment.
10. List federal, private, and international organizations that set standards for rescue equipment.
11. Describe a scenario that would result in a catastrophic failure when using a knife in the vertical environment.

Key Terms

ASTM An international organization that creates standards through a "full consensus" method. Among the ASTM standards that apply to the high angle environment are ones relating to search and rescue, recreational climbing equipment, and arboriculture equipment.

CE The European Union standards setting authority (European Committee for Standardization). Standards cover a wide range of products including ones for recreational climbing, industrial fall protection, and rope access.

Chest Harness A type of harness worn around the chest for upper body support. In the high angle environment, it should never be used as the only source of support but always in combination with a seat harness.

Emergency Seat Harness A temporary, tied harness to be used when a manufactured, sewn seat harness is not available.

Full Body Harness A type of harness that offers both pelvic and upper body support as one unit.

Helmet Head covering that protects against head injury both from falling objects and from head impact. When used in this book, "helmet" indicates head protection specifically designed for high angle work.

NFPA National Fire Protection Association, a national organization that sets safety standards, among them life safety equipment for firefighters.

Safety Belt A belt-like harness worn around the waist to prevent falls from elevated positions. It should never be used as sole means of suspension.

key Terms—cont'd ▼

Seat Harness A system of nylon or polyester webbing that wraps and supports the pelvic region to attach the wearer to the rope or other protection in the high angle environment.

UIAA The Union of International Alpine Associations. An organization that sets performance standards for ropes, harnesses, ice axes, helmets, and carabiners to be used by climbers and mountaineers.

CLOTHING, FITNESS AND HEALTH, AND PERSONAL EQUIPMENT

The correct choices of clothing and personal equipment you use in the high angle environment can give you a greater margin of safety, add to your comfort, and enable you, the high angle rope technician, to perform your job more effectively and more efficiently.

Headgear

One of the most critical pieces of personal protective equipment is the *helmet.* This can protect you not only from falling objects, such as rocks or climbing hardware, but also can reduce the severity of brain injury should you fall and hit your head.

You should purchase only helmets specifically designed for high angle activities. Other types of helmets may provide only an illusion of protection. In the end, they can actually be dangerous to the wearer. For example, *construction-type or motorcycle helmets are not suitable for high angle work.* They are not designed to offer protection from the forces that may be applied to the head in the high angle environment. They also may be uncomfortable or inconvenient to wear in the high angle environment. Motorcycle helmets, for example, tend to be very uncomfortable during hot weather and can reduce hearing. Many construction helmets offer only minimum protection at best and tend to slip off the head when you need protection most.

It is very important that helmets have a secure chin strap. Helmets with elastic chin straps are not suitable for high angle work. As the elastic chin strap stretches, the helmet may flip off the head, leaving the wearer without head protection. This often occurs when the helmet is stressed, such as when the wearer falls or is hit by falling objects.

Any helmet used in high angle work should also have what is called a *three-point suspension.* This means that besides support points on each side of the helmet, there is a third one at the rear. The third suspension point helps prevent the helmet from falling forward over your eyes. The chin straps on many construction-type helmets are designed to easily release when the helmet snags on something. A good high angle helmet should have a chin strap that requires much greater force to release. This helps the helmet stay on the user's head in a tumbling fall.

The shells of helmets used in high angle rescue are constructed of materials such as glass-reinforced polyamide or fiberglass composites. This shell should have the rigidity that resists impacts delivered to the helmet and penetration by sharp objects. At the same time, the shell should have some "give" to absorb some of the blow that otherwise would be directly transmitted to the skull and spine. The design of the helmet should protect the head against objects falling from above and hitting from the side.

The inside suspension of the helmet should hold the shell away from the skull during blows to the helmet and provide air circulation and comfort, particularly during hot weather.

A slight brim helps prevent rainwater or spray from dripping into the face. But the helmet should have a profile that is narrow enough so that the wearer has a good upward field of vision and so that the back of the helmet does not catch on a pack when you raise your head.

Helmets that have passed *UIAA* or CE certification are usually adequate for high angle work. Helmets with the *NFPA* certification have good impact resistance, but many fire helmets are inadequate for high angle rope work. Those with extended rear brims are cumbersome in the high angle environment. Their bulky nature tends to obstruct vision, makes it difficult to maneuver in the sometimes cluttered and confined high angle environment, and can be very uncomfortable in hot weather.

Don't purchase an inexpensive helmet for high angle work. A few extra dollars for a helmet with good suspension and impact absorption is cheap compared with the cost of ending up brain dead.

Hydration

The human body is made up of 80% water. For the body to function efficiently there must be little variation from this norm. Body fluid transports nutrients and oxygen to muscles and the brain. It also is responsible for lubrication and temperature control. Studies have shown that most people doing physical labor in extreme temperatures become dehydrated.

Some ways dehydration will affect you include:

◆ It will be harder for you to stay warm.
◆ You cannot think at full efficiency. Even moderate dehydration greatly affects your ability to do complex problem solving.
◆ Your energy reserves will be low.
◆ Dehydration causes electrolyte shifts that affect your fine motor skills.
◆ Dehydration can cause disabling headaches and muscle cramps.

Dehydration lowers body function and can cause a dangerous loss of judgment. This is very insidious because most people drink fluids only when thirsty, and thirst is a poor indication of the need for hydration. A more reliable indicator of hydration is urine output.

Clear or lightly colored urine usually shows you are adequately hydrated.

Dehydration is not just a problem in hot environments. It is common in cold environments, because people are less motivated to drink fluid. The important thing is to constantly drink fluids, even if not thirsty, so that you have clear or lightly colored urine.

Urination, particularly in social situations such as rescue, may seem inconvenient and embarrassing. But if you are not urinating regularly, you are not hydrated.

Keep at least 2 L of water in your pack, particularly if there are not group water sources available. The best fluid to drink for hydration is plain water.

Protection from Heat and Cold

Humans are physically weak and vulnerable compared with many other creatures on earth. It is our brain that has enabled us to survive and prevail. If our brain function is threatened then our survival is at risk.

One of the greatest weaknesses of the human body is that it was designed to survive only in a narrow temperature range. Being outside this range, either too hot or too cold for a long time, will progressively inhibit our body from functioning, cause dangerous mental confusion, and eventually, death.

We lack the natural defenses of animals, for example, having fur to stay warm and panting to lose heat, so we must create artificial defenses to protect ourselves from temperature extremes.

The human body loses or gains heat in four different ways:

1. Conduction (direct contact with cold or hot object):
   ◆ Example of heat loss through conduction: Sitting or lying on a cold metal structure.
   ◆ Example of heat gain through conduction: Sitting or lying on hot rock slabs.
2. Convection (air currents rob body heat or overload it):
   ◆ Example of loss of heat through conduction: Standing on a tower where cold wind is blowing.
   ◆ Example of gain of heat through conduction: Working in a containment vessel on hot day.
3. Radiation (radiant heat robs body of heat or adds heat):
   ◆ Example of gain of heat through radiation: Working in the sunshine on a hot day.
   ◆ Example of loss of heat through radiation: Working with head uncovered in cold environment.
4. Respiration (body is cooled or heated through respiratory system):
   ◆ Example of loss of heat through respiration: Cool air is inhaled and warmed by the respiratory system before being exhaled.
   ◆ Example of gain of heat through respiration: Hot, ambient air raises body temperature through respiration.

One secret to maintaining a temperature equilibrium is being adaptable to changes in temperature and weather. This means adding or removing clothing and other protection whatever the heat or cold challenge.

Clothing

The principle of clothing protection is to maintain warmth when needed, but also allow the body to lose warmth before becoming overheated. The principle of insulation is the ability to retain air in the fibers of the garment. The great danger to insulation is wetness both from the outside (rain, snow) or from the inside (perspiration). Wetness will quickly sap body heat.

One important piece of clothing that protects from outside wetness is the "shell" made of waterproof material such as coated nylon or Gore-Tex. This can protect both against precipitation and the cooling effects of wind. But remember that with intense physical activity, the lack of air circulation under the shell can result in the production of large amounts of perspiration. This may result in the interior of the shell being as saturated as the outside. Therefore there must be some way for "venting" heat away from the body before perspiration begins. One way of doing this is with a zipper down the front of the garment. Some outdoor clothing has zippers along the side or under the armpits to help release the body heat before it produces perspiration.

There are now several types of fabric, such as Gore-Tex, designed to allow body perspiration to escape while protecting from precipitation. How well this concept works, however, still depends on specific climate conditions and use by the wearer. Some users have found that under incessant and heavy rain the fabric allows wetness to soak through. Also, production of large amounts of perspiration can overwhelm the fabric system and inhibit its function.

But whatever the specific type of rain wear you use, if you can stand for half an hour under a shower and still not get soaked through, then it will probably protect you in the outdoor high angle environment.

There should be an insulating layer of clothing under the shell. This provides warmth but it must also protect the wearer against chilling even when wet, either from outside precipitation or from perspiration. The key for insulation value is the ability to retain air in the fibers and not get wet from outside or inside the garment.

Cotton is the least desirable fabric in wet and cold environments because it tends to lose its insulating qualities when wet. The traditional choice for a fabric that retains warmth when wet is wool. A more recent development, and a fabric that is more comfortable next to the skin, is polyester pile. Both fabrics, particularly pile, offer little shielding from wind, so they need to be worn in combination with an outer windbreaker shell.

For the outdoors, underwear made of synthetic materials such as polypropylene has become common. Its advantages are that it dries quickly and tends to draw moisture away from the skin, which prevent it from having a cooling effect on the body.

Clothing should protect the high angle rope technician against adverse environmental conditions and provide maximum comfort for any activity. Shirts and pants must be sized so they will not bind when arms are extended above the head or when legs are raised.

Footwear

Among the requirements for footwear are comfort, protection, and adhesion. Although boots are increasingly being partially or completely fabricated of materials such as Gore-Tex or plastic, leather is still the material having the qualities most needed in a high angle, multipurpose boot.

Boots should provide support to the ankles and protect the feet from scrapes, cuts, and bruises. Yet they should be pliable enough to be comfortable after hours of standing or walking. The soles should not be "slick" like street shoes but should have adhesion to help the wearer maintain balance against surfaces found in the high angle environment. Rubber boots, such as those commonly used in the fire service, are not appropriate for high angle operations. They do not have the needed foot protection and they encumber the feet and legs.

Lug soles, particularly those made from Vibram, have been very much in fashion but they may not be required as long as the boot sole provides adhesion. Furthermore, in some cases a lug sole may actually be a disadvantage. Some types of lug soles may become dangerously slick once they are wet or caked with mud.

For specialized rock climbing, technical climbing boots with soles constructed of special rubber compounds may adhere to the rock better. Many of these climbing boots have little or no welt, so they may be better for certain climbing techniques such as "edging" along the rock. They are specifically made for climbing, so they are not comfortable for walking or standing for long periods of time.

A good choice of socks is important for warmth, comfort, and prevention of injury such as blisters. A two-sock combination can reduce friction on the skin that causes blisters. An inner sock, made of a synthetic such as polypropylene, wicks moisture away from the foot so that it stays dry. A thick outer sock, made of a material such as wool, increases the warmth and provides some protection for the foot.

Gloves

Gloves are worn in the high angle environment to protect hands against the weather and, more importantly, to protect them against burns and abrasions from a running rope. Gloves shield the hands and prevent discomfort that might cause the high angle rope technician to lose control of the rope.

While providing protection, gloves must allow the hands to retain a sense of feeling so that the fingers can manipulate equipment. Therefore gloves constructed of soft leather, such as deerskin or goat skin, offer the best compromise. Heavily insulated gloves, such as those sometimes worn by firefighters, should not be used in ropework. They tend to prevent the proper feel of the rope when rappelling or rope handling.

Commercial versions of rope handling gloves are available, which have added protection across the palm, but with thinner material on the fingers so they allow the hands to retain a sense of feeling.

Some gloves with extra heat protection for what is called *fast rope* handling of the rope are sometimes used in tactical operations. However, if you need gloves with such extra heat protection (more than a few layers of leather) you are rappelling too fast for rescue ropework.

Seat Harnesses

Seat harnesses are among the most important pieces of equipment for high angle activities. It is essential that you choose a harness for safety, security, and comfort.

High angle seat harnesses are constructed of nylon or polyester webbing. The webbing wraps the pelvic region to support it and attaches the rescuer to the rope or other protection (see Figure 2-1 for an example of a sewn, manufactured seat harness).

An unsuitable *seat harness*, or one that is badly fitted, can result in such severe discomfort that it can inhibit the wearer from performing a task. Even worse, it can be dangerous to the wearer.

The most secure and comfortable of the seat harnesses are those that are presewn and manufactured.

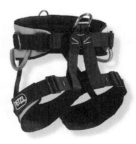

FIGURE 2-1
Manufactured sewn seat harness.

Life belts, ladder belts, pompier belts, and similar *safety belts* with support only around the waist must not be used as the single point of support in high angle activities.

These types of equipment are designed only as a safety element to help prevent falls from ladders or other elevated positions. When a person hangs free in them, the belts can constrict the waist and rib cage to impair breathing and cause possible damage to internal organs. They can also slip up under the armpits to cause permanent damage to nerves and result in permanent paralysis to the arms. Their use, in place of a seat harness, as the single support can result in injury, permanent disability, or death.

Although the tied *emergency seat harnesses* may be used in a pinch (two types are described in this chapter), they are no substitute for a well-designed, sewn, manufactured harness.

It is extremely difficult to make a tied seat harness that is as secure and comfortable as a well-designed and carefully manufactured product. One reason for this is that it takes a great deal of skill to tie secure knots in a tied seat harness. Another reason is that the narrow webbing usually employed in tied harnesses does not give the support of the wider material used in manufactured harnesses. This narrow material, along with the knots, causes constricted blood circulation and severe discomfort to body parts.

Even more critical is a well-engineered harness design. The harness should support your pelvic girdle so your weight does not create pressure points on the nerves and arteries in the groin and back.

In a high angle rescue situation, a person may have to be hanging in the harness for a relatively long period. Twenty minutes is not an unusual time, and periods of more than an hour are a possibility. Although there is no harness that will be totally comfortable in these conditions, the tied seat harness tends to cause greater discomfort and possible circulatory problems.

While hanging in an inadequate seat harness, the wearer's discomfort begins as the narrow webbing or rope compresses the kidneys and thighs. This becomes even more painful as circulation to the legs is constricted. After only a few minutes, leg muscles are deprived of perfusion and become useless. Ultimately, the person may be threatened from dangerous blood pressure changes and buildup of blood toxins.

Foot Supports

For those situations where you may be suspended in a seat harness for long periods, especially in a free drop (not in contact with a wall), even the best harness will become uncomfortable. The use of foot loops, stirrups,

or etrier (short ladder made of webbing) to stand in momentarily will provide relief by restoring circulation.

You can attach the foot supports with a Prusik hitch or ascender on the rope above your rappel device or rope attachment point (see Chapter 10, Ascending, for information on Prusiks and ascenders). You can also attach them directly to your seat harness main attachment points.

Requirements and qualities for a secure and comfortable seat harness include the following:

- The webbing should be wide (at least 2 inches) for comfort at critical points such as waist and thighs. Padding can make the webbing even more comfortable.
- Stitching should be sewn securely and evenly and be of contrasting color so that abrasion and wear can be detected.
- The harness should have leg and thigh supports, such as leg loops. These add comfort and support by spreading the body weight, or the force of a fall, over other portions of the body, such as the thighs and buttocks.
- The harness should allow you freedom of movement both when hanging in it and when wearing it on the ground.
- The harness should be easy to put on and to adjust.
- The harness should not slip down when you walk around.
- When you fall and are caught by the harness, it should allow you to easily return yourself upright.
- The harness must not allow you to fall out when you are upside down.
- The harness should have a front tie-in point designed so that you maintain a correct center of gravity whatever activity you are performing.
- The stress points such as the tie-in should be faced with extra webbing and/or use heavy duty metal connectors.
- Depending on how it is being used, the harness should be certified by appropriate standards, such as UIAA, NFPA, CE, *ASTM*, or ANSI.

Because of the variations in anatomy and because there are different kinds of activity in the high angle environment, no one seat harness design is suitable for everyone. Before selecting a particular seat harness and investing the money, you should try several different designs to see which one is best for you.

Differences Between Climbing and Rescue Harnesses

Most climbing harnesses are made to be lighter weight, are often cut for ease of movement, and are made for recovering from leader falls. Harnesses specifically designed for rescue are usually heavier and bulkier because they have wider webbing and padding for comfort while sitting in them for long periods. They are not designed for lead climbing. Rescue harnesses generally have a metal attachment point

A seat harness by itself should not be used as the only tie-in point for swift water operations. If you are attached only to a seat harness in swift water, the force of the current can easily force your upper body back over into the water, making it impossible for you to right yourself and resulting in your drowning. Swift water technicians usually employ a tie-in point higher on the body, such as a *chest harness*. Obtain instructions on this procedure from a qualified, swift water technician.

into which carabiners are directly clipped. Climbing harnesses have a reinforced webbing loop to directly attach the belay rope. The rope is usually attached directly to the harness with a loop created from a figure **8** follow through (Flemish bend).

Climbing and rescue harnesses are also designed to meet test standards for different organizations. Climbing harnesses are generally designed to meet the UIAA, CE, and ASTM (F08) standards. Rescue harnesses are designed to meet standards developed by NFPA and ANSI. There is also a rescue/industrial standard by CE.

Rescue Harnesses

Rescue harnesses are specifically designed for rescue use. Rescue harnesses often feature wider webbing and optional padding for increased comfort. They are usually heavier and bulkier than climbing harnesses. Some rescue harnesses also have a large **D** ring for front attachment point. These types of harnesses are not designed for absorbing shock loading and should not be used for lead climbing activities.

Full Body Harnesses

In certain circumstances, a *full body harness,* or a combination of a seat harness with a chest harness, may be preferable to only a seat harness. These may include the following situations:

◆ When a person is involved in a dangerous activity requiring constantly being held upright. One example would be where a person is entering a confined space and is equipped with a harness attached to a retrieval line.
◆ When wearing equipment that makes one top heavy, such as breathing apparatus. The chest portion of the harness helps distribute the extra weight of the apparatus on the body.
◆ Persons of greater than average weight. The higher tie in point helps them stay upright.
◆ During certain climbing/mountaineering activities when it is necessary to be held upright should a fall occur. An example would be when wearing a heavy pack that would make it difficult for you to right yourself (see Figure 2-2 for an example of a

seat/chest harness combination and Figure 2-3 for an example of a full body harness).

◆ To be placed on a subject in certain rescue situations (see Chapter 13).

In these situations a full body harness, or a combination seat/chest harness, may provide needed security, but in some circumstances a full body harness may be a disadvantage. In certain rescue situations, some persons may find the full body harness too con-

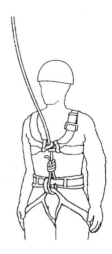

FIGURE 2-2
Combination seat/chest harness.

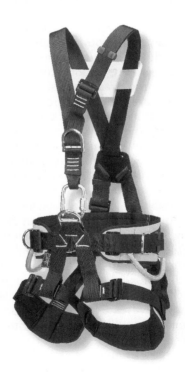

FIGURE 2-3
Full body harness.

straining, thus preventing the range of motion needed for rescue activities.

Seat/Chest Harness

The seat/chest harness combination may be preferable for some rescuers because it allows the wearer to choose options based on the specific conditions. A chest harness, worn with a seat harness, can be quickly connected or disconnected to the system, depending on the needs of the user. Should the wearer need to be held upright without using upper body strength, then he or she can quickly connect it. If it is too constraining, then he or she can unclip it but continue wearing it. An added advantage to a rescuer carrying a chest harness is that he or she can use it to hold a rescue subject upright in certain types of operations.

Chest Harnesses

Chest harnesses are comfortable, easily adjusted, easily combined with a seat harness, and easy to put on and take off. A chest harness must not be used alone for high angle activities but always in combination with a seat harness.

OSHA, ANSI, ASTM, NFPA, UIAA, and CE Standards

Standards from the Federal Occupational Safety and Health Administration (OSHA), ASTM (F08), the American National Standards Institute (ANSI), the National Fire Protection Association (NFPA), European Committee for Standardization, and the International Union of Alpine Associations (UIAA) apply to the construction and use of some harnesses.

Each of these standards applies to a specific group of users, but *in no case does any standard apply to everyone who uses high angle equipment.* OSHA and ANSI standards apply to certain workplace activities, while NFPA standards apply to firefighters. ASTM (F08), UIAA, and some CE standards apply to mountaineers.

For specific information on any standard, contact the responsible organization. See Appendix A for mailing addresses of standards setting organizations.

SECURING HARDWARE IN THE HIGH ANGLE ENVIRONMENT

High angle hardware, such as carabiners, is easily lost when working in the high angle environment. Even worse, hardware can easily be dropped and injure another person who happens to be in the path of its fall. When working in the high angle environment, keep all equipment attached to something secure. One convenient place is the equipment loops that many harnesses have (Figure 2-4).

If equipment slings or loops are not manufactured into the harness, they can be easily created with the use of utility cord.

Shoulder Slings

Shoulder slings for equipment are preferred by some persons. These may work well particularly if the equipment carried is not bulky and does not interfere with high angle activities. However, some strangulation deaths have occurred when climbers have fallen and accidentally snagged the shoulder slings.

LIGHT SOURCES

High angle operations, particularly in rescue, often take place at night or in enclosed areas with no light. Consequently, all personnel should have with them a reliable source of light. You will need both hands to be free during high angle operations, so these light sources should be in the form of headlamps (Figure 2-5). A headlamp follows the movement of your head, usually placing the light where you are looking.

Choose a headlamp that is easily adjustable and field serviceable. Always carry extra batteries and a spare bulb. Many headlamps have battery packs to the rear of the head, which help balance weight on your helmet. When choosing this kind of lamp, you must be certain that it will remain stable on the head and not easily fall off.

Some traditional headlamps have a belt battery pack attached by a cord to the headlamp. Although this may provide a sufficient source of light, high angle technicians sometimes find that the cord snags and either becomes entangled or breaks. This is particularly a problem in confined spaces. One possible solution is to wear the cord inside clothing, but should the wire short, then the wearer may discover a whole new meaning to the term *hot wired.*

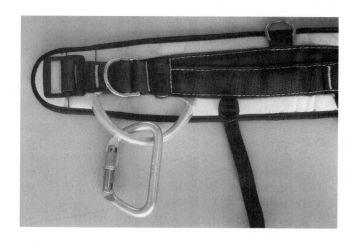

FIGURE 2-4

Seat harness equipment loops.

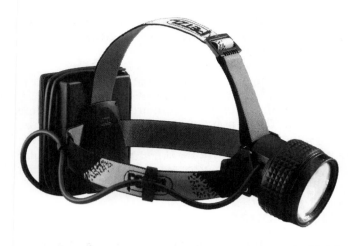

FIGURE 2-5
Headlamp.

The lamp should have an adjustable beam and a secure switch so that the light cannot be turned on accidentally when in storage.

The battery type that has the longest shelf life and is resistant to the effects of cold is the lithium cell. However, it is also the most expensive and has been known to cause explosions by venting gas. After the lithium cell, the alkaline battery is the next most desirable in terms of long life and operating temperature and is not as expensive as the lithium.

The halogen bulb gives a brighter light than the standard bulb but will drain batteries much quicker. Some rescuers carry both the standard and halogen bulbs. They use the standard normally to save the batteries then switch to the halogen when they need extra light.

Persons entering potentially explosive atmospheres must use light sources that are intrinsically safe for the particular conditions. This means that the design of the lighting equipment safeguards it against ignition in a hazardous atmosphere. There are several levels or classes of hazards, so lamps that are certified for one level might not be safe in others.

KNIVES IN THE HIGH ANGLE ENVIRONMENT

Carrying knives in the high angle environment has almost become a custom for some. But the careless use of knives can have terrible consequences. Knives in the high angle environment, other than presenting the real danger of personal injury, are a threat to life because of the ease with which they destroy life-supporting equipment.

A naked knife blade is a particular danger to ropes loaded with the weight of one or more persons. When stretched, as they are when supporting weight, rope yarns are very susceptible to being cut by any sharp object.

Typically a person would want to reach for a knife when his or her tee shirt or hair has gotten sucked into the rappel device and is stranded. However, in such a situation the person is likely to be under stress, possibly in pain, and have limited freedom of movement. It would be very difficult to cut his or her way out without touching the knife edge to the rope.

One alternative to a knife is the tool used by emergency services personnel to cut seat belts. This instrument has a recessed blade so that it does not accidentally cut a lifeline as easily as a naked knife blade.

Even better than cutting is the use of advanced skills and optional equipment to extricate yourself from a jammed rappel device and similar situations. One alternative is to use a Prusik knot or an ascender to take the weight off the rappel device and extricate you from such a predicament. The skills and equipment required for this procedure are described in Chapter 10.

Evaluation Exercises

◆ COGNITIVE AND AFFECTIVE EXERCISES ◆

1. **A helmet worn in the high angle environment does all of the following,** *except:*
   A. Decreases the risk of significant skull fracture.
   B. Decreases the risk of severe brain injury.
   C. Decreases the risk of accidents.
   D. Protects from falling objects.
2. **A helmet for the high angle rescue environment should include which of the following:**
   A. Chin strap.
   B. Certification from appropriate agency.
   C. Three-point suspension system.
   D. All of the above.
3. **All of the following are appropriate foot wear for high angle ropework,** *except:*
   A. Heavy mountaineering boots.
   B. Rubber, fire service boots.
   C. Vibram soled light-weight hiking boot with good ankle protection.
   D. Heavy-weight leather hiking boots.
4. **Footwear worn by the high angle technician should have which of the following characteristics:**
   A. Comfort.
   B. Good sole-to-terrain adhesion.
   C. Good ankle protection.
   D. All of the above.
5. **Wearing gloves helps a person maintain control of the rope in the high angle environment because they:**
   A. Protect the wearer from dirt and grime.
   B. Limit feeling the heat of the rope.
   C. Protect against burns and abrasions.
   D. Improve grip on materials.

6. **Which of the following may cause life-threatening complications if used as a single point of suspension in the vertical environment:**
   A. Life belts.
   B. Ladder belts.
   C. Pompier belts.
   D. All of the above.

7. **A person who is hanging for a long period in an unsuitable seat harness in the high angle environment might experience all of the following,** *except:*
   A. Euphoria.
   B. Syncope (fainting).
   C. Pain.
   D. Hypotension.

8. **An international organization involved in seat harness standard setting is:**
   A. UNICEF
   B. AMGA
   C. UIAA
   D. OSHA

9. **A U.S. organization involved in setting standards for rope rescue equipment is:**
   A. USIA
   B. NFPA
   C. IODA
   D. USDOT

10. **The best strategy for relieving pressure on your lower body while hanging for long periods in a seat harness would be:**
    A. Prusik a foot loop to the rope above the harness.
    B. Hand hang.
    C. Weight on to the belay line.
    D. Foot loops to the harness.

11. **All of the following situations would require a rope to your seat harness,** *except:*
    A. Rappelling.
    B. Attending a litter in vertical terrain.
    C. Entering the water during a swift water rescue.
    D. Belay or safety line close to cliff edge.

12. **A convenient place to store rigging hardware while rigging a rescue is:**
    A. On your seat harness utility loops.
    B. On the litter.
    C. In your pack.
    D. On the ground at the site.

13. **Which of the following represents a situation in which the use of a knife might lead to disaster?**
    A. Catching a tee shirt in a rappel device.
    B. Freeing the working rope of a fused Prusik.
    C. Cutting brush away from the edge during a rope operation.
    D. All of the above.

▼ PSYCHOMOTOR EXERCISES ▼

14. **When in a comfortable, well-lighted room, perform the following:**
    a) Tie a quick-don harness ("Swiss seat").
    b) Tie a "mountaineer" harness.

15. **Put on your foul weather clothing and headlamp, enter the full, running cold shower at your home or station, and perform the following tasks:**
    a) Tie a ring bend.
    b) Tie a figure 8 on a bight.
    c) Tie a quick-don harness ("Swiss seat").
    d) Tie a "mountaineer" harness.
    e) Tie into a rope, once you have tied an emergency harness.

16. **Set up a rope in a classroom or garage secured to the ceiling then perform the following:**
    a) Hang 3 feet off the floor in your sit harness for 20 minutes to locate the pressure points and tight areas of your harness.
    b) Hang 3 feet off the floor in your harness attached to a rappel device, then rig a Prusik above your device and attach a foot loop to it and stand to relieve pressure on your lower body. Then return to a rappel position.

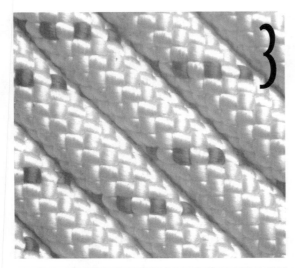

3 Rope and Related Equipment

Objectives ▼

At the completion of this chapter, you should be able to:

1. List the type of rope used in climbing verses that used in rescue situations.
2. Describe the considerations for rope construction to create a low stretch rope versus a dynamic rope.
3. Identify the design, weakness, and limitations of the rope currently used by your organization or group.
4. Given a system and problem, determine the safety factor.
5. Given a scenario, determine the fall factor for a rescuer.

Key Terms ▼

Abrasion The damaging wear on rope and other gear caused by rubbing against abrasive material.

Dynamic Rope A type of rope designed for high stretch to reduce the shock on the climber and anchor system. Usually used in rock climbing and mountaineering.

Fall Factor The distance fallen in relationship to the amount of rope used to catch the fall. The fall factor calculation is used to estimate the impact force on a rope when it is subjected to stopping a falling mass.

Kernmantle A rope design consisting of two elements: an interior core (kern) that usually supports the major portion of the load on the rope and an outer sheath (mantle) that serves primarily to protect the core, which may also support a minor portion of the load.

Kevlar Trade name for a type of Aramid fiber manufactured by the Dupont Corporation, which has high tensile strength, low elongation, and high resistance to heat.

Laid Rope A rope design that consists of fiber bundles twisted around one another.

Low Stretch Rope A type of rope designed to be used in applications such as rescue, rappelling, and ascending where high stretch would be a disadvantage and where no falls, or very short falls, are expected before being caught by the rope. The term *low stretch rope* can refer to ropes with slightly more elongation than the traditional static ropes or to both types of ropes (see static rope).*

*The Cordage Institute Standard on *Low Stretch and Static Kernmantle Life Stafety Ropes* has recently attempted to divide what were once known as static ropes into two categories. One is now known as *static kernmantle* and the other is known as *low stretch*. Low stretch ropes built to the Cordage Institute Standard will have more elongation than static ropes built to the same standard. More elongation provides lower impact forces when the rope is used to arrest sudden load. In this text, the terms *static* and *low stretch*, as well as the associated rope application, can be used interchangeably.

key Terms—cont'd ▼

Nylon 6 A type of nylon used in rope manufacturing. Because of type 6 nylon's shock absorbing qualities, it is found in most climbing ropes. One trade name for this nylon type is *Perlon*.

Nylon 6,6 A type of nylon used in rope manufacturing. With its resistance to wear and less elongation under load, most static ropes are constructed of type 6,6. In North America it is manufactured by Dupont and Monsanto.

Perlon A trade name for one type of nylon type 6.

Polyester A type of fiber used in some rope manufacturing. Also known by the trade name *Dacron*.

Polyolefins A group of fiber types used in manufacturing ropes that are often used in water applications. In this group are polypropylene and polyethylene.

Safety Factor The ratio between the maximum load expected on high angle system, or on its components such as rope and hardware, to their breaking strengths. The larger the ratio, the greater the safety factor.

Software A category of high angle equipment that is not hardware. In this category are rope and webbing.

Spectra Trade name for a high modulus polyethylene fiber with high tensile strength.

Static Rope A type of rope designed to be used in applications such as rescue, rappelling, and ascending where high stretch would be a disadvantage and where no falls, or very short falls, are expected before being caught by the rope. Static ropes have slightly less elongation than low stretch ropes built to the same standard. Less elongation prevents loss of system efficiency due to rope stretch (see low stretch rope)*

Tensile Strength A measurement of the greatest lengthwise stress under slow pull conditions that a rope can resist without failing.

DETERMINING THE RIGHT ROPE FOR THE JOB

Rope is the universal link in high angle activities and in rope rescue. During the past years, there have been great strides in the technology and manufacture of rope. But rope is only as good as how it is used and will perform only as well as the care you give it.

There are many different kinds of rope for high angle activities. Each kind has a specific design and fiber that determine how it will react to natural and human forces. Before choosing a rope, you must decide whether it will be used for climbing rock or ice, for rappelling or ascending, for rescue, for swift water, or for another specialized activity. The incorrect use of a rope can result in severe problems for the user and, in some cases, tragedy.

Ropes for Technical Climbing and Mountaineering

Ropes for climbers and mountaineers are designed to catch the user if he or she falls while climbing. Ropes for lead climbing must have stretch to absorb the energy of the fall without causing harm to the climber. A good climbing rope, besides protecting the climber, helps reduce force from being transmitted to anchors and "protection" and causing them to fail. This kind of rope is called *dynamic,* a term that relates to the use of force in motion. **Dynamic ropes** are also called *high stretch*.

Most of the stretch in a dynamic rope is built into it during manufacture and is achieved through various designs that elongate under load, much like a spring (Figure 3-1).

Another characteristic of dynamic ropes for climbing and mountaineering is that they are soft and pliable. These qualities are necessary in climbing because the rope is constantly being moved, knotted and unknotted, and run through hardware. This quality of being soft and pliable is called *hand*. It is achieved in part by manufacturing climbing ropes with a sheath, or outer surface, which is loose and thin.

Standards for climbing ropes have been established by the UIAA, CEN, and ASTM (see Appendix A, Standards Setting Organizations).

Ropes for Rappelling and Ascending

The rope, when used for rappelling or ascending, does not act as a safety for the person on the rope but as a means of travel. This is known as *single rope technique (SRT)*. The user actually travels down the rope using a rappel device or travels up the rope using ascenders. One example of SRT is vertical caving.

In SRT, the stretch of a dynamic rope would be a disadvantage and its thin sheath would be susceptible to **abrasion**.

For these kinds of activities, many prefer to use a *static rope,* which has very little stretch. In static ropes, the interior fiber bundles are constructed nearly parallel to one another so that most of the stretch is through the inherent stretch in the nylon (Figure 3-2). Static ropes typically stretch only about 18% to 20% before breaking.

In addition, static ropes characteristically have a thicker and tighter sheath to offer greater protection to

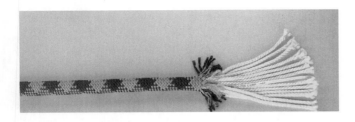

FIGURE 3-1
Typical dynamic rope core.

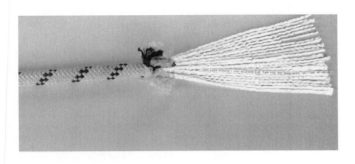

FIGURE 3-2
Typical static rope core.

the core. The result of this construction is that static ropes do not have the ease of handling of dynamic ropes and may be slightly more difficult for tying knots.

Ropes for Rescue Use

Ropes designed for rescue share some characteristics with ropes designed for SRT: low stretch and high resistance to damage from abrasion.

In rescue, the quality of **low stretch** means greater control of the rope for those persons performing a rescue. One example of this would be rescuers using rope to lower a litter. As the litter is eased over the edge of a vertical face, a greater load suddenly comes onto the rope. If a dynamic rope were being used, then there would be a great deal of stretch, with a significant drop in the litter. With a static rope there would be less stretch and therefore more control.

In addition, there is not as much "creep" in a system using a static rope. When a rope is first weighted, there is the initial stretch. But additional stretch, known as creep, will slowly come into the rope over a length of time, as it remains loaded. This creep tends to be greater in a dynamic rope. In a rescue situation, creep would be a disadvantage. It would, for example, make it more difficult for a dynamic rope to hold a litter in a constant position on a vertical face while a patient is loaded into the stretcher.

THE ROLE OF THE FALL FACTOR

One method of estimating the forces at work on a rope is by computing a measurement known as the **fall factor** (Figure 3-3). As shown in the first part of the illustration, a person is attached to a rope that will catch him or her in a fall, but will keep him or her from hitting the ground. The other end of the rope is directly attached to a point of "protection" that will not come loose. The fall factor is calculated by dividing the distance the person on the rope falls by the length of the rope between him or her and the point of protection.

$$\frac{\text{Distance person falls}}{\text{Length of rope}} = \text{Fall factor}$$

In the first example, consider that the length of rope is 100 feet (Figure 3-3, *A*). If the person were climbing up from below and slipped just before reaching the point of protection and fell exactly 100 feet, then the calculation would be:

$$\frac{\text{Distance fallen: 100 feet}}{\text{Length of rope: 100 feet}} = \text{Fall factor: 1}$$

If the person were climbing up from below and fell before reaching the point of protection, then it would be less than a factor 1 fall (Figure 3-3, *B*). For example, if the fall were only 50 feet:

$$\frac{\text{Distance fallen: 50 feet}}{\text{Length of rope: 100 feet}} = \text{Fall factor: 0.5}$$

Now, note the third part of the illustration. The figure has now climbed up above the point of protection by a full rope length (Figure 3-3, *C*). If he or she were to fall now:

$$\frac{\text{Distance fallen: 200 feet}}{\text{Length of rope: 100 feet}} = \text{Fall factor: 2}$$

Any fall from above the point of protection would be more than a factor 1 fall (Figure 3-3, *D*). If, for example, he or she fell 50 feet above the protection:

$$\frac{\text{Distance fallen: 150 feet}}{\text{Length of rope: 100 feet}} = \text{Fall factor: 1.5}$$

As the fall factor approaches and moves above 1, the severity becomes much worse. Note that it is not just the length of fall that matters, but the length of fall in relationship with both the amount of rope and the point of protection.

FIBERS USED TO MAKE ROPE
Natural Fibers

For many years, ropes made of natural fibers, such as sisal, hemp, and manila were standard. Then at about the time of World War II, mass production began of rope made of synthetic fibers such as *nylon* or *polyester.*

Today, synthetic fiber ropes are considered standard for situations where the safety of a person is "on the

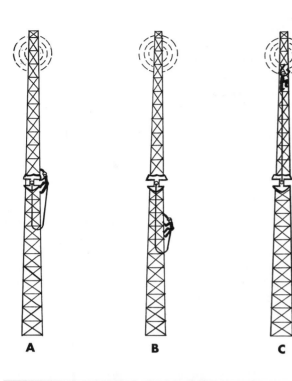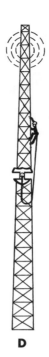

A   **B**   **C**   **D**

FIGURE 3-3
Comparison of fall factors.

! Warning

Although calculating the fall factor is useful in obtaining general estimates of the forces on a rope in a fall, these situations shown in Figure 3-3 above are ideal ones. Other factors will often enter into the situation to alter the results. They include the following:

◆ The rope may be running through intermediate points of protection or it may be rubbing against rock or other surfaces. This creates drag that may slow the rope's ability to stretch. This in turn effectively shortens the length of rope available to absorb the energy of the fall. The net result would be a much higher fall factor and greater impact forces on the person and parts of the system such as the anchors.

◆ In most climbing situations, a fall is not completely in free air. The fall factor is of little importance if the person taking the fall slams into the ground or is bashed against the wall on the way down.

line." In vertical sport activities such as climbing or vertical caving, synthetic fiber ropes have long since displaced those made of natural fibers. Synthetic fiber ropes are also considered the standard for rescue ropes. National organizations such as the International Association of Fire Fighters (IAFF), the International Society of Fire Service Instructors (ISFI), and the National Fire Protection Association (NFPA) have all condemned the use of natural fiber rope in life safety applications for the following reasons:

◆ Low resistance to abrasion.
◆ Limited ability to absorb shock loading.
◆ Will degrade in strength even with the best care.
◆ Can rot without outward visible signs.
◆ Have lower breaking strengths than ropes of the same diameter made of synthetic fibers such as nylon or polyester.
◆ Does not have strands that are continuous along its entire length because natural fibers are never more than a few feet long.

Synthetic Fiber Ropes

Among the advantages that synthetic fiber ropes have over natural fiber ropes are:
◆ Do not rot.
◆ Do not age as quickly as natural fiber rope.
◆ Can be made into more advanced rope designs than natural fibers.

There are several different synthetic fibers used in making ropes. Each fiber has distinct characteristics that make it suitable for certain uses and unsuitable for others.

Polyolefins (Polypropylene)
Advantages: Cheap
◆ Do not absorb water.
◆ Float (specific gravity of 0.91). Consequently, they are useful in activities on the water.
◆ Good chemical resistance (pH 2 to 12).
Disadvantages:
◆ Relatively low tensile strength (6 to 6.5 g per denier).
◆ Poor abrasion resistance.
◆ Low melting points (150° to 200° F).

◆ Poor shock absorbing capability.
◆ Poor resistance to damage from sunlight.

Polypropylene or polyethylene ropes are often found in water activities. But because of the low tensile strength, low abrasion resistance, and low melting point they should not be direct loading in life-support operations. For example, polyolefin ropes are unsuitable for rappelling and rescue lowering and hauling systems.

HMPE (*Extended Chain, High Modulus Polyethylene*)

Advantages:
◆ High tensile strength (30 to 35 g per denier breaking tenacity).
◆ Will float (0.97 specific gravity).

Disadvantages:
◆ Low melting point (around 150° to 200° F).
◆ Poor shock absorbing qualities (2.7% to 3.5% elongation at break).
◆ Material is very slippery, so it may require special knots to hold when tied.

Among the HMPE group is *Spectra,* a polyethylene yarn. Spectra is found in climbers' slings and runners. Spectra is very slippery and does not hold knots very well. Because Spectra has poor shock absorbing qualities, slings and runners made of this material should be used with dynamic rope or other energy absorbers in the rope system to absorb impact loads.

Aramids

Advantages:
◆ Resistance to high temperatures (350° F working limit).
◆ High tensile strength (18 to 26.5 g per denier).

Disadvantages:
◆ Easily damaged by abrasion.
◆ Easily damaged by continued small radius flexing (as in knotting).
◆ Poor shock-loading capability (1.5% to 3.6% elongation at break).

Kevlar

As with any new material, there has been considerable controversy over the best uses of *Kevlar* rope. However, there seems to be a consensus that it might have uses where it is not subject to continued small radius bending. For example, rock climbers have used Kevlar cord successfully as protection sling material, where it remains continually knotted, and when used with dynamic rope or other shock absorbers. But the consensus seems to be that current designs of Kevlar rope should not be used where it will be subjected to abrasion and continued small radius flexing (as in repeated knotting and unknotting). It is generally considered unsuitable for such activities as rappelling, ascending, belaying, and rescue lowering and hauling systems.

Polyester

Advantages:
◆ High tensile strength even when wet (7 to 10 g per denier).
◆ Good abrasion resistance.
◆ Melting point of about 480° F (high temperature working limit of 275° F).
◆ Resistant to damage from acids (pH of 3.5 to 7.5).

Disadvantages:
◆ Cannot handle shock loading as well as nylon (12% to 15% elongation at break).
◆ Susceptible to damage from alkalis.
◆ Does not float (specific gravity of 1.38).

Polyester fibers are found in a number of life safety applications. But because polyester does not handle shock loading as well as nylon, it is generally not found in climbing ropes.

An example of polyester is *Dacron,* the Dupont trade name for a type of polyester.

Nylon

There are actually several different types of nylon. The two most commonly used in life safety ropes are *nylon 6,* also known as *Perlon,* and *nylon 6,6* (Box 3-1).

Advantages:
◆ About 10% stronger than polyester in ropes of comparable diameter when dry (7.8 to 10.4 g per denier breaking tenacity).
◆ Good shock loading capability (15% to 28% elongation at break).
◆ Melting point of around 480° F, 250° C (type 6,6) (high temperature working limit of 250° F).
◆ Good chemical resistance to alkalis (pH 6.5 to 10.5).

Disadvantages:
◆ May lose 10% to 15% of its strength when wet (will regain the deficiency when dry).
◆ Susceptible to certain strong acids, such as those used in storage batteries.

Ropes made of nylon yarn are commonly used in life support applications including climbing, vertical caving, rescue, and tactical operations.

 Box 3-1 Nylon Type 6

Nylon type 6, also known by its European trade name, *Perlon,* has better elongation qualities than 6,6, which gives it better shock absorbing qualities. Consequently, nylon type 6 is found in most climbing ropes.

Type 6,6 has a slightly higher melting point and a slightly higher breaking point than type 6. In addition, nylon type 6,6 has slightly better resistance to wear and less elongation under load. This is why most static ropes are constructed of type 6,6. Whether these differences in the nylon actually appear in the rope depend in large part on the individual rope design.

Nylon type 6,6 is found in some ropes manufactured in North America. The Dupont and Monsanto corporations manufacture the type 6,6 yarn.

ROPE CONSTRUCTION

The choice of a rope for a specific job depends not only in part on the fiber it is made from but also on the manner in which it is constructed.

Laid

Laid construction, also known as *twisted* or *hawser lay*, means twisting small fiber bundles of material and then combining them in larger bundles, which are twisted around one another, usually in groups of three (Figure 3-4). This type of rope construction resembles the designs of older types of rope constructed of natural fibers.

Characteristics:
◆ When loaded, the fibers tend to untwist slightly thus causing spin and kinking. Many modern laid ropes are of balanced construction in an effort to limit this problem. Even so, this type of rope has a good bit of inherent twist.
◆ Because each fiber may appear at the surface of the rope somewhere along its length, the load-bearing fibers are more susceptible to damage by abrasion.
◆ Tend to be very stretchy.
◆ Tend to kink unless carefully handled.

Those persons still using laid rope in life support operations usually employ the tighter lay, or "mountain lay," design. The "marine lay" design is looser and more susceptible to damage by abrasion. However, the mountain lay is more difficult to find than the marine lay.

Ropes of laid construction have been displaced in most high angle work by other designs.

Plaited

Plaited ropes usually consist of bundles of fibers plaited together (Figure 3-5).
Advantages:
◆ Tend to be soft and pliable.
Disadvantages:
◆ Prone to "picking" (the snagging and pulling out of fiber bundles).

Braided

Braided ropes are found in two different types:
1. Solid braid (Figure 3-6). In this type of design, the rope is constructed entirely of a single weave of three or more fiber bundles. The design is sometimes called a *clothesline braid*. Because the load-supporting fiber bundles in single braid construction are vulnerable to destruction when the rope is being used, single braid construction ropes have limited use in high angle operations.
2. Hollow braid. This is essentially a very thick sheath. It sometimes is found with a "filler" such as scrap yarn or filament plastic. It typically is found in inexpensive hardware store type rope, not in life safety line.

Double Braid

Double braid ropes are essentially a solid braid covered with a hollow braid combined into one construction (Figure 3-7). One braid acts as the rope core, while a second braid is constructed around it to act as a sheath and help protect the inner braid.

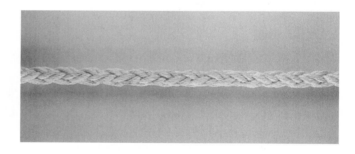

FIGURE 3-5
Plaited construction.

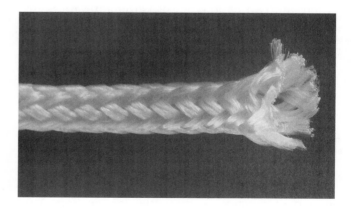

FIGURE 3-6
Solid braid construction.

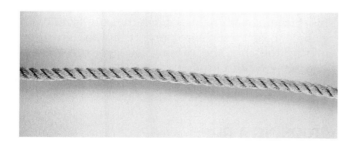

FIGURE 3-4
Typical laid rope construction.

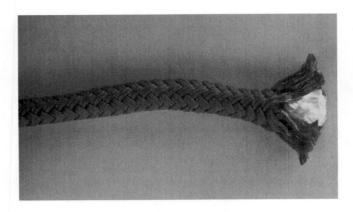

FIGURE 3-7
Double braid construction.

Advantages:
 ◆ Soft and flexible.
Disadvantages:
 ◆ Susceptible to contamination of core by grit and dirt.
 ◆ Susceptible to "picking."
 ◆ Susceptible to abrasion.
 ◆ When cut around its diameter, sheath tends to slip down on core.

Kernmantle

This term comes from a compound German word, *kern* or *core* and *mantle* or *sheath* (cover). The **kernmantle** rope design consists of a central core (kern) of fibers that support the major portion of the load on the rope. This core is covered by a woven sheath (mantle), which supports a lesser portion of the load. But the tight weave of the mantle protects the core from abrasion, dirt, and environmental effects, such as sunlight. The kernmantle construction results in a rope that is strong and resists damage but is easy to handle. It also does not have the drawback of severe twisting that affects other rope designs, such as laid. There are two basic types of kernmantle ropes: dynamic kernmantle and static kernmantle.

Dynamic Kernmantle

The term *dynamic* indicates a rope with high stretch. This is meant to act as sort of a shock absorber when a falling climber is caught by the rope. Some dynamic kernmantle ropes stretch by as much as 60% before breaking.

This stretch is created with a rope core that mechanically lets out under load, much as a spring does. The design of the core varies slightly from one manufacturer to another. Figure 3-8 illustrates one design of dynamic kernmantle construction. Most dynamic rope cores are constructed of a group of twisted bundles. A small percentage of dynamic ropes have braided cores.

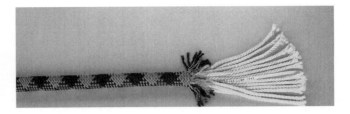

FIGURE 3-8
Dynamic kernmantle construction.

When compared with static kernmantle rope, the sheath, or mantle, of dynamic kernmantle ropes tend to be relatively thin, but with more fiber bundles over the same area. This means that the sheath will cover the core better when the rope is stretched or bent.

Advantages of Dynamic Kernmantle Ropes:
 ◆ The elasticity is an advantage for climbing situations where long falls are possible.
 ◆ Very easy to handle and tie knots in.
Disadvantages of Dynamic Kernmantle Ropes:
 ◆ Thin sheath makes them susceptible to damage from abrasion and to contamination from dirt and grit.
 ◆ Their elasticity makes them less suitable for activities such as rappelling and ascending and for many rescue operations.

Static Kernmantle

This is also known as *low stretch* kernmantle. The term static indicates a type of rope with very low stretch (no more than 20% of its length at break). Manufacturing a rope core of fiber bundles that are nearly parallel to one another creates this low stretch (Figure 3-9). In some static ropes there is so little stretch that what there is results largely from the inherent stretch of the nylon.

Because there is so little stretch, static ropes provide a more sudden stop when catching a fall. This sudden stop subjects the climber's body, the equipment in the system, and the anchors to greater impact loading than would be seen if a dynamic rope were used.

Most static kernmantle ropes also have a thicker and tighter sheath than dynamic kernmantle ropes. This thicker sheath helps protect the core from damage by abrasion and helps prevent dirt and grit from entering the core and causing damage to the inner fibers. One result of a tighter sheath is a rope that is stiffer and not as easy to handle as the dynamic kernmantle with its thinner sheath.

CHOOSING A ROPE

A rope is the one essential element in the high angle system. It is in essence a tool, and, as with all tools, the correct rope should be chosen to fit the job.

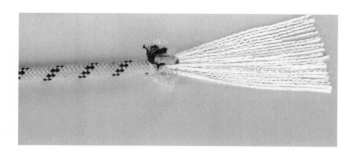

FIGURE 3-9
Static kernmantle construction.

All references in this book to dynamic rope or static rope are to very specific constructions of rope. A dynamic rope is one specifically built for climbing or mountaineering and is not just a stretchy rope. A static rope is a rescue static rope made especially for rope rescue, or a sport static rope made for personal ascending or rappelling.

These special ropes will normally not be found at the average hardware store. They should be purchased only from reputable dealers and manufacturers who sell their products for these specific uses.

Dynamic versus Static Ropes

If you are going to be doing exclusively recreational rock climbing or mountaineering, the choice will be a dynamic rope. There are many types of dynamic ropes that can be used depending on the climbing environment and the style of climbing. For this, you should consult an instructional manual on climbing or any of several catalogues from companies that specialize in climbing equipment.

Also, if the rope is going to be used as a belay for falls that result in severe shock loading, then a dynamic rope will be more appropriate. There is considerable debate on at what point the fall becomes severe enough to require a dynamic rope. Much of this will depend on local conditions such as the climbing environment, the equipment used, and the experience of the people involved. But certainly if a fall approaching the severity of a factor 0.25 is expected, then a dynamic rope should be used. This is not so much for the sake of the rope, but to reduce the impact loads on the person attached to the rope and on the anchors.

If the activities were going to be restricted to rappelling and ascending, particularly under harsh conditions, then a static rope would probably be preferable. Most rescue personnel now use static rope in their operations.

Size and Strength

If the choice is a static rope, and the decision has been made on the type of rope fiber and construction, then there must be a decision on how strong a rope is needed, or on the **tensile strength.** The tensile strength of a rope depends very much on its cross section of material or the amount of yarn used per foot of length.

There may be a temptation to choose the largest diameter rope available (usually ⅝ inch for a synthetic fiber, life-support rope), but this could be a serious mistake and could actually hinder activity with the rope.

Presently, most rescue teams select ⁷⁄₁₆ or ½ inch static kernmantle construction ropes for their main rescue lines. But each team should make their own decision based on such factors as rescue needs, environment, and nature of their team.

Problems with Large Diameter Ropes

There are several problems in using large diameter ropes, including the following:
- ◆ Higher costs because of more material in the rope.
- ◆ The larger the diameter of a rope, the more it weighs. This means difficulty in carrying the rope to where it is needed (usually up hill or up flights of stairs).
- ◆ Handling problems. When the rope is hanging vertically, the higher weight will mean more difficulty in rappelling and in handling the rope.
- ◆ Incompatibility with other equipment. Many types of high angle equipment are not made for use with ropes over ½-inch diameter.

The one obvious advantage to very large diameter ropes is their overall strength. However, in normal field use, larger diameter ropes have only slight abrasion and cut resistance over ⁷⁄₁₆ and ½ inch ropes.

Determining the Safety Factor

The most realistic way to determine the needed tensile strength of the rope, and therefore the diameter, is by calculating the safety factor. The *safety factor* estimates conditions you are expected to encounter in the local high angle environment, plus a realistic margin of safety.

The first step in determining the safety factor is to estimate what will be the maximum load you expect to be on the rope. If this will only be the weight of one person, as in a recreational situation, plus high angle equipment, then the total weight may only be 200 lb. If the rope is to be used in rescue, then the estimated weight will probably be more. If, for example, there will be a rescue subject plus a rescuer and a litter with assorted gear, the total weight might be 600 lb.

If 600 lb is the expected load, then obviously the breaking strength of the rope cannot be exactly

600 lb. The rope will be subjected to shock loading, to reduce strength through knots and sharp bends and because of wear. So it is necessary to have a strength several times greater than 600 lb as a margin of safety or a safety factor.

In industry and construction, where a load on the rope is to be equipment or materials but not people, a common safety factor is 5:1. But a safety factor of 5:1 or less is unacceptable when a person is on the rope.

Some individuals and groups accept a safety factor of 10:1. The 10:1 safety factor is accepted among some mountain and wilderness rescue groups. These mountain and wilderness rescue units use the 10:1 safety factor for several reasons. First of all, they may have to carry rope for long distances, so weight is an important factor. But mountain rescuers also feel they have better control of their equipment and are very knowledgeable about its history. They also may be skilled enough to assess equipment limitations such as potential overloading and other damaging factors. For these reasons, they feel they do not need a safety factor greater than 10:1.

Some rescue disciplines feel they need a greater safety factor. For example, a safety factor for rescue rope that is widely published in written standards and commonly used in the fire service is 15:1.

Therefore if 600 lb is the expected maximum load, with a safety factor of 10:1, the rope should have a minimum breaking strength of 6,000 lb. If a safety factor of 15:1 is employed, then the minimum breaking strength should be 9,000 lb.

The NFPA has now set guidelines for life safety rope and rates them either as single person or two person life safety ropes. The NFPA standards consider a single-person load as 300 lb and a two-person load as 600 lb.

The NFPA Standards for Rope and Related Equipment (NFPA 1983-95) provide a separate set of standards for a personal escape rope (bailout line). Under the bailout line section of the standards, a 10:1 safety standard is acceptable. Thus, because most individuals and equipment weigh less than 300 lb, a bailout rope for most individuals could have a tensile strength of 3,000 lb.

Breaking Strength of Rope

The breaking strength of a rope is measured as *tensile strength at break*. On the face of it, this may seem like a very simple idea. But there are many different ways of conducting tests that will result in different test results on the same piece of rope. Among the different factors that will affect the outcome of a tensile test include the following:

- ◆ Speed of the pull. A rope pulled apart slowly will register a higher breaking strength than one pulled apart at a faster speed. (Results may be different in dynamic drop tests, depending on rope materials and construction.)

- ◆ Diameter of the object that rope is attached to when it is pulled. A rope pulled to failure by a small diameter object will break at a lower tensile strength than a rope pulled with a larger diameter object. Similarly, a rope pulled with a knot in it will break at a lower strength than one without a knot. (This is because whenever a rope is placed under load in a sharp bend, some strength is lost. See Chapter 4, Care and Use of Rope and Related Equipment on page 34.)

Rope Tensile Test Standards

There is one test standard developed by the U.S. Federal Government that can be used for comparisons among the rope manufacturers who use it. This is the *Federal Test Method 191A, Method 6016*. This guide specifies guidelines such as what the rope is tied to during the test and the rate of pull, along with other criteria.

In addition, certain NFPA standards apply to rope that is used by those who adhered to NFPA standards. Contact the NFPA for specific information on these standards. See Appendix C for addresses of standards setting organizations.

Rope Colors

Although many people choose a rope color for aesthetic reasons, the color of a rope can also serve a functional purpose. If, for example, there are several ropes being used together, the differing colors can help distinguish one line from another, so that the user can immediately know which rope to haul or lower.

Another way to use color is to buy a different colored rope for each year to quickly tell the age. Or one might use varying colors for different sizes of rope.

Process for Coloring Ropes

Nylon, when manufactured, is off-white, so any color for a rope has to be added at some point during its manufacture. Any color added to the rope material will somewhat affect the rope strength and, in some cases, affect its resistance to damage by sunlight. How much these properties are affected depends on the method for adding the dye to rope material and, in some cases, the dye material itself.

There are two basic methods of adding color to a rope. One technique for dying a rope is known as *solution dying*. In this technique, the color is added to the raw material as the yarn is being manufactured. The second method of coloring is *surface-applied dying*, in which the color is added to the synthetic yarn after it has been manufactured or added to the rope after it has been braided.

Solution dying usually causes slightly more strength loss in the rope than surface-applied dying. Also, the strength loss will vary from color to color because of chemical differences among the various dyes.

Accessory Cord

Accessory cord is smaller diameter rope used for a variety of tasks where the regular rope would be too bulky. Two types of accessory cord parallel main line ropes:

1. Rescue accessory cord:
   - It has a static kernmantle construction, with low stretch.
   - It is heavier duty and longer lasting but does not knot and grip as well as climber's accessory cord. Consequently it does not work well with friction knots such as Prusiks.
   - It typically ranges in diameter from 4 to 7 mm.
2. Climber's accessory cord:
   - It is softer and more flexible (like climbing rope).
   - It is not as resistant to wear as rescue accessory cord but it is easier to knot and grips better in friction knots such as Prusiks.
   - It is usually found in sizes up to 9 mm.

Webbing

Webbing, because of its special characteristics, is sometimes preferable to rope for certain situations. For example, webbing is more comfortable than rope against the body for seat harnesses. Webbing is commonly used for anchoring because it is less expensive than rope. And due to its wide, flat surface it can be more abrasion resistant in some rigging applications.

One drawback to webbing is that it does not absorb shock loading as well as many ropes. This means that when webbing is used for anchors, it will tend to transmit the shock loading to the anchor points. This is one reason why some people prefer rope to webbing in anchoring.

There are fewer secure knots for webbing than for rope. Because webbing has a slick surface, knots can pull out if they are not carefully tied, safetied, and monitored. Consequently, you may prefer webbing anchor loops that are presewn at the factory.

Materials

Most webbing is made of nylon or polyester, which are materials that have the same characteristics as those used to manufacture rope. Some webbing is made from Spectra, which has high tensile strength

but does not absorb shock loading as well as nylon or polyester. For this reason, webbing made of Spectra should be used with dynamic rope or other energy absorbers in the rope system to absorb impact loads.

Construction

Flat Webbing. Flat webbing is constructed of a single layer of material, the same as seat belt webbing. It is less expensive but stiffer and more difficult to work with than tubular webbing.

Tubular Webbing. Because tubular webbing is more supple and easier to work with, it is more often used in the high angle environment. The tubular shape is obvious if you look at it from one end and squeeze the two edges together. There are two types of tubular webbing: edge-stitched and spiral weave.

Edge-stitched webbing. Edge-stitched webbing is formed by folding over flat webbing lengthwise and stitching the two edges together (Figure 3-10). You should be careful when purchasing edge-stitched webbing and buy it only from a reputable dealer. Because webbing is susceptible to abrasion along its edges, some types of edge-stitched webbing may become unstitched when the thread is broken. The better design of edge-stitched webbing locks the stitches under one another so they are not as prone to coming unstitched.

Spiral weave. Spiral weave is also known as *shuttle loom construction.* This design of tubular webbing is traditionally more common in high angle operations (Figure 3-11). It is constructed by weaving a tube as a unit.

There are hundreds of sizes and types of webbing in the marketplace. Many types are unsuitable for high angle operations. You should buy webbing for life-support applications only from quality suppliers who publish tensile strengths and specifications. Be particularly cautious about the use of surplus webbing that usually has no information about tensile strength, material, specifications, date of manufacture, or history of

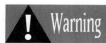 **Warning**

Climbers accessory cord does not use the same high stretch core yarns as dynamic climbing rope and should never be used in place of those ropes for impact load situations.

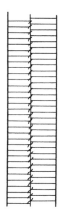

FIGURE 3-10
Edge-stitched webbing.

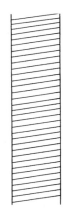

FIGURE 3-11
Spiral weave webbing.

use. Use the same procedure for deciding the safety factor for webbing as for rope and other equipment.

Webbing Size

There are various widths for webbing ranging from ½ inch up to 2 inches. The most common size used in high angle work is the 1-inch width. For seat harnesses, the larger widths are more comfortable.

Webbing Strength

Although there are hundreds of sizes and styles of webbing products, the most common webbing sold by suppliers of high angle equipment include the following:
◆ 1-inch tubular nylon: Most common is Mil-W-5625, which has a tensile strength of about 4,000 lb.
◆ 1-inch solid nylon: Most common is Mil-W-4088, type 18, which has a tensile strength of about 6,000 lb.
◆ 1^{15}/16-inch or 2-inch solid seatbelt-type webbing, nylon or polyester: It has a tensile strength of 4,500 to 6,000 lb, depending on material and type.
◆ 1^{23}/32-inch flat nylon webbing, Mil-W-4088: It has a tensile strength of about 9,500 lb.

Evaluation Exercises

◆ COGNITIVE AND AFFECTIVE EXERCISES ◆

1. **Dynamic ropes are designed to stretch because:**
   A. Stretch is required for knots.
   B. It allows energy to be absorbed during shock loading.
   C. It allows for a "weak" link.
   D. It allows systems to bend.

2. **Static ropes are designed not to stretch because:**
   A. It reduces stretch in mechanical advantage, rappelling, and ascending situations.
   B. It allows for energy absorption.
   C. It allows the climber to absorb the kinetic energy.
   D. It allows for easier knot placement.

3. **A climber is connected at the top of a 1,200 foot cliff with a 100-foot length of rope to a secure point of protection. While at this point of protection, he or she falls the full length of the rope. This is a factor _____ fall.**
   A. 1.5
   B. 2
   C. 1
   D. 0.5

4. **A rescuer is connected 200 feet up a 700-foot tower with a 100-foot length rope to a secure point of protection. He or she climbs up past the point of protection by 100 feet and falls past the point of protection the full length of the rope before being caught by the rope. This is a factor _____ fall.**
   A. 0.5
   B. 1
   C. 1.5
   D. 2

5. **A rescuer is climbing a 300-foot wall and is being belayed on a 200-foot dynamic rope. The belay point is 200 feet up the cliff. The climber starts climbing again at the belay point and has climbed 100 feet up from the belay point when he falls. He falls free and is caught by the belay. This would be a factor _____ fall.**
   A. 0.5
   B. 1
   C. 1.5
   D. 2

6. **Advantages of synthetic fiber rope for high angle activities include all of the following, *except*:**
   A. They have higher temperature resistance.
   B. Each fiber runs the entire length of the rope.
   C. They have low resistance to abrasion.
   D. They do not rot.

7. **The nylon types commonly used in rope for high angle activities include:**
   A. Polyester and nylon 6.
   B. Nylon 6.6 and nylon 6.
   C. Perlon and Kevlar.
   D. Nylon 6.6 and polyolefins.

8. **The advantage(s) of plaited rope is/are:**
   A. Softness and pliability.
   B. Picking.
   C. Abrasion resistance.
   D. Stiffness.

9. **Single braid rope is generally not adequate for high angle operations because:**
   A. It is constructed of three fiber bundles.

B. It is braided as a "clothesline braid."
C. It is vulnerable to destruction.
D. All of the above.

10. The term *kernmantle* refers to:
  A. The core and sheath construction.
  B. The solid braid over a single braid.
  C. The eight bundles of fibers plaited together.
  D. The three fiber bundles twisted together.

11. You are about to make a traverse to a subject who is trapped on a ledge, approximately 100 feet away. The subject is approximately 200 feet above the ground and you are on the same elevation with the subject. You would choose which of the following ropes to use for protection during your traverse:
  A. Plaited rope.
  B. Dynamic kernmantle.
  C. Single braid.
  D. Static kernmantle.

12. You have reached the subject in the above situation and you want to set a rope to the bottom for other rescuers to ascend. You would choose which of the following ropes for the ascent rope:
  A. Plaited rope.
  B. Single braid.
  C. Static kernmantle.
  D. Dynamic kernmantle.

13. The safety factor of a rescue rope with a breaking strength of 4,500 lb and with a 600-lb load would be:
  A. 15:1
  B. 7.5
  C. 12.5:1
  D. 10:1

14. Using a safety factor of 15:1, the minimum tensile strength rope to be used where the expected load will be 600 lb would be:
  A. 4,500 lb
  B. 6,000 lb
  C. 7,500 lb
  D. 9,000 lb

15. Flat weave webbing is typically considered to have a breaking strength of:
  A. 2,500 lb
  B. 4,000 lb
  C. 5,000 lb
  D. 6,000 lb

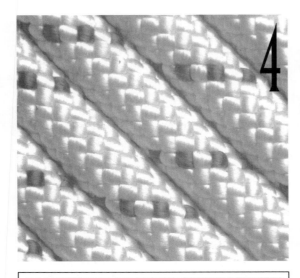

4 Care and Use of Rescue Rope and Related Equipment

Key Terms

Abrasion The damaging wear on rope and other gear caused by rubbing against abrasive material.

Laid Rope A rope design that consists of fiber bundles twisted around one another.

Polyester A type of fiber used in some rope manufacturing. Also known by the trade name D*acron*.

Static Rope A type of rope designed for low stretch. It is used in applications such as rescue, rappelling, and ascending where high stretch would be a disadvantage and where no falls, or very short falls, are expected before being caught by the rope. Also called *low stretch*.

Tensile Strength A measurement of the greatest lengthwise stress under slow pull conditions that a rope can resist without failing.

Objectives

At the completion of this chapter, you should be able to:

1. List the elements of a rope log.
2. Identify the storage situations that could harm a stored rope.
3. List the advantages to bagging a rope for storage and transport.
4. List the situations or substances that may damage a working rope.
5. Cite several methods for protecting a working rope.
6. Define the 4:1 rule.
7. List the steps for inspecting a rope.
8. List the reasons for retiring a rope.
9. List several strategies for avoiding the tangling of a working rope.
10. Describe the process for throwing or dropping a rope down a face or wall.

CARE OF ROPES

The modern high angle rescue rope is a marvel of design and engineering. But a rope's performance, how long it lasts, and its safety still depend on how well it is cared for. The condition of a rope ultimately depends on its history: the age of the rope, the conditions to which it has been subjected, and the care it has received.

If a rope is owned and used by only one person, then that person probably knows the history of the rope. However, if more than one person is using the rope, then there has to be a system of tracking that rope's history. Each rope must have a rope history log.

Keeping a Rope History Log

To track each rope's history, it must have its own log card with pertinent information on the manufacturer, diameter, design, **tensile strength,** date of purchase, and so on. There should be space on the log card for indicating each time the rope was used and the activity it was used in. There must be specific entries made whenever the rope was subjected to abuse that could affect its performance or safety. Figure 4-1 shows an example of a rope history log.

It is essential that entries for each rope be made every time it is returned to storage after use. This discipline must be followed by every user, otherwise the rope history will be incomplete.

Tagging a Rope

Because most groups with high angle rescue gear have ropes of similar color, length, and diameter, there must be some way of distinguishing each individual rope so that its history can be kept. Each rope should have some distinguishing identification such as a number or letter that corresponds with its card. This identifying mark must be placed on the rope so that it is unmistakable and so that it cannot be eradicated or lost. Some examples of tagging a rope include the following (Figure 4-2):

- ◆ Hot stamping the end of the rope.
- ◆ Marking the circumference at the end of the rope and protecting the mark with clear plastic tape, clear heat shrink tubing, or a protective coating such as Whip End Dip.

Storage of Rope

In short, a life support rope must be stored in a place of its own where it is protected from harm. You can *damage* your rope if you do the following:

- ◆ Leave it in sunlight. (All fibers used in life safety ropes, including nylon and *polyester,* will degrade under prolonged exposure to sunlight.)
- ◆ Expose it to vehicle exhaust systems or to fumes or residues from storage batteries. (Both of these vehicle components produce substances damaging to rope.)
- ◆ Leave it on the floor. (Concrete floors are alkaline but they may contain damaging substances from materials used in sealants and from acids used in cleaning. Stepping on rope grinds in dirt and grit. Also, damaging substances can be dropped onto the rope.)
- ◆ Store the rope in wet or damp areas. (This will promote the growth of mold or mildew on the rope.)
- ◆ Store rope in areas of high temperature. (Prolonged exposure to temperatures higher than humans can tolerate will promote degradation of rope.)
- ◆ Contaminate it with dirt and grit. (Dirt and grit work into the core and damage the yarn. Avoid needlessly dragging a rope on the ground and *never* step on a rope.)

ROPE USAGE & HISTORY

SERIAL NUMBER	I.D. MARKING	LENGTH	DIAMETER

DATE OF MFG.	ISSUE DATE	DATE IN SERVICE

FIBER	COLOR	CONSTRUCTION	MFG SLOT NUMBER

INSPECT ROPE FOR DAMAGE OR EXCESSIVE WEAR EACH TIME IT IS DEPLOYED AND AGAIN AFTER EACH USE.
IMMEDIATELY RETIRE ALL SUSPECT ROPES

DATE USED	INCIDENT LOCATION	TYPE OF USE	ROPE EXPOSURE	DATE INSPECTED	INSPECTORS INITIALS	ROPE CONDITION & COMMENTS

FIGURE 4-1
Rope history log.

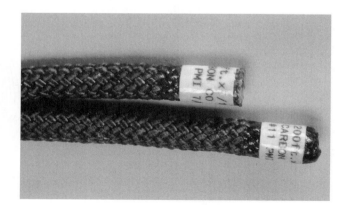

FIGURE 4-2
Rope tagging example.

Bagging Ropes

One of the most convenient ways of storing, transporting, and protecting the rope, is called *bagging* (Figure 4-4).

Some of the advantages of bagging include the following:

◆ The bag helps protect the rope from damage while keeping it clean.

◆ You can usually flake rope into a bag quicker than you can coil it. Figure 4-4 shows a fast technique for bagging a rope.

◆ If the bag has a shoulder strap or pack straps, it is a convenient way in which to carry the rope.

◆ A bagged rope is easy to deploy. Simply secure the upper end of the rope and drop the bag over the edge. In most cases, the rope will flake out

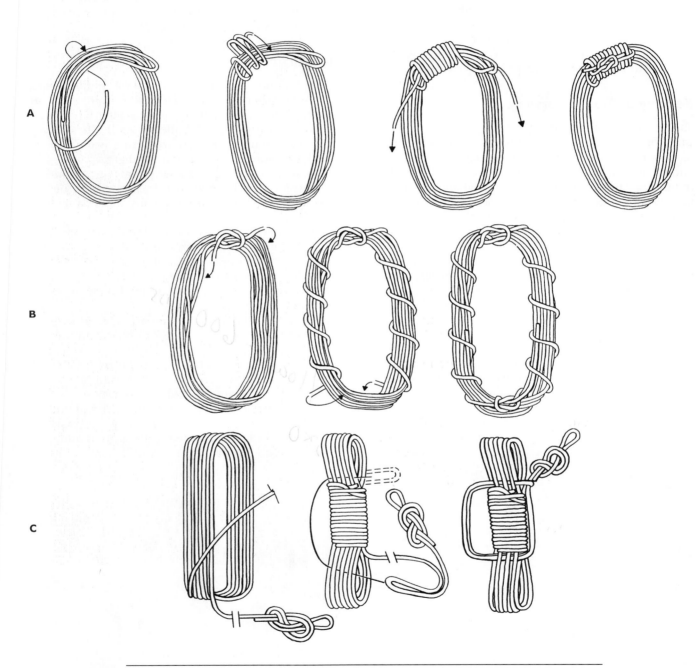

FIGURE 4-3

A, Mountaineer coil, a traditional climbers' coil, can be quickly made. **B,** Cavers coil is designed to be carried through caves without snagging. **C,** Butterfly coil is useful for paying out rope, such as dropping down a face. Also, the ends can be secured so the coil can be carried on a person like a backpack.

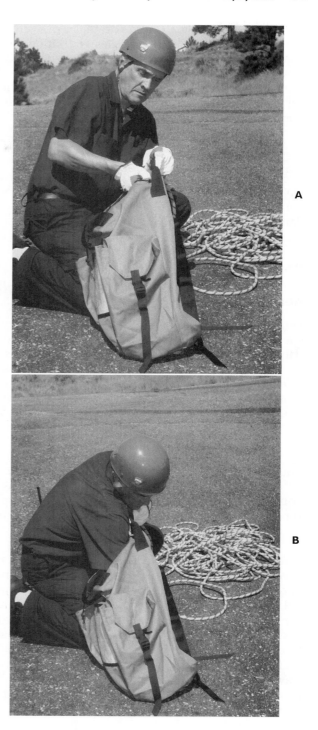

> ⚠️ **Warning**
>
> To avoid damage to the rope, use common sense in dropping bagged rope. Do not, for example, drop a bag with 600 feet of rope down 100 feet. The 500 feet remaining in the bag when the bag hits bottom may be damaged by the impact. Match the amount of rope to the distance of the drop.

of the bag without tangles. Secure the bottom end of the rope to the bottom of the bag so that the bag is not lost when you drop it.

Techniques for Bagging Rope

1. If you are wearing a seat harness, clip a carabiner into the harness and run the end of the rope through the carabiner and into the bag. If you are not wearing a harness, begin with the next step.
2. Grasp the top edge of the bag and hold the bag open and upright with your nondominant hand *(left hand for right-handed people).*
3. Lightly trap the rope between your thumb and index finger as it enters the bag.
4. With your dominant hand *(right hand for right-handed people)* below the other hand, grasp the rope and pull it into the bottom of the bag.
5. Slide the dominant hand back up to the other hand, take another length of rope, and pull it down into the bag.
6. Continue with these short strokes until the rope is bagged.

Coiling

Before bagging became common practice, coiling was commonly used for storing and transporting ropes. The specific type of coil will depend on the circumstances or environment in which the rope is to be used. Figure 4-3 shows some basic types of coils: mountaineer coil, cavers coil, and butterfly coil.

HOW ROPES ARE DAMAGED
Harmful Substances

The following list includes some of the common substances that can destroy or deteriorate certain kinds of rope.
Damaging to Nylon:
   ◆ Acids, particularly those found in storage batteries.
   ◆ Bleaches.
Damaging to Polyester:
   ◆ Alkali (such as found in soot).
Damaging to Nylon and Polyester:
   ◆ Many other strong chemicals. (Avoid any contact with a chemical unless you know for sure it is harmless to rope fiber.)

FIGURE 4-4

Bagging a rope.

Overloading a Rope

Overloading a rope creates internal damage that could endanger those people who use the ropes in the future. Damage from overloading usually occurs when a rope is used in activities for which it was not intended and when the load greatly exceeds the rope's safe working load. Some examples of overloading a rope include towing vehicles and lifting heavy objects.

A separate set of ropes, for utility use only, must be used for activities such as these two examples. These utility lines must be stored separately from life support ropes and distinctly marked, for example, "utility line, *not for life support operations.*"

Damage from Falling Objects

Objects such as rocks or tools that fall on the rope, particularly when it is under load, can cause serious damage. Any time that heavy or sharp objects have been seen falling on a rope, or when the rope has been used in a rock fall zone, then it should be inspected for damage.

Abrasion

One of the most common ways of destroying a rope, or shortening its life, is through **abrasion**. This kind of damage is usually avoidable. Damage from abrasion commonly occurs when the rope is under tension and is lowered and raised across a rock or over the edge of a building. Abrasion often happens when a person is doing "bouncy" rappels or ascending, causing the rope to "saw" back and forth across a rock or hard object.

Techniques for Avoiding Abrasion

There are numerous ways for avoiding abrasion on rope, many of them using simple and inexpensive equipment. Every person and every team that owns a rope should carry equipment for preventing edge abrasion.

Rope Pads. Rope pads are among the simplest and least expensive techniques for protecting rope from abrasion. They work best for fixed ropes, such as rappel lines. Among the commonly used types of pads are canvas pads (heavy-duty canvas can easily be made into protective pads). For greater protection and durability, a square of heavy-duty canvas can be folded twice, stitched around the edge to prevent fraying, and then cross-stitched (Figure 4-5). For added convenience, large grommets can be set in two corners. These grommets can be used to attach the pad so it will not slide away as the rope is moving. A complete edge protection kit should include a variety of pads ranging from approximately 2 x 3 feet to 2 x 6 feet or larger.

Several commercially made canvas rope pads are also available, which include fire hoses and improvised rope pads.

Fire Hose. Sections of discarded fire hose can also be converted to effective rope pads. In order to avoid having to feed the rope through the hose, modify the hose in the following manner:

1. Split the hose down the center.

2. To prevent the rope from slipping out, secure the edges of the hose with a closure such as snaps or Velcro (Figure 4-6).
3. Set a hole or grommet in each end so the hose can be anchored to prevent it from slipping down the rope.

Improvised Techniques. If no premade edge protection is available, then other materials may be pressed into service to protect the rope from abrasion. Some examples of improvised rope pads are:

- ◆ Packs
- ◆ Turnout coats
- ◆ Clothing
- ◆ Blankets
- ◆ Carpet squares

Note that wool carpet squares are preferable because synthetic material carpet may melt under heat fusion with the rope.

Commercial Rope Protectors

There are a number of different rope protection devices on the market. They usually fall into two categories:

1. Metal devices: Often used in lowering or hauling operations.

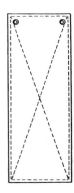

FIGURE 4-5

Canvas rope pad.

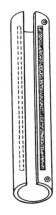

FIGURE 4-6

Fire hose rope pad.

Advantages:
- ◆ Offer greater protection.
- ◆ Reduce friction, particularly in hauling.

Disadvantages:
- ◆ More expensive.
- ◆ Heavier.
- ◆ Prone to tipping over unless carefully anchored.

2. Soft protection (canvas and other fabrics): Often used where the rope is not moving, such as a rappel rope.

Advantages:
- ◆ Less expensive than metal devices.
- ◆ Weighs less.

Disadvantages:
- ◆ Offers less protection.
- ◆ Does not reduce friction as much as metal devices.

Commercial Soft Protection. Commercial soft edge protection may be similar to canvas edge pads or similar to the fire hose pads. Some fabrics may be coated canvas or other fabrics such as PVC coated nylon (Figure 4-7). Some are made with closures so the pad stays wrapped around the rope.

Mechanical Rope Protection Devices

Edge Rollers. Edge rollers are one of the most effective techniques for protecting ropes from abrasion. They are usually more expensive than soft edge protection but they have the added advantage of greatly reducing friction of rope over an edge. This is particularly important in hauling systems, where edge friction makes the tasks of raising much more difficult and puts great stress on equipment. Edge rollers may tip over if they are not carefully anchored.

Edge rollers are available in three main types:
1. Single unit rollers. A single roller is set into a frame with a flat base (Figure 4-8). It usually takes two or more of these single units to provide adequate edge protection. They generally must be stabilized by anchoring them with their attachment points. When they are stabilized, these units perform well on irregular surfaces, such as cliffs and other natural situations.

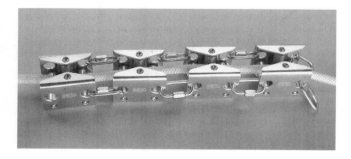

FIGURE 4-7
Commercial rope protector.

2. Roof rollers. The roof roller consists of a unit of two rollers set in a 90-degree frame (Figure 4-9). They are designed for edge protection on buildings and other structures where 90-degree angles are present.
3. Roll module. This has rollers on the side as well as the bottom, so if it tips over, it still offers protection. The four modules are linked together with screw links and can conform to a variety of surfaces.

Other Mechanical Edge Protection. Other mechanical edge protection devices include those with smooth metal bars that can be clipped together. One

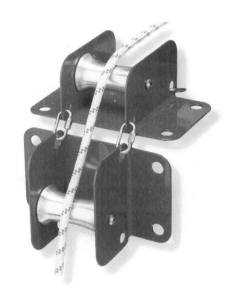

FIGURE 4-8
Edge roller.

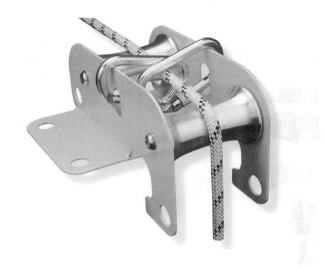

FIGURE 4-9
Roof roller.

example is the Terrain Protector. The bars in the Terrain Protector do not rotate; they do not reduce friction as much as edge rollers but they reduce it more and provide more protection than with soft protection. They are also lighter weight and less expensive than most edge rollers. The Terrain Protector is versatile because you only use as many sections as is necessary to provide protection. You can connect the individual sections of the Terrain Protector with screw links, carabiners, or accessory cord.

Heat Fusion

Heat fusion results when two pieces of synthetic material rub together. It is very destructive to rope and can cut a line as surely as if it were cut with a knife. Heat fusion usually happens when one rope runs across another rope or across webbing, or when one line moves quickly across one spot in a second line that remains stationary. Heat fusion occurs in the following situations:

- Two ropes under tension where one remains stationary while the other, being lowered, runs across the first.
- A loaded rope running across an anchor rope or webbing also under load.
- A rappeler holding a rope against his or her seat harness webbing while performing a rapid rappel.

Damage to ropes because of heat fusion can happen quickly, without warning, and can be catastrophic. Everyone working in the high angle environment must constantly be on the alert for heat fusion and take steps to avoid it.

Some ways to prevent heat fusion due to rope cross include:

- Rigging ropes so that they do not make a contact to create heat fusion.
- Holding ropes away from one another with pulleys or edge rollers.
- Padding the stationary rope where one rope runs across it.
- Never placing a moving rope and a stationary rope in the same edge protection device, such as edge rollers (use separate rollers or devices).

Note that heat fusion occurs when one rope is stationary and the other moves across it *in one spot* so that the heat builds up. If both ropes are moving constantly so that one spot is not subjected to heat buildup, then

destructive heat fusion is not likely to occur. In a Munter hitch (see page 90), for example, the rope is running across itself, but all surfaces are moving. So when correctly used, the Munter hitch is not likely to cause heat fusion.

Rope Damage through "Flash" Rappels

All rappel devices operate through friction of the rope across the device. This results in heat buildup that increases with the speed of the rappel. Fast rappels must be avoided because they can damage rope through heat buildup. Such "flash" rappels also indicate poor technique and/or lack of control on the part of the rappeler.

Rotate Ropes Used in Rappel Training

Ropes that are in constant use for rappel training and that are always anchored on the same end will eventually change handling characteristics due to sheath bunching at the lower end. When a rope is used for many rappels, alternate ends of the rope as anchors to avoid potential change in characteristics.

Strength Loss through Knots

All knots reduce the overall strength of rope, but some knots cause a greater loss than others. The general rule is this: knots with tight bends, such as bowlines, cause greater strength loss than knots with more open bends, such as the figure 8 family of knots.

Effects of Bending a Rope. Whenever a rope is placed under load in a sharp bend, some strength is lost (Figure 4-10). The rope fibers on the outside of the bend receive a greater share of the load, while those on the inside of the bend receive very little of the load or none at all.

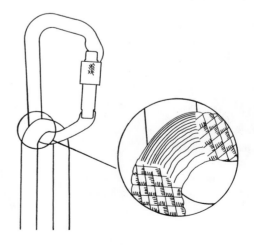

FIGURE 4-10
Effect of bending rope.

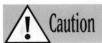

Whenever you use more than one rope on edge protection devices, be on guard for heat fusion (see page 33). Never use both a stationary and moving rope on the same edge protection device. This can cause the moving rope to cut through the stationary rope. This can happen quickly and without warning.

Common situations where ropes receive this kind of stress include ropes that have knots or kinks when they run over a sharp bend, such as in a carabiner or small diameter pulley.

The 4:1 Rule. Rope users have long estimated rope strength loss with what is known as the *4:1 rule*. This means that strength loss in rope does not become significant until the rope has a bend less than four times the diameter of the rope. The 4:1 rule applies more to natural fiber and to a few synthetics than it does to nylon rope, where loss may not be significant until it gets below a 2:1 ratio.

The 4:1 ratio is still used as a guideline by many users of nylon rope, in part because it includes a safety margin. The 4:1 rule is used when choosing mechanical devices such as pulleys to assure there will be little strength loss when using the devices.

The other reason to use the 4:1 ratio as a guide relates to efficiency. Very small pulleys mean low efficiencies as the rope turns around them. By using the 4:1 guide, there will be fewer problems with efficiency.

To choose a pulley using the 4:1 rule, compare the diameter of the rope with the diameter of the pulley sheave. If the rope diameter is ½ inch, then the pulley should have a diameter of at least 2 inches.

INSPECTING A ROPE

Rope inspection is an ongoing process to be done before, during, and after rope use. You inspect rope in two ways: *looking and feeling*. After each use, inspect your rope thoroughly by looking and feeling along every inch of its length.

Visually inspect the rope, looking for the following:

◆ Discoloration: An obvious change from the rope's original color. Discoloration, particularly brown, gray, black, or green, could indicate chemical damage.
◆ Glossy marks: Could indicate heat fusion damage.
◆ Exposed core fibers (white in most **static rope**): Indicates damage to the sheath.
◆ Lack of uniformity in diameter and size: May indicate broken sheath bundles.
◆ Inconsistency in texture and stiffness (hold the rope in a loop and see if it is a uniform radius around the entire bend): An inconsistency in the bend may be the result of a soft spot that indicates core damage.

Run the rope slowly through the bare hands, feeling for the following:

◆ Stiffened fibers
◆ Obvious changes in diameter
◆ Soft or hollow spots
◆ Contamination with dirt and grit

If enough strands are broken, there will be a localized change in the diameter of the rope usually indicated by a depression or hourglass shape that can be felt. Some types of damage will result in "puffs," or core fibers protruding from the sheath. If rope is contaminated with dirt, it should be washed.

Establishing Responsibility

As with other life safety devices, such as breathing apparatus, ropes used by a team must be assigned a *chain of responsibility*. Someone must be responsible for knowing where they are, how they have been used, who has used them, and what condition they are in. Someone must be responsible for inspecting them after each use, for keeping a log for each rope, and, where appropriate, for removing them from service.

RETIRING A ROPE

Unfortunately, the only tests that currently exist to reliably measure rope strength will also destroy the rope. Therefore it is essential to be able to determine if a rope should be retired. That ability is the result of education in rope use and construction combined with experience and good judgment (Box 4-1).

 Box 4-1 Guidelines for Retiring a Rope

The following are general guidelines that can assist in deciding when to retire a rope:

SHEATH WEAR
More than half of the outer sheath yarns are broken

SHOCK LOADING
The rope has been subjected to severe shock loading.

OVERLOADING
The rope has been subjected to the kind of overload for which it was not designed. Examples of overloading for life support rope would include towing a vehicle or hauling heavy equipment or materials.

CHEMICAL CONTAMINATION
Unless you specifically know the chemical is *harmless*, consider it a contaminant.

LACK OF UNIFORMITY IN TEXTURE
Soft, mushy places or hard spots.

AGE
The rope is simply "worn out" from use.

LACK OF UNIFORM DIAMETER
The rope necks down to a smaller diameter similar to an hourglass shape.

LOSS OF FAITH
The rope was used by persons you suspect may not have taken proper care of it.

But the bottom line is this: *When in doubt, throw it out.*

Rope, compared with many other types of equipment, is an inexpensive tool. The cost of replacing a rope is certainly less expensive than a severe injury or loss of life.

WASHING ROPE

All ropes eventually will become dirty after use. Using your rope when it is dirty will shorten its life. So one element of a rope inspection program should be to decide when the rope needs a bath. Although soiling most obviously affects the appearance of rope, the most serious effect of soiling is more serious and hidden. Particles of grit and dirt eventually work their way into the core of the rope to damage the load-supporting yarn as it stretches and flexes. (Stepping on a rope forces more of this damaging material into the rope core.) Furthermore, the dirt on the surface of a rope will accelerate wear on hardware, such as rappel devices, much as would sandpaper.

Also damaging to rope are aluminum particles, which are forced into rope as it runs through metal hardware such as rappel devices. Correct washing of your rope can also remove much of these damaging particles.

Rope Washing Devices

Commercial devices are available that are specifically designed for washing ropes. Some operate very much like the hose-washing devices that are used by fire departments. As water jets spray into the center of the device, the rope is pulled slowly through it. One model has a built-in brush to help scrub away the surface dirt (Figure 4-11). It will adjust to various rope diameters up to ¾ inch.

Rope washing devices are most effective against larger particles of dirt but may not make the surface of the rope appear completely clean. This can be done only with further steps.

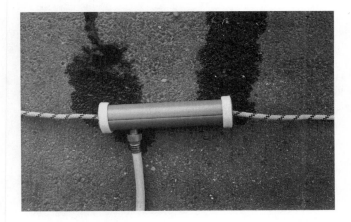

FIGURE 4-11
Rope washer.

Cleaning Ropes with a Washing Machine

Washing machines can thoroughly and effectively clean rope, but you must use them with care and with certain specific precautions to prevent damage to the rope.

Front-loading, tumbling-type machines are preferable. Their tumbling-type action usually causes less tangling of the rope than the agitator action of top-loading machines. The machine should not have a plastic window because in a spin cycle the rope could be damaged by heat fusion from striking the plastic. Most commercial machines are now top loading machines. But use caution with top loading washers because they can damage the rope through tangling with the agitator.

If you must use a top-loading machine, make certain the agitator is not going to rub back and forth on the rope, using the following techniques:

- Coil the rope to prevent tangling. One commonly used coil for washing is the *chain coil* (Figure 4-12).
- To prevent tangling or abrasion on the agitator, place the rope in a mesh bag. Such bags are used to wash delicate fabrics in washing machines. Or you could use a scuba equipment mesh bag. Close the bag securely before placing the bagged rope in the machine.
- Use gentle soaps and follow package directions for their use. Soaps that indicate they are "safe for all synthetics" will most likely be safe for rope cleaning. Still, to make certain, some rope owners use only the gentlest cleaners such as Woolite or Ivory Flakes (not dishwashing liquid detergent).
- Do not use bleaches or bleach substitutes.
- Use the "cold water" setting.
- Rinse thoroughly to remove all soap traces.
- Carefully dry the rope without heat. Hang the rope loosely out of direct sunlight and allow it to air-dry.

Fabric Softeners

Some people use fabric softeners to give a soft feel to the rope sheath. Ropes rinsed with a fabric softener solution that is mixed according to the fabric softener manufacturer's directions should actually perform better than ropes washed only with soap and water. Fabric softeners can make it easier to tie knots by delaying the rope stiffness that comes with age. The lubricants in fabric softeners can help replace the lubricants originally furnished on the yarns by the manufacturer, which were removed by repeated washing of the rope. Replacing the lubricants helps the yarns load more evenly, which might raise the tensile strength slightly in older, well-washed ropes.

Special Cleaning Problems

Despite careful handling, ropes may become spotted with oil, grease, or mildew. There is no indication that any of these substances destroy rope fiber but they are unattractive and may stain clothing or high angle gear. Petroleum substances may cause other contaminants to stick to the rope.

⚠ Warning

Treating ropes with fabric softener can make them more slippery, which means there will be less friction on the descender and possibly more difficulty in controlling a rappel or lowering line.

One study indicates that the soaking of rope in a *heavy concentrated solution* of fabric softener may be destructive to the rope yarn and cause significant strength loss to the rope.

These substances can often be removed by soaking the rope in cool, soapy water and scrubbing the affected areas with a fingernail brush.

Avoid strong solvent-based cleaners. Many solvents that loosen grease and grime will also dissolve nylon. Contact the rope's manufacturer for specific types of cleaning problems.

DRESSING ROPE ENDS

Cut rope ends should always be carefully dressed. Frayed ends have a sloppy, unprofessional appearance, become snagged, and eventually grow in size. This is particularly true with *laid rope.*

The most effective method of cutting synthetic fiber rope is using an electric hot cutter (Figure 4-13). Before the rope is cut, the spot where it is to be severed should be firmly taped.

If you do not have a hot cutter, then take the following steps:

1. Firmly tape the spot to be cut to prevent fraying.
2. Cut down the center of the tape.
3. Immediately fuse the cut ends with heat, such as a lighter or other small flame. Taper the shape of the melt slightly (Figure 4-14). It should not be in the shape of a mushroom, which would get snagged when pulled through hardware or rock.

⚠ Caution

Molten nylon will burn your fingers. (An alternative to melting the rope ends is to seal them with a liquid vinyl material such as Whip End Dip.)

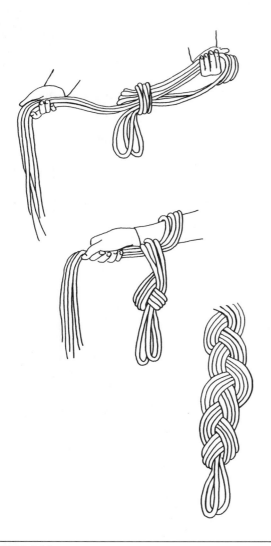

FIGURE 4-12
Chain coil.

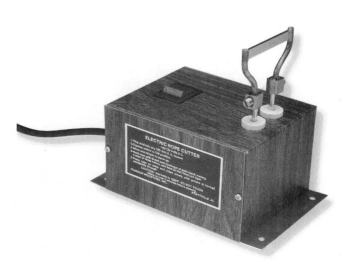

FIGURE 4-13
Hot cutter.

CARE OF WEBBING

In general, webbing should have the same care as rope: (1) protect it from abrasion and damaging substances and (2) inspect it after each use.

Note that webbing is more susceptible to damage than rope from shock loading. As with rope, webbing should be protected from friction heat damage.

HINTS FOR ROPE HANDLERS
Avoiding Tangles

Rope will not usually come out of a coil without tangling. To ensure that the line runs smoothly in the operation, it should first be "stacked." This simply consists of taking the rope off the coil and laying it on the ground on top of itself with the end to be used first on the top (Figure 4-15). The stack should be completed out of the way of the operation but located so that the rope will run off to where it is needed without entangling debris, other rope, or persons. Rope stacked in this manner will usually slide off the pile smoothly. But it is a good idea to assign a rope handler to feed the rope to the person using it to ensure there are no tangles or kinks.

Bagged rope is less likely to tangle. But friction devices such as figure 8 descenders will twist the rope, creating tangles between the 8 and the bag, which will increase as more rope is fed through the descender.

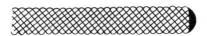

FIGURE 4-14
Shape of melted rope end.

Therefore when using devices such as the figure 8 that twist the rope, pull the rope out of the bag and stack it on the ground. Friction devices such as the brake bar rack twist the rope very little, so the rope can be left in the bag when using "racks."

Throwing and Dropping Rope

There are many situations where it is not easy to get rope from the top of a drop to the bottom. As mentioned before, large bags of rope should not be dropped because of potential damage to rope. Many times, the face of the drop may not be completely vertical but broken. Also, you may not have the rope in a bag but in a coil.

Most coils will not automatically feed out when dropped over the edge. To get a rope over the edge without tangles, do the following:

1. Stack the rope as described earlier. Be sure that the top end (at the bottom of the stack) is secured so it will not slip over the edge.
2. Tie a bulky knot, such as a figure 8 on a bight in the bottom end of the rope. This will help prevent rappeling off the end. This is a particular concern in the dark or when you cannot see the end of the rope.
3. At the bottom end of the rope (top of the stack) take several loose coils in your throwing hand (Figure 4-16).
4. Add three or four loose coils in the opposite hand. The remainder of the rope should be coming off the top of the stack.
5. Loudly shout, "rope!" so that any persons below will be warned of falling rope.
6. With a side arm motion pitch the loose coils in your throwing hand out horizontally. Note that if the wind is blowing, it may blow the rope off target or back up the cliff. You may have to throw the rope in a downward motion.

A

B

C

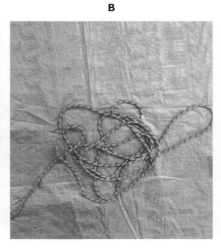
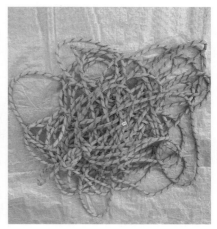

FIGURE 4-15
Stacking rope.

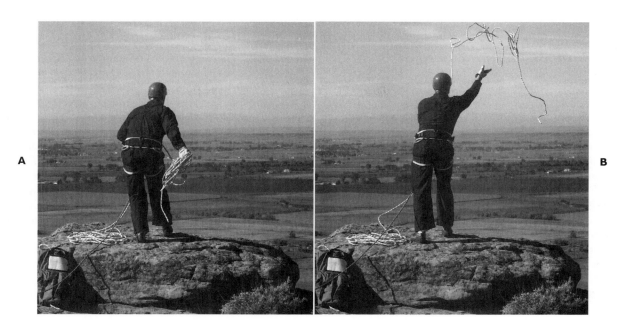

FIGURE 4-16
Throwing rope.

7. Allow the momentum of the falling rope to take the coils from your second hand. The rope should now pay out as it is pulled down by its own weight. Be sure to control the rope's speed through your *gloved* hand or, on very long drops, through a descender or belay device.

Evaluation Exercises

◆ COGNITIVE AND AFFECTIVE EXERCISES ◆

1. **Which of the following are conditions in which rope should *not* be stored?**
   A. Near vehicle batteries.
   B. In direct sunlight.
   C. In contact with a concrete floor.
   D. All of the above.
2. **Advantages to bagging rope, over coiling it, include all of the following, *except*:**
   A. Bagging can be accomplished quicker than coiling.
   B. Bagged rope is more convenient to carry.
   C. Bagged rope is easier to deploy.
   D. Bagging protects the rope from heat damage.
3. **You will damage an 11mm static rope by doing any of the following, *except*:**
   A. Using it to lower a 600 lb rescue load.
   B. Pulling all of the stretch out of the rope during highline operations.

   C. Lifting heavy objects.
   D. Towing a vehicle.
4. **Techniques for reducing rope damage from abrasion include:**
   A. Use of canvas pads.
   B. Use of a fire hose.
   C. Use of edge rollers.
   D. All of the above.
5. **A trainee is rappelling down the group's rope but is going very fast. You discuss with the trainee not to continue that practice because of the risk of:**
   A. Heat fission.
   B. Heat fusion.
   C. Kinking.
   D. Piling.
6. **All of the following are examples of dangerous heat fusion situations, *except*:**
   A. A rappeler moving very fast with his rope against his or her seat harness webbing.
   B. A loaded rope running over the anchor rope.
   C. A belay using a Munter hitch.
   D. Two ropes running under tension, but one is stationary, with the other running over it.
7. **All of the following are ways to prevent heat fusion, *except*:**
   A. Holding rope away from another rope, using webbing to pull the moving rope.
   B. Rigging ropes so that they do not make contact.
   C. Holding ropes away from one another with pulleys or edge rollers.
   D. Padding stationary ropes where another runs over it.

8. **Using the 4:1 rule, what is the smallest bend that can occur in a ½-inch rope before it begins to reduce strength of the rope:**
   A. 2 inch
   B. 1.5 inch
   C. 1 inch
   D. 0.5 inch

9. **Which of the following are guides for determining when a rope should be retired:**
   A. Chemical contamination.
   B. Overloading.
   C. Sheath wear.
   D. All of the above.

10. **Precautions to take when cleaning a rope in a washing machine include all of the following, *except:***
    A. Use a front-loading machine.
    B. Use any manufactured soap.
    C. Chain coil the rope.
    D. Use cool water.

▼ PSYCHOMOTOR EXERCISES ▼

11. **Using an 11 mm x 50 m dynamic climbing rope, coil the rope in each of the following methods:**
    a) Mountaineer coil.
    b) Cavers coil.
    c) Butterfly coil.

12. **Place a 3-m piece of rope over a sturdy table edge and hold moderate pressure on both ends. Using various edge protection devices, place the devices under the rope to protect it and practice securing them in place to compensate for rope movement, both vertical and horizontal.**

13. **Acquire four 3-m sections of 11 mm and ½ inch rope; two sections with various damage and two new sections. Use these to allow all group members to practice rope inspection.**

14. **Using a 100 m static rope, practice "stacking" or "flaking" the rope out to prevent tangling.**

15. **Using a 100-m static rope, practice dropping and throwing the rope down a face. Assure that all personnel are secured to the top with anchor and harness attachment.**

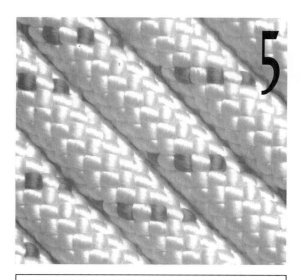

5 Basic High Angle Hardware

Objectives

At the completion of this chapter, you should be able to:

1. Describe how a carabiner design can influence its strength.
2. Given a diagram, identify the parts of a carabiner.
3. Given a scenario, identify the appropriate carabiner to use.
4. Given a scenario, identify the appropriate descender device to use.
5. Identify the different types of ascenders and the important considerations in their selection.
6. Describe a scenario using ascenders that may result in a catastrophic failure.
7. Describe the purpose and situations in which the following rock protection would be used:
   ◆ Natural anchors
   ◆ Stoppers
   ◆ Active and passive cams
   ◆ Pitons
   ◆ Bolts
8. Define belaying.
9. Describe the disadvantages to body belaying.
10. Identify the basic types of devices.
11. Describe the use of the Munter hitch (Italian hitch).
12. List the uses for pulleys in the high angle environment.
13. Given a scenario, select the best pulley to use.
14. List two main functions of edge rollers.

Key Terms

Ascenders Rope grab devices used by individuals to ascend a fixed rope or, with specific types of ascenders, used in the creation of hauling systems. There are basically two categories of ascenders: (1) *personal ascenders*, which are normally used for no more than one person's body weight and (2) *general-use ascenders*, used as personal ascenders and in hauling systems for progress capture devices and as rope grabs.

Bolts Metal devices used to create permanent anchors on a rock surface by drilling a hole in the rock and setting the device in the hole. Most bolts have a mechanical means for expanding to jam themselves in the drilled hole. A *hanger* is usually attached to the bolt so that the bolt can be used as an anchor point.

Brake Bar Rack A descending device consisting of a U-shaped metal bar to which several metal bars are attached that create friction on the rope. Some "racks" are restricted to use for personal rappelling, while others may also be used for lowering rescue loads. Also commonly known as *rappel rack*.

Cams Devices used in climbing for protection or in anchoring that lodge in a rock crack. There are "active" cams with springs to help adjust to the width of the crack. There are also "passive" cams (nuts, stoppers, and chocks) that wedge to fit the crack.

Descenders Metal devices that, through friction with the rope, create braking action for a controlled rappel or lowering.

Edge Rollers In-line, free-turning rollers that are anchored at an edge of a wall or cliff face to reduce rope friction.

key Terms—cont'd

Figure 8 Descender A device used for rappelling and, in some cases, for lowering. It is in the general shape of an 8, with a large ring to create friction on the rope and a smaller ring for attaching to a seat harness.

Locking Carabiner A carabiner with a locking sleeve on its gate side that secures the gate shut.

Manner of Function The method in which a particular piece of equipment was designed to be used.

Nonlocking Carabiner A carabiner without a means of securing its gate shut.

Piton A slender metal wedge, with an eye for attachment, that is driven into a rock crack for climbing protection or for anchoring.

Prusik A soft rope grab constructed of rope of a diameter smaller than the rope it grabs.

Pulley A device with a free-turning, grooved metal wheel (sheave) used to reduce rope friction, and with side plates to which a carabiner may be attached.

Rappel Rack See Brake Bar Rack.

Rope Grab Devices that grip the rope. There are two types: (1) mechanical rope grabs, usually made of metal, which grip the rope with a camming action and (2) rope or webbing rope grabs that use a hitch to grip the rope.

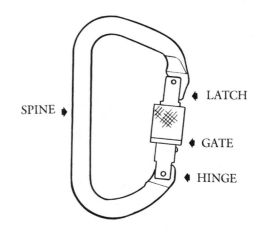

FIGURE 5-1

Basic parts of a carabiner.

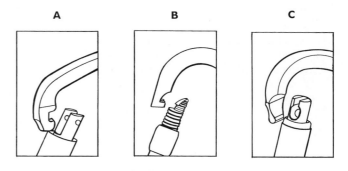

FIGURE 5-2

Examples of carabiner latches.

HARDWARE AND THE HIGH ANGLE SYSTEM

Rope, webbing, and other software are critical to the high angle system. But another vital link in the system is the category of equipment known as *hardware*. Hardware includes a variety of gear, usually constructed of metal, which performs specific functions in the high angle environment.

Carabiners

Carabiners are metal connectors that link the elements of the high angle system. They are also sometimes called *biners, snap links,* and *krabs.* (In Europe, the United Kingdom, and some parts of Canada carabiner is spelled "karabiner" with a "k.") The basic parts of a carabiner include the spine, hinge, gate, nose, and latch (Figure 5-1).

Carabiner latches, depending on the manufacturer, are designed in a variety of ways. However, there are three basic types (Figure 5-2). One style of carabiner latch consists of a pin in the top of the gate that slips into a slot in the nose (Figure 5-2, *A*). When the carabiner is loaded, the pin is trapped in the slot. This adds overall strength to the loaded carabiner.

Another basic type of latch consists of a claw on the gate that slips into a slot on the nose (Figure 5-2, *B*). In some versions of this design, the locking mechanism does not completely engage, and the carabiner can fail at very low loads.

The third type of latch consists of a keyhole-shaped slot in the top of the gate that slips into a matching key-shaped area of the nose (Figure 5-2, *C*). When loaded, the "keylock" design engages firmly to contribute to its strength. One advantage of the keylock carabiner is that the notch does not snag soft material, such as rope and webbing, as much as other carabiner designs.

Basic Carabiner Shapes

Carabiners are manufactured in a wide variety of shapes and are usually designed for specific uses.

They were originally designed as a simple oval shape (Figure 5-3, *A*). When the oval carabiner is placed under load, the stress is the same on both sides, equally on the spine and the gate. The problem is that in any carabiner the weakest part is the side with the gate.

The design that takes most advantage of the strength of the spine is the D-shaped carabiner (Figure 5-3, *B*). Note that the spine side of the carabiner is longer than the gate side, with the top and bottom of the carabiner flaring toward the spine. The purpose of this design is so that when under load, materials such as a rope clipped into the carabiner will slip into position on the spine side. The result is greater stress on the stronger side of the carabiner.

Since the development of the D-carabiner, there have been other designs such as the "modified D" (Figure 5-3, *C*). One carabiner designed for a special use is the HMS (Figure 5-3, *D*). This pear-shaped cara-

biner is designed for use with the Munter hitch (see Chapter 8). The term *HMS* is the abbreviation for the German word *Halbmastwurfsicherung*.

Carabiner Sizes and Strengths

Because climbers must carry their equipment with them, they have a great concern for weight. Consequently, carabiners made primarily for rock climbers tend to be lightweight. Some of these are constructed of hollow aluminum and have strength ratings as low as 3,000 lb (20 Kilonewtons [kN]).

Carabiners, for more demanding use and where more than one person's body weight may be involved, such as rescue, need higher strength ratings. These carabiners are made of solid aluminum or steel.

Another difference among carabiners relates to size. Again, because climbers place a premium on weight and bulk, their carabiners tend to be relatively small. But in situations where large amounts of material must be connected inside the carabiner, such as in rescue activities, the carabiner will need to be larger.

Carabiner Gate Opening

Along with differences in carabiner sizes and weights, there are also differences in the widths of gate openings. For some activities, the carabiner gate opening will have to be larger than normal. In rescue activities, for example, a carabiner may have to be clipped over a litter rail, which can be as large as 1 inch in diameter. Only a few carabiner designs have gates that will open this wide.

Accidental Gate Opening. The main job of a carabiner is to maintain its link with the other elements of

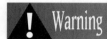

! Warning

Strength ratings for carabiners usually represent the ideal situation, such as in a D carabiner when material pulls only on a small area of the carabiner next to the spine. If material pulls across a wide area of the carabiner top or bottom (such as wide webbing does) then there could be greater stress on the gate side of the carabiner. Consequently, the carabiner may fail at a load lower than its rated strength.

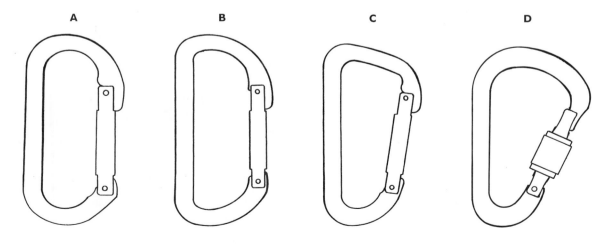

FIGURE 5-3

Carabiner designs. **A**, Oval. **B**, D-shaped. **C**, Modified D. **D**, HMS.

the high angle system. To do this, the carabiner gate must remain securely closed. If it does not remain closed, then the connecting elements will come unlinked and the system will fail.

There are several ways in which carabiner gates may come open accidentally. Among the most common are situations where:

- The carabiner is pressed against an edge of a wall or rock, forcing the gate open (Figure 5-4).
- A rope or piece of webbing is pulled across the carabiner gate, forcing it open (Figure 5-5).

If there is any chance that a carabiner gate may come open and only *nonlocking carabiners* are available, then two carabiners should be set together reversed and opposed. That is, the pair of carabiners should be set with their gates reversed to one another and their tops and bottoms opposed to one another (Figure 5-6).

Locking Carabiners

Although two reversed and opposed carabiners are usually very secure, it is often quicker and more convenient to use a single locking carabiner (Figure 5-7). Although specific designs will vary with the manufac-

turer, *locking carabiners* usually fall into the following categories:

- A locking sleeve moves on screw threads over the nose of the carabiner to ensure closure.
- A sleeve turns around a pin on the gate to move up and close over the nose.
- A spring-loaded sleeve makes a quarter turn to unlock. (This is a very convenient carabiner to use but it should be employed with caution because some versions come open very easily. Therefore some manufacturers incorporate various safety features into these carabiners. Safety features include moving the sleeve up before turning or pressing a lock button before turning it.)
- A sleeve moves downward over the hinge to hold the gate locked. (These hinge-locking carabiners are now rarely seen.)

Carabiner Strength. Not all carabiners are as strong with the locking knobs in the unlocked position as when they are locked. Some carabiner designs need the locking knob to hold the claw-type latch together in the locked position for the carabiner to have its full-rated strength. Tests have shown that some of

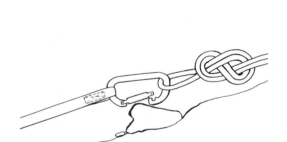

FIGURE 5-4
Gate opened by rock/building edge.

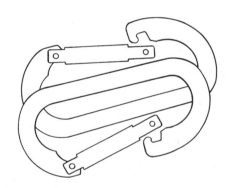

FIGURE 5-6
Carabiner reversed and opposed.

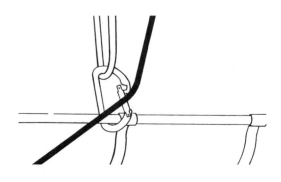

FIGURE 5-5
Gate opened by rope/webbing.

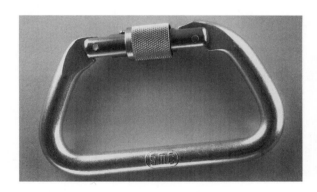

FIGURE 5-7
Locking carabiner.

these types of carabiners can fail at a much lower rating than their advertised strength if the gate is unlocked.

Besides the long-axis locked strength of a carabiner, you should also know its long-axis unlocked strength, long-axis gate open strength, and the short-axis (gate cross-loaded) strength.

Whatever type of carabiner is used, it is the responsibility of those using it to maintain vigilance to make certain that the carabiner stays closed.

Additional Concerns for Locking Carabiners. If a carabiner chronically becomes unlocked without cause, then it should be retired from service.

Older-design carabiners can become jammed if the locking knob is overtightened. This is because the older-designed locking sleeve would ramp up hard against the frame when tightened. If the sleeve were slightly turned while the carabiner was loaded, the spring in the frame would jam the sleeve when weight was released. This makes it difficult or impossible to turn the sleeve without reweighting the carabiner. The newer designs leave a gap between the sleeve on the gate and the nose of the frame when the sleeve is screwed completely closed. To check and see if a carabiner is of the newer design, screw it all the way closed. There should remain a slight amount of play in the gate.

If a carabiner locking mechanism is of the older design and becomes "frozen" through overtightening, then the following procedures may release it:

1. If the carabiner is not already on a seat harness, attach it to one. Have the wearer move to a secure position, away from the edge of any drop.

2. Attach the carabiner via a sling to a convenient anchor.
3. Reload the carabiner by sitting down with it attached to the anchor point.
4. Often, the locking nut can then be easily loosened.
5. If it still cannot be loosened, try tightly wrapping a short piece of webbing around the lock nut to gain leverage.
6. If this does not work, then the careful use of a pair of pliers may be the only remaining option.

Aluminum versus Steel Carabiners

Carabiners are constructed from one of two metals:
1. Aluminum alloy.
Advantages:
 ◆ Significantly lighter weight.
 ◆ Does not rust (but can suffer some forms of corrosion).
 ◆ Less expensive than steel.
Disadvantages:
 ◆ Locking mechanism on some aluminum designs may eventually wear out.
 ◆ May suffer permanent damage as the result of severe shock loading.
 ◆ Some aluminum carabiners are not as strong as comparable steel designs.
2. Steel.
Advantages:
 ◆ Locking mechanism on some steel-locking carabiners may hold up better than the locking mechanism on aluminum carabiners.
 ◆ May hold up better under severe shock loading.
Disadvantages:
 ◆ It's heavier. This becomes a significant factor when one has to carry more than a few carabiners for any distance.
 ◆ More expensive than aluminum.
 ◆ Unless plated, it will rust. Consequently, most steel carabiners require more maintenance.

Some steel carabiners are plated to resist rusting. If you plan to purchase plated carabiners, make certain they have stainless steel hinge springs. Unless they are stainless, the springs could rust and break. Consequently, the gates will not stay locked, making the carabiner dangerous to use.

If you work in high angle environments exposed to salt spray, such as near the ocean, choose carabiners constructed of all stainless steel (currently manufactured by SMC).

Carabiner Standard Labeling

There are currently two labeling systems for carabiners sold in the United States, with an additional one being developed.

CE and UIAA. Carabiners that pass standards established by the UIAA (Union of International Alpine Associations) and CE (European Committee for Standardization) are labeled with specific markings. These

---

⚠ Warning

Locking carabiners can and do come open after being locked. The following are common ways they can come open, along with possible countermeasures:
 ◆ Carabiner gate unlocks by rubbing against wall or cliff face.
Countermeasure:
Turn carabiner away from face.
 ◆ With some carabiner designs, vibration can cause the locking sleeve to unscrew.
Countermeasure:
Place carabiner so the gate is at the bottom and gravity keeps the locking screw closed. (This may not be an ultimate solution in high vibration environments, such as helicopters.)
 ◆ Gate is opened by rope or webbing running across it.
Countermeasure:
Move carabiner out of contact with the line or place padding between it and the rope or webbing.

carabiners will be stamped with major axis, minor axis, and gate opening strengths shown in kilonewtons (kN) (Figure 5-8). (Newtons are a force measurement, with 1 N equal to about 0.225 lbf. One kN is 1,000 N, or about 225-lb force.)

NFPA. Carabiners that meet the NFPA 1983-85 standard on Life Safety Rope and Auxiliary Equipment also carry special markings (Figure 5-9). These carabiners will be marked "Meets NFPA 1983, '95 ED." They will carry the name or logo of the manufacturer, along with the label of the third party that certifies that the product meets the standard.

In addition, NFPA-certified carabiners will have either a "P" or "G" stamped into the frame. The letter "P" shows that the carabiner is for *personal* use and designed for one person loads, with a major axis minimum breaking strength, with gate closed, of 6,000 lbf (26.67 kN).

The letter "G" on NFPA-certified carabiners shows that it is for *general* rescue use, with a minimum major axis breaking strength, with gate closed, of 9,000 lbf (40 kN).

Other Labeling. At the present time there are two other carabiner standards under development. One standard for rescue carabiners is being developed by the ASTM F32 (Search and Rescue) Committee. A second standard, for recreational carabiners, is being developed by the ASTM F08 Committee.

General Points on Buying Carabiners

Some carabiners carry no labeling and may not be tested to any standard. If the carabiner does not carry NFPA, CE, UIAA, or ATSM labeling you may not be able to be certain about the carabiner qualities such as open gate strength, along with minor and major axis strengths and other qualities.

It is up to you, *the user,* to find out information from the manufacturer.

Using Carabiners in Their Manner of Function

The carabiner manner of function is designed for being loaded along its long axis, or lengthwise (Figure 5-10). As mentioned earlier, the weakest point of a carabiner is the gate. Consequently, side loading stresses the gate and places an unnatural force on the carabiner, severely reducing its strength, which may cause it to fail.

Hard Linking

Another possible cause of carabiner failure is *hard linking.* Hard linking occurs when a carabiner is rigged so that it cannot rotate with forces placed on it. This twisting force can cause the carabiner to break. Some examples of hard linking include:
- Clipped into eyebolts on walls.
- Clipped into a second carabiner that cannot rotate.
- Clipped into a vehicle tow hook.

To solve hard linking, rig a soft link between the hard links. An example of a soft link would be a section of webbing or rope.

Carabiner Brake Bars

To avoid cross loading, you should avoid using carabiner brake bar systems (Figure 5-11). Brake bars are solid bars of metal, with a hole drilled in one end and a slot cut in the other end. They are sometimes fitted to oval carabiners to create rappel systems and, on occasion, lowering systems. Carabiner brake bar systems are not as common as they once were but are still found among some persons in the high angle environment. Because they subject carabiners to forces for which they were not designed, carabiner brake bar systems should be avoided. (Brake bars are used on brake bar racks [see page 50]. When brake bars are used for brake bar racks, for which they were designed, they do not create an unnatural stress on the "rack.")

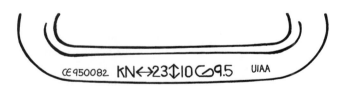

FIGURE 5-8
UIAA/CE markings for carabiners.

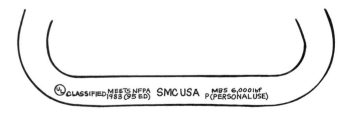

FIGURE 5-9
NFPA markings for carabiners.

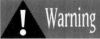

⚠ Warning

All equipment used in the high angle environment is designed to be used in a specific *manner of function.* This is particularly true of carabiners. Any equipment, such as carabiners, not used in the manner of function may result in failure of the equipment and in severe injury or death. Details on carabiner manner of function are explained next.

Three-Way Loading

As mentioned before, carabiners are designed for loading along their long axis. However, some designs of seat harnesses have tie-in points consisting of right and left attachments. When a carabiner is clipped into these attachments and then loaded through a rope to a descender or other point, the carabiner becomes loaded from three directions. This can place potentially dangerous side-loading forces on the gate (Box 5-1).

Screw Links

Triangular or semicircular screw links are increasingly being used in the place of carabiners where three-way loading is necessary. In the place of the swing-open gate found on carabiners, screw links have a screw-locking sleeve that closes the opening (Figure 5-12). When the screw link is screwed closed completely, it has the same strength regardless of the direction(s) of loading.

Advantages:
- ◆ Strong regardless of direction of load.
- ◆ Inexpensive.

Disadvantages:
- ◆ Must be screwed all the way closed for strength. Because of the number of turns required to close the locking sleeve, they are slow to open and close.

Care and Inspection of Carabiners

Inspect each carabiner after use. Check the gate for signs of excessive side loading, such as rough pivoting

Box 5-1 Possible Solutions to Three-Way Loading

Use a large pear-shaped carabiner for the seat harness. Place the two harness attachment points in the large end of the carabiner and the third point, such as the descender, in the small end. You must still be careful that the carabiner does not rotate out of this configuration and become sideways so it loads the gate. Use a triangular or semicircular screw link in place of the seat harness carabiner. These devices are designed for loading from any direction. They are described in the next section.

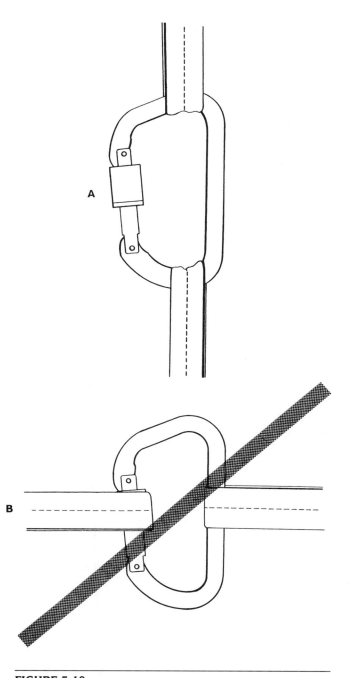

FIGURE 5-10

A, Acceptable loading. **B,** Unacceptable loading.

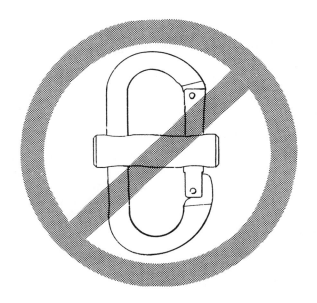

FIGURE 5-11

Carabiner brake bars.

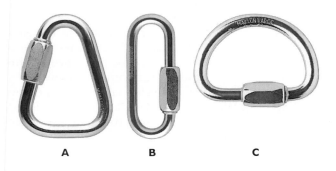

FIGURE 5-12

Screw links. **A,** Triangular screwlink. **B,** Oval screwlink. **C,** Semi-circle screwlink.

action and bent tabs. Pay particular attention to hinge pins and latches. Make certain that what may look like a scratch is not actually a crack. A deep scratch gouge in a carabiner can reduce the cross-sectional area needed for strength. Scratches can also provide an entry point for corrosion. Corrosion is particularly critical in hinge pins, latches, springs, and locking knobs.

If your carabiners have gotten wet, dry them in a warm place. Use a preservative and lubricant such as LPS-1 or WD-40 on critical areas such as hinge pins, springs, latches, and locking knobs to help prevent development of corrosion. Wipe off excess lubricant before storing the carabiners. Box 5-2 gives solutions for various carabiner problems.

Descenders

Note that a more complete discussion of the *use* of *descenders* is included in Chapter 9, Rappelling. The following section is a brief review of the equipment used in rappelling and lowering.

Descenders, also generally called *rappel devices,* are braking devices. The user places one on the rope and attaches it to the seat harness to descend the rope at a controlled speed. Some of the same equipment can also be used as braking devices to lower people or equipment under control. Such lowering operations may be required during rescue activities. Although there are many different descenders on the market, they all work on the same principle: they create friction by the rope running through them to create a controlled descent (Box 5-3). In most cases, the user controls the speed of the descent by pulling on the section of rope that is below the descender.

Types of Descenders

Figure 8s. *Figure 8 descenders* are one-person rappel devices roughly in the shape of an **8** but with rings of unequal size. The smaller ring, or lower one when in use, is clipped into a seat harness with a carabiner or screw link. The larger ring, or upper

Box 5-2 Troubleshooting

PROBLEM

Sticking gates or gates that close sluggishly.

SOLUTION

This may be due to contamination by dirt or to corrosion. The mechanism may be cleaned by blowing it with an air hose. *Do not use oil or grease-based lubricants* because they will attract more dirt and grit. Lubricate the gate mechanism with LPS-1 or WD-40.

PROBLEM

Carabiner gate with broken spring.

SOLUTION

Carabiner should be discarded.

PROBLEM

Broken latch mechanism.

SOLUTION

Carabiner should be discarded.

PROBLEM

Carabiner is bent (usually the result of being loaded with gate not completely closed, or subjected to overloading).

SOLUTION

Carabiner should be discarded.

one, is the one through which the rope passes to create friction (Figure 5-13). All figure 8s are fabricated of metal. Most are either of machined or forged-aluminum alloy, which is then anodized for greater resistance against wear from the rope.

Some figure 8s are constructed of steel. Their primary advantage is their resistance to wear. They will outlast several aluminum figure 8s, so they are particularly appropriate for heavy-duty uses such as in training departments. Their disadvantages are that they weigh much more than the aluminum 8s and they cost more.

Figure 8s are made by a number of different manufacturers and come in a variety of shapes and sizes. They are also a commonly used rappel device and are relatively inexpensive compared with some more complicated devices.

Disadvantages:
   ◆ In all models, once on the rope, the rappeller cannot create a wide range of friction in the device.
   ◆ In all models, long rappels (over approximately 150 feet) are more difficult to control.

Conventional Figure 8s. These are mostly found in small sizes and typically have a rounded or slightly squared large ring. They are mostly used in recreational activities such as climbing.

Advantages:
   ◆ Fairly compact and lightweight. Generally favored by climbers and others for whom size and weight are primary considerations.

Disadvantages:
   ◆ Smaller models will not dissipate heat easily.

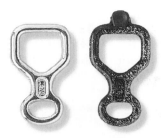

FIGURE 5-13
Conventional figure 8 descender.

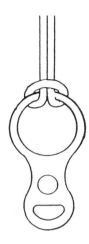

FIGURE 5-14
Figure 8 with girth hitch.

Box 5-3 Guidelines for Purchasing a Descender

- Be certain the descender is sized properly for the diameter of rope you will be using.
- The descender should create enough friction so that you have absolute control over the descent without using brute strength. You should be able to go as slowly as you like and be able to stop at any time.
- Keep in mind that in a real situation, hardware and equipment will make you significantly heavier than your "street weight." You may also be wearing gloves.
- It must have a lock-off function so that you can secure yourself and remain stopped on the rope with hands off the device.
- It must be strong enough to have an adequate safety factor (see page 23 for information on how to calculate a safety factor).
- It must be adequate for the length of descent needed.
- If desired, it must double as a lowering device.

- Smaller models will not take larger diameter ropes.
- All models will twist the rope.
- In conventional models, rope can slip around the large ring to form a girth hitch (Figure 5-14). If this occurs during a rappel, it may trap the user on the rope.
- This is a situation difficult to extricate oneself from alone. (See Chapter 9, Rappelling, for ways to prevent this from happening and Chapter 10, Ascending, for possible ways to extricate oneself from this kind of problem.)

Figure 8 with "Ears." The "ears" in a figure 8 are projections fabricated into the large ring (Figure 5-15) and are sometimes called *rescue 8s*. They are specifically designed so that the rope contours better around the large ring and does not slip over it to form a girth hitch. This type of figure 8 is found in larger sizes.

Advantages:
- Rope will not slip around large ring to form girth hitch.
- Because these models are in larger sizes, they dissipate heat better.

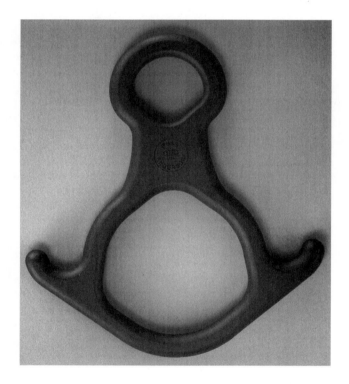

FIGURE 5-15
Figure 8 with ears.

- Will accept large-size ropes.
- Easier to lock off.

Disadvantages:
- Bulkier and slightly heavier than the smaller models of the conventional figure 8.
- As with all figure 8s, will twist rope.
- As with all figure 8s, once rappeler is on rope, he or she cannot create a wide range of friction.

♦ As with all figure 8s, more difficult to control on longer rappels.

Brake Bar Racks. *Brake bar racks* (also called *Cole racks* or **rappel racks**) are descending devices that offer a great amount of control and the ability to vary greatly the amount of friction (Figure 5-16). They can also be used for very long rappels. The brake bar rack consists of two primary elements:

1. An inverted U-shaped frame, one leg of which is longer than the other leg. Most frames are made of cold-rolled steel. There are also titanium versions. The titanium models are very light in weight but are more expensive. The end of the longer leg has an eye through which a carabiner can be clipped.
2. A series of bars with a hole drilled in one end so that they slide freely on the long side of the frame. On their other end, the bars are notched so that the end of the bar will clip into the short side of the frame. The rope is woven through the bars. Under tension, the rope keeps the bars in place on the frame.

Friction for rappelling may be controlled by the control hand on the rope below the rack, by varying the bar spacing with the other hand and by varying the number of bars engaged on the rope. (For more detailed information concerning the use of the rack for rappelling, see Chapter 9.)

The bars, when used correctly, are the only elements of the device that wear out. They must be replaced from time to time and depending on the bar's requirements for friction, they can be purchased in a variety of sizes and materials:

Larger Bars:
♦ Create greater friction.

Hollow Steel Bars:
♦ Dissipate heat better.
♦ Last longer.
♦ Are more expensive.
♦ Give less friction.
♦ Are prone to rusting (unless they are stainless steel).

Aluminum Bars (most commonly used):
♦ Give more friction than steel.
♦ Are less expensive than steel.
♦ Wear out sooner than steel.
♦ Leave aluminum marks on rope.

In the most common configuration, the rack is arranged with a 1-inch diameter grooved "top bar" at the top to keep the rope in the middle of the bars as it runs through the device. Usually five additional aluminum ¾-inch diameter bars fill out the remainder of the rack.

A short version of the rack is available with five bars. It is designed to be compact for persons, such as cavers, with limited space. It is not recommended for rescue work because it provides less friction and has less versatility than the six bar rack.

For rappelling, the brake bar rack works most efficiently with the open side of the rack towards the ground. Some seat harnesses have a horizontal D ring as a clip-in point that will cause the open side of the rack to be facing the rappeler's side. To adapt to this there are versions of the rack with a quarter turn in the eye so that the rack will remain with the open

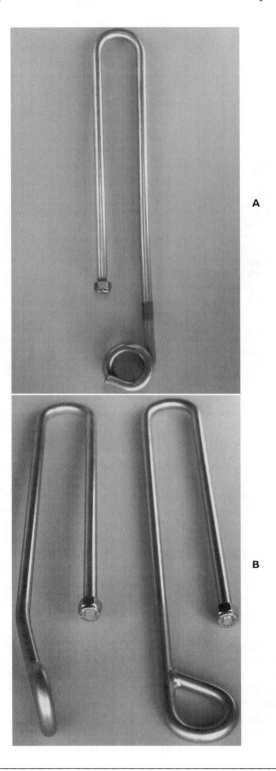

FIGURE 5-16

Brake bar rack. **A,** Twisted eye. **B,** Welded eye.

side toward the ground when you are wearing this design of harness.

Personal versus rescue versions of the rack. The rack frames are designed in differing configurations for the specific needs of the user. In some personal versions of the rack, the eye at the end of the long side is formed by twisting the steel bar around itself (Figure 5-17). Because large loads could cause this type of eye to untwist, this style of rack should not be used for loads of more than one person.

For larger loads, such as in rescue operations, there is the rack with the welded eye (see Figure 5-16, *A* on page 50).

Other types of brake bar racks. There is another version of the rack. This rack is designed with the legs of the U of equal length. In use, this type has the ends of the U pointing up and secured with nuts, while the attachment to the seat harness is in the curve of the U. The most common type has three fixed and three slotted bars. The primary reason for this design is that the rack remains straight when loaded. The major disadvantage is that, when loaded, you cannot vary friction by disengaging or engaging bars (Box 5-4).

Other Descenders. There are hundreds of other descenders available. Among them are:

- ◆ Stop (Petzl)
- ◆ Sidewinder (Lirakis)
- ◆ Ruapehu (Ruapehu Mountain Equipment Co.)
- ◆ Sky Genie (Descent Control)

As with all gear you use in the high angle environment, it is your responsibility to obtain specific information on the characteristics of each device and training in its use.

Emergency Descent. Emergencies may occur in the high angle environment where it is necessary to descend immediately, although a person has no hardware specifically designed for rappelling. One improvisation that has commonly been used in the past is the "carabiner wrap." This consists of wrapping the rope several turns around the carabiner to create friction and attaching the carabiner to the seat harness.

The carabiner wrap *is not recommended* as a rappelling technique. There have been many injuries and some deaths in rappelling attempts using the carabiner wrap. These failures have often been the result of the rope wraps slipping out of the carabiner gate.

There are other alternatives for emergency descent that are preferable to the carabiner wrap. For a review of emergency rappel techniques, see Chapter 9, Rappelling.

Rope Grabs

Rope grabs are devices that grip the rope when needed for a variety of needs in the high angle environment.

In this book, "rope grab" refers to devices used for personal safety, in ascending the rope, and for hauling systems. (In industry and construction, types of rope grabs are also used for personal fall protection.)

Many rope grabs are mechanical devices fabricated from metal that use a camming action to grip the rope. (They are sometimes called **hard cams.**) Rope grabs can also be rope or webbing formed into a hitch that grips the rope. (They are sometimes called *soft cams.*) The most commonly used of these is the **Prusik,** but there are several other hitches that can be used as rope grabs.

Personal Ascenders

Personal ascenders (also called *ascent devices*) are rope grab devices used to travel up ("ascend") a fixed rope. They all work on the same principle: when correctly attached to the rope, their gripping action allows you

 Box 5-4 Characteristics of the Standard Rack

ADVANTAGES

Friction can be varied greatly even after the rappel has begun.
- ◆ Welded eye version is very strong.
- ◆ Can be used as a lowering device.
- ◆ Does not twist rope.
- ◆ Can be easily attached to rope without detaching the rack from the seat harness.
- ◆ Will take large-size ropes.
- ◆ Can use two ropes at the same time.

DISADVANTAGES

Bulkier and heavier than some other rappel devices.
- ◆ May take slightly longer to lace onto rope.

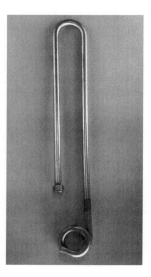

FIGURE 5-17
The brake bar rack (coiled eye).

to slide the ascender freely in one direction (up). They then lock in place when you correctly apply a downward force, such as body weight, to them.

For this system to work, you usually must use at least two *ascenders.* You attach the ascenders to yourself with rope or webbing sling. You ascend the rope by raising one ascender while being supported by the other ascender as it locks on the rope. By alternating this action, you are able to proceed up the rope.

This is the basic principle of ascending. There are dozens of variations in this technique, many using three ascenders for added security. (See Chapter 10, Ascending, for specific details on ascending techniques.)

Personal ascenders are designed for ascending with only one person's body weight (not for hauling systems where forces are multiplied). They work in part through a cam action, which pivots inside the ascender frame and also grips the rope with a toothed cam (Figure 5-18). Many personal ascenders have a handle that is equipped with a safety catch that releases the cam so that the ascender can be placed on a rope using one hand.

Many personal ascenders are used in pairs, usually with right- and left-handled models. For additional security, many people also include a third ascender in their system. Most personal ascenders cannot be used on rope above ½-inch diameter.

Among the personal ascenders currently being manufactured are:

◆ Clog (Wales). The frame is fabricated from rolled aluminum.
◆ CMI (W. Va.), which has two models:
1. Ultrascender (large): accommodates ropes from ¼ inch (6 mm) to ⅝ inch (16 mm) and has molded hand grip.

2. Ultrascender (small): A small version without molded handgrip. Both models are constructed of extruded aluminum and have toothed cams.
◆ Jumar (Switzerland). The frame is fabricated from cast aluminum.
◆ Petzl (France). All Petzl models are fabricated from rolled aluminum and have three models:
1. Ascension.
2. Basic: a compact, handleless design but with a toothed cam. Available only in a right-hand model.
3. Croll: a model with a toothed cam, designed to lie flat against the chest attached between a seat harness and a chest harness.
◆ SRT (Australia). The frame is machined from extruded aluminum. There are several models made for different-size ropes:
1. 8 to 11 mm rope.
2. 8 to 16 mm rope.

See Box 5-5 for a list of questions to ask when purchasing personal ascenders.

General-Use Ascenders

General-use ascenders operate primarily by the force of a cam action wedging the rope against the inside of the shell (Figure 5-19). The load is attached directly to the ascenders, and when the ascender is loaded, it activates the cam to grip the rope. Initially you may find general-use ascenders to be a little more difficult to operate than other types of ascenders because they must be taken apart to be placed on the rope. But once you have assembled them on the rope, they tend to stay there.

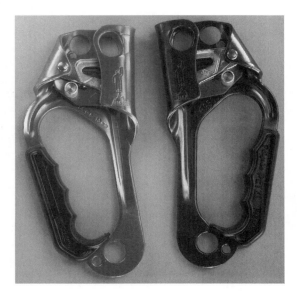

FIGURE 5-18
Typical personal ascender.

Box 5-5 Questions to Ask When Purchasing Personal Ascenders

◆ What size rope are they designed for?
◆ What is their strength rating and how is that determined?
◆ Can they be operated easily (placed on and taken off the rope) with one hand?
◆ Do they have a secure safety catch to prevent them from accidentally coming off the rope?
◆ Can they be easily used while wearing gloves?
◆ Are they comfortable in the hand while using them as a rope grab device?

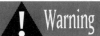 **Warning**

Personal ascenders may cut through rope sheath when loaded with as little as 1,200 lb. Consequently, personal ascenders should never be loaded with more than the weight of one person and should never be shock loaded.

General-use ascenders tend to hold better on wet, muddy, or icy ropes than do other types of ascenders. The teeth on the cams are designed to hold well on the rope while causing a minimum of damage to the rope sheath. Any general-use ascender, under high loads or severe shock loading, may cause damage to rope.

The two most commonly used of the general-use ascenders are the Gibbs (Gibbs, Inc., Salt Lake City, Utah) and the Rescucender (Thompson Manufacturing, Inc., Centerville, Utah). The Rescucender, developed after the Gibbs, was designed to cause less damage to rope than the Gibbs under the stress of rescue and hauling systems. Some newer models of the Gibbs have since been designed to be less damaging to the rope.

The Gibbs is available in two basic types:
1. "Free running" (there is no spring involved in the mechanism).
2. Spring loaded (spring action assists in setting the cam).

Recent improvements in the spring design have made it more durable and easier to manipulate than the older design. However, the older model spring-loaded Gibbs was designed so that its spring could be disengaged so the cam could be used free running; the newer model spring-loaded Gibbs does not have this option.

The Gibbs is available in two sizes:
1. Regular: for rope diameters ½ inch (12.7 mm) and smaller.
2. Large: for rope diameters ⅝ to ¾ inch.

The Gibbs is available in a variety of metals:
1. Cast cams, aluminum shell (lightweight, for recreational activities).

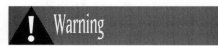

Any cam-type ascender can cut the rope at much less than the rated strength of the rope or of the cam.

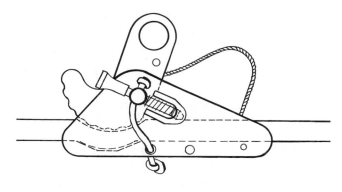

FIGURE 5-19
Typical general-use ascender.

2. Forged cams, stainless steel shells (heavy duty, longer wear).

Characteristics of General-Use Ascenders
Advantages:
- Hold better than other ascenders on wet, icy, or muddy ropes.
- Strong.
- Cam action does not tear rope sheaths as easily as some other types of ascenders.

Disadvantages:
- Must be taken apart to be put on and taken off rope.
- Takes two hands to put on and take off rope.

Rope Grab Devices for Belaying and Hauling. Many personal ascenders should not be used in hauling systems and other rescue rigging where there are loads greater than one person's body weight. Most general-use ascenders should not be used as belay devices because they tend to damage the rope under high weight loading and under shock loading. See Chapter 12, Rescue Belaying, and Chapter 16, Hauling Systems, for a discussion of rope grab devices used for rescue.

Hardware for Anchoring
Rock Anchors (Artificial Anchors)

Artificial anchors comprise a family of hardware used to create anchors where there are no natural anchors (such as trees or rocks) around which rope or webbing can be placed.

Artificial anchors go directly *into* the rock (and in some cases, into ice or snow). Most often, they are placed in cracks or gaps in the rock but in some cases they are physically driven into the rock to become permanent emplacements.

The ability to place reliable artificial anchors is an art involving a number of subtleties, such as the character of the rock itself, the nature of the cracks or gaps in the rock, and the direction of loading on the anchor. This kind of knowledge is dependent very much on hands-on instruction and experience. These finer points of placing artificial anchors are beyond the scope of this book. Those wishing to develop these skills should seek qualified instruction manuals and literature (some of which is listed in Appendix A).

Pitons

Pitons have been used in mountaineering for many years as a means of anchoring. They are a thin, metal spike with an eye to which a carabiner or webbing can be attached (Figure 15-20). Pitons are driven into a rock crack with a hammer.

Bolts

Bolts are a means of establishing a permanent anchor in a wall, usually when no other anchors are feasible.

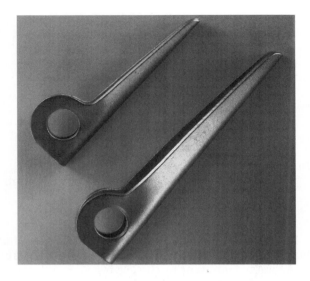

FIGURE 5-20
Typical piton.

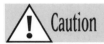

It is very difficult to drive pitons without permanently defacing the rock. Consequently, in some areas such as in state and federal managed parks, the use of pitons is prohibited. Also, many in the rock-climbing community consider the use of pitons to be bad etiquette.

Although there are different designs of bolts, most work on the same principle (Figure 5-21).

1. First, a hole is driven into the rock using either a separate drill or, in some designs (called *self-driving*), a drill that uses a part of the bolt itself as the bit.
2. The bolt is set in the hole by causing an element in it to expand, either through a screw-like action or by hammering on it. Some bolting systems use glue for greater security.
3. A "hanger" is attached to the bolt through which a carabiner can be attached.

For strength and long life, all bolts and components should be made of stainless steel. (CE standard on bolts requires that they be of stainless steel.)

"Clean" Hardware

Other types of anchoring hardware have been developed, partly because pitons and bolts deface the rock. This was initially known collectively as "clean" hardware. Although clean hardware generally does not deface rock, it may not be as secure as pitons and bolts.

When performing rescues, environmental concerns take a secondary role to the rescue needs and safety for the rescuers. Consequently, there may be little

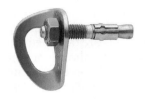

FIGURE 5-21
Typical bolt.

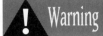

The setting of a bolt creates a permanent change to the rock. Either the bolt remains fixed in place or is broken out (chopped), which defaces the rock. In many managed areas, such as state and federal parks, the setting of bolts is forbidden. Also, many in the rock-climbing community consider the improper use of bolts to be bad etiquette.

Bolts set previously by unknown persons and at an unknown time are, as a result, an unknown factor. Because of the varying techniques for setting bolts and because the rock may weather around them, bolts of unknown quality should not be trusted for anchors.

choice as to location or types of anchoring used by rescuers. The most solid anchor in the safest location may be what you have to choose in rescue.

These devices are manufactured by a number of different companies and some may have very specialized uses. Some with very similar designs may go by different names. Some of the basic types of "clean" hardware for anchoring include the following:

♦ Nuts, chocks, or stoppers work by being wedged in a rock crack that bottlenecks (Figure 5-22).
♦ Hexcentrics can work both by a wedging and a cam action (Figure 5-23).
♦ Spring-loaded camming devices (Friends, Camalots) work by a spring-loaded, opposed cam action (Figure 5-24).

Belaying

To belay is to protect a person from falling by managing an unloaded rope (the belay rope) in a way that secures him or her from falling in case their main line rope or support fails. The belay rope is attached to the person being belayed and is controlled by the belayer. The difference in belaying techniques relates mainly to the manner in which the rope is held, or belayed.

The oldest of the belay techniques is the *body belay.* This involves the running of rope around the body of the belayer, usually around his or her waist. In this

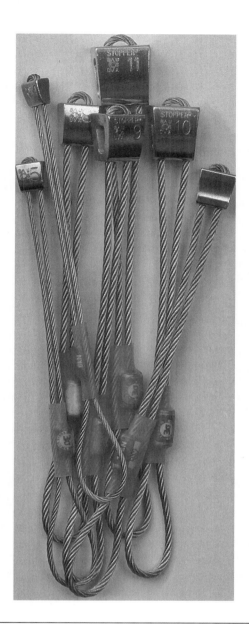

FIGURE 5-22

Stoppers.

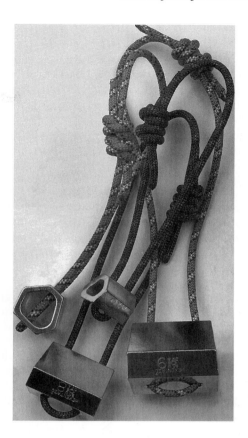

FIGURE 5-23

Hexcentrics.

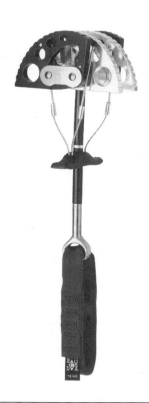

FIGURE 5-24

Spring-loaded camming device.

way, the rope can be brought tight when the person on the end of the rope (the climber, rappeller, worker, or rescuer) falls. The rope is held by friction around the belayer's body. There are significant disadvantages to body belaying:

- ◆ The force of the fall may cause the belayer to lose control of the rope and drop the climber.
- ◆ The force of the fall can easily injure the belayer.
- ◆ The belayer can become entangled in the rope. If the belayer does catch the climber, he or she must hold the climber until the climber can become secure.

Because of these problems, alternatives to body belaying have been developed and are preferable.

Personal Belay Devices

Personal belay devices are equipment used to belay a person exposed to falling. In most personal belay devices, a bight of rope is fed through the unit. One end of the rope goes to the climber or the persons who might fall. The other end of the rope is controlled by the belayer.

Some personal belay devices work through friction caused by the device pressing the rope against a carabiner. One example of this type is the belay plate. It consists of a small, metal plate with one or two holes. A bight of rope is fed through the plate and secured with a carabiner on the opposite side. The carabiner is then clipped into an anchor. When the two strands of rope are pulled apart, a high degree of friction is created on the rope. This stops the fall of the climber.

One example of a brake plate is a Sticht (Salewa, Austria). The oldest of the belay plate designs is a *Sticht plate,* which has almost become a generic term. It comes in several different configurations, depending on the specific needs of the user.

Another example of a personal belay device that works through friction is an Air Traffic Controller (ATC) by Black Diamond (Figure 5-25). The ATC can be used with ropes from 8.5 to 11mm in diameter.

Another type of personal belay device works through a camming action on the rope. One example of a camming belay device is the Grigri (Petzl, France).

Other Belay Alternatives

Another system for belaying requires only a large locking carabiner, something to anchor it to, and a rope. This is called the Munter hitch (also known as the *Italian hitch*).

The Munter hitch is used by some rescue people who believe they can successfully catch rescue loads using the device. Recent data suggest that a rescue load may be difficult to catch when it is *hanging in free air,* which is when the rescue load and the rope do not touch an edge, face, or directionals. These elements in a high angle system add friction and thus help absorb the force of a falling load.

No belay device or technique is perfect for all rescue loads and in every rescue environment. You should use great caution in choosing any belay device for rescue loads. Before you put the device to use, test it under realistic conditions that you will encounter in your own rescues. (See Chapter 8, Belaying of One-Person Loads, for more information concerning the Munter hitch.)

One belay system often used in rescue belaying is the *tandem Prusik belay* (see Chapter 12).

Pulleys

Pulleys are designed primarily to reduce rope friction. But this quality makes them useful in a number of functions in the high angle environment:

◆ To change direction of a running rope. Among the ways this may be useful are:
1. To position a rope more conveniently, such as to an area where people using the rope will be less exposed to falling, where there is less rock fall, and where they might have more room.
2. To reduce abrasion on a rope. A pulley could be used to hold a rope up from a rock or to bring it away from other rope or webbing.

◆ In hauling systems to develop mechanical advantage (see Chapter 15).

In certain situations, such as "big wall" climbing, lightweight pulleys are often used for such activities as hauling gear bags. Because weight is a primary consideration and the pulley is used for low-stress activities, these lightweight pulleys are often made of plastic or nylon.

But in certain high angle systems, and particularly in rescue hauling, the rope is under such stress that

---

⚠ Warning

A personal belay device may *not* be the most appropriate device for catching loads of more than one person's body weight.

Before using any device or system to belay a rescue load, you should test it under conditions similar to those you will encounter in an actual rescue situation. This ensures that you will be able to catch the load when it falls (see an example of the belay practice system on page 44).See Chapter 12, Rescue Belaying, for further information.

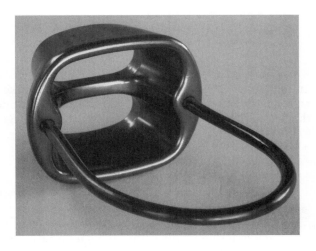

FIGURE 5-25
Typical personal belay device.

heat friction can cause a pulley to melt and fail. So where such life support is involved, only all-metal pulleys should be used.

Other Characteristics of Pulleys for High Angle Activities (Figure 5-26)

◆ The *sheave* (wheel) should have a diameter that is at least four times the diameter of the rope. (See Chapter 3, Rope, for a discussion of the 4:1 rule.)

◆ *Sideplates* should be movable so the pulley can be placed on the rope anywhere along its length without having to feed the end of the rope through the pulley.

The sideplates should extend beyond the edge of the sheave far enough to protect the rope from abrasion.

Sideplates are generally the weakest part of a pulley. Consequently, pulleys for higher tensile strength rope (above ½ inch) should have stronger sideplates. Pound for pound, steel sideplates are stronger than the aluminum ones.

◆ *Axles* should have rounded bolt heads that will not snag rope, other gear, or rock.

◆ *Bearings.* Most pulleys for high angle work have one of two types:

1. Bronze bushing.

Advantages:
◆ Less expensive than ball bearing.
◆ Can be taken apart to be cleaned.
◆ Very strong.

Disadvantages:
◆ Can be contaminated by dirt and grit.

2. Ball bearing.

Advantages:
◆ Turns slightly freer than does the bronze bushing.
◆ Some are sealed to protect from contamination by dirt and grit.

Disadvantages:
◆ Slightly more expensive.
◆ Does not take stress, such as sudden blows, as well as the bronze bushing. They become damaged when the hardened steel balls dent the bearing races (technically called *brinelling*).

Specialized Pulleys

There are a number of pulleys for the high angle environment that are designed for specific tasks. One of them is called the *knot-passing pulley* (Figure 5-27). Their large sheaves are designed so those knots that connect lengths of rope will easily pass over them. Other specialized pulleys include the Kootney Carriage, tandem pulleys, and Prusik minding pulley.

Edge Rollers

Edge rollers are important in reducing friction of rope over an edge. This not only helps with the work being done, as in hauling systems, but also helps prevent abrasion damage to the rope.

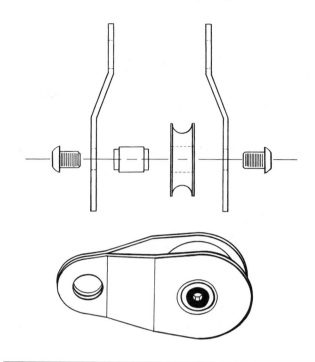

FIGURE 5-26
Parts of a pulley.

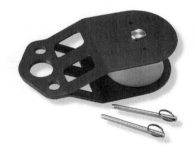

FIGURE 5-27
Knot-passing pulley.

See Chapter 4, Care and Use of Rope and Related Equipment, for descriptions of edge rollers and other rope protection equipment.

Evaluation Exercises

◆ COGNITIVE AND AFFECTIVE EXERCISES ◆

1. **All of the following would be situations that the rope would come out of a nonlocking carabiner, *except*:**
   A. The carabiner presses against a rock.
   B. A rope or piece of webbing pulls across the gate.

C. The carabiner is reversed and opposed with another.

D. The carabiner presses against the edge of a wall or cliff.

2. **When you wish to decrease the risk of rope coming out of a gate in the nonlocking carabiner, you should use which technique:**
   A. Opposition and alignment.
   B. Reversed and opposed.
   C. Reversed and aligned.
   D. Munter.

3. **All of the following are stronger along their spine than along their gate,** *except:*
   A. Locking oval carabiner.
   B. Nonlocking D carabiner.
   C. Locking modified D carabiner.
   D. Locking D carabiner.

4. **The locking carabiner can come unlocked in which of the following situations?**
   A. Rubbing against the cliff face.
   B. Vibration.
   C. Rope running across the gate.
   D. All of the above.

5. **The carabiner "manner of function" refers to its design to load along the long axis of the carabiner:**
   A. False
   B. True
   C. Only in Klingon warships
   D. Say what?

6. **Solutions to three-way loading of a carabiner on a seat harness include:**
   A. Using a pear-shaped locking carabiner, placing the harness points in the large end and the device or rope in the small end.
   B. Using a triangular screw link.
   C. Tying into the rope directly.
   D. All of the above.

7. **A carabiner loaded with the gate open is a problem due to all of the following,** *except:*
   A. The locking mechanism may jam.
   B. Rope may slip out.
   C. A device (rappel or ascent) may slip out.
   D. The carabiner may fail completely.

8. **Advantages to using a figure 8 descender include:**
   A. Will not dissipate heat rapidly.
   B. Smaller models will not take larger diameter ropes.
   C. Fairly compact and light weight.
   D. Rope can slip around ring and into a girth hitch.

9. **Disadvantages to the brake bar rack include:**
   A. Friction can be varied even after use has begun.
   B. Will not twist rope.
   C. Bulkier and heavier than a figure 8.
   D. Can be used as a lowering device.

10. **The personal ascender should not be used for which of the following purposes?**
    A. Personal ascent of a rope.
    B. As a cam in a mechanical advantage system.
    C. As a personal grab device on a fixed line.
    D. Hauling a 75-lb pack up a face.

11. **Examples of artificial anchors include all of the following,** *except:*
    A. Rock horn
    B. Stoppers
    C. Bolts
    D. Pitons

12. **Disadvantages of using bolts include:**
    A. Creates a permanent change in the rock.
    B. Bolts set by unknown persons may not be secure.
    C. Bolts may have to be "chopped" to remove them.
    D. All of the above.

13. **Some anchoring devices are known as "clean." These include all of the following,** *except:*
    A. Pitons
    B. Passive cams
    C. Active cams
    D. Stoppers

14. **Disadvantages of body belaying include all of the following,** *except:*
    A. The force of the fall may result in the loss of control.
    B. The belay is quicker than other methods.
    C. The belayer may become entangled in the rope.
    D. The force of the fall may injure the belayer.

15. **Which of the following might be an alternative to body belaying?**
    A. Use of a bowline knot.
    B. Use of a figure 8 device in reverse.
    C. Use of a Munter (Italian) hitch.
    D. Use of carabiner brake bar system.

16. **Pulleys may serve all of the following functions,** *except:*
    A. Change of direction.
    B. Use in mechanical advantage systems.
    C. To reduce abrasion on a rope.
    D. Belay device.

▼ **PSYCHOMOTOR EXERCISES** ▼

17. **Using a locking carabiner, attach it between two ropes and load it along its long axis.**

18. **With a locking carabiner in front of you, identify the following:**
    a) Spine
    b) Latch
    c) Gate
    d) Hinge

19. **Using a conventional figure 8, attach it to the rope appropriately.**

20. **Using a six bar brake rack, attach it to the rope appropriately.**

21. **Properly place all of the following into cracks at ground level, in a cliff face (wear your helmet):**
    a) Stopper
    b) Passive cam
    c) Active cam

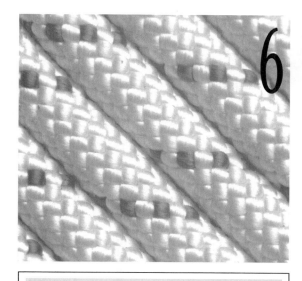

6 Knots

Objectives ▼

At the completion of this chapter, you should be able to:

1. Describe why it is necessary to have proficient knot skills before entering the high angle environment.
2. Discuss why it is necessary to continually practice knot tying.
3. Describe the qualities of a good knot.
4. List the ways in which knots affect rope strength.
5. Describe the functions of the following knots:

◆ Simple overhand.
◆ Simple figure 8.
◆ Figure 8 on a bight.
◆ Figure 8 follow through.
◆ Figure 8 bend.
◆ Ring bend (water knot).
◆ Double overhand backup knot.
◆ Grapevine ("double fisherman's") knot.

6. Tie the following knots correctly:

◆ Simple overhand.
◆ Simple figure 8.
◆ Figure 8 on a bight.
◆ Figure 8 follow through.
◆ Figure 8 bend.
◆ Ring bend (water knot).
◆ Double overhand backup knot.
◆ Grapevine ("double fisherman's") knot.

Key Terms ▼

Back-Up Knot A second knot used to secure the tail of a primary knot. Also known as a *safety* or *keeper knot*.

Bend A class of knot that joins two ropes or webbing pieces together.

Bight The open loop in a rope formed when it is doubled back on itself.

Foundation Knot A simple knot that is tied as the first step in tying a more complicated knot. Examples of foundation knots include the overhand and the simple figure 8.

Knot A fastening made by tying together rope or webbing in a prescribed way. Knots include bights, bends, and hitches.

Safety Knot See Back-Up Knot.

Stopper Knot A knot tied in a rope to help provide bulk. Examples are a simple figure 8 tied in the bottom end of a rope to prevent a person from rappelling off the end, or tied in the top of the rope to prevent it from accidentally slipping through equipment.

The ability to tie knots correctly, confidently, and without hesitation, and to know how they are used, are necessary skills for the high angle technician. If you go into the high angle environment without these knot skills you may be a danger to yourself and others around you.

Knots are the link for many elements in the high angle system. The following list includes some of the situations in which knots are used in the high angle environment:

◆ For anchoring.
◆ For tying ropes together.
◆ For tying webbing together.
◆ For tying loops in rope and webbing.
◆ For tying people directly into ropes.
◆ For certain belay systems.
◆ For emergency situations, such as emergency seat harnesses.
◆ For backing up other knots.
◆ To keep rope ends from pulling out of equipment.
◆ For personal safety, such as to keep from rappelling off the end of a rope.
◆ To create emergency ascenders.
◆ For tying safety lines.
◆ For improvisation, where other elements of the system fail.
◆ To extricate yourself from unexpected difficulties.

Knots must be continually practiced so that you remain proficient at knot tying and can tie a specific knot instantly when it is necessary. To maintain good high angle skills, you should own at least two lengths of rope, each several feet long, so that you can continually practice knot tying.

Group training sessions typically should begin with a review of knots. Those persons who do not maintain their knot-tying skills should be denied group certification and not be allowed in the high angle environment. The failure to learn simple but essential skills such as knot tying may indicate lack of motivation.

Because many activities take place under severe environmental conditions, every high angle rope technician should be able to tie knots under stress, in the dark, when cold, using only one hand, and with diminished physical ability.

There are thousands of knots, but the number of knots explored in this chapter is reduced to that necessary for major situations encountered in the high angle environment.

Note that certain specialized knots are not reviewed in this chapter, but are reviewed in sections associated with the special skills that use the knot. For example, the Munter hitch ("Italian hitch") is reviewed in Chapter 8, Belaying of One-Person Loads, and the Prusik is included in Chapter 10, Ascending, and in Chapter 12, Rescue Belaying.

THE QUALITIES OF A GOOD KNOT

Although knots vary in their specific use, all good knots have certain characteristics in common, which include:

◆ They are relatively easy to tie.
◆ You can easily determine if they are tied correctly.
◆ Once tied correctly, they remain tied.
◆ They have a minimal effect on rope strength.
◆ They are relatively easy to untie after loading.

HOW KNOTS AFFECT ROPES

Every knot diminishes the strength of rope somewhat. The reason for this is that in any sharp bend of a rope (less than four times the diameter of the rope), the rope fibers on the outside of the bend carry most of the load on the rope. The fibers on the inside of the bend will carry very little of the load or none at all (Figure 6-1). (See the discussion of the 4:1 rule in Chapter 4, page 35).

Some knots, such as bowlines, have sharper bends and cause more of a strength loss in a rope than knots such as figure 8s, which have more open bends. Ultimately, the strengths of knots, along with other elements of a high angle system, must be taken into consideration when deciding on a safety factor for a rope. (See Chapter 3, Rope and Related Equipment, regarding safety factors.)

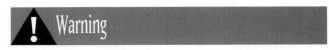

An improperly tied knot, or the incorrect application of a knot, could result in serious injury or death.

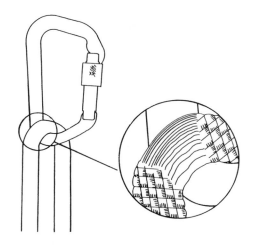

FIGURE 6-1
Effect of bending rope.

Knots should be removed from a rope before the rope is put away and stored, for the following reasons:

♦ If a knot has been loaded and left in the rope over a long period, it may cause a permanent loss of strength in the rope.
♦ If knots are left in the rope over a long period, they will tend to "set" and become more difficult to untie.

BACKING UP KNOTS

It is good practice to back up knots with a *backup (safety) knot*. Although an overhand knot is often used as a backup, a more secure backup is the double overhand knot (see page 65 for instructions on tying a double overhand backup knot). A backup knot is a particular concern when the rope is stiffer, such as static kernmantle ropes, or if the knot is going to be flexed a great deal. The backup should be tied as close as possible to the main knot it is safetying.*

DRESSING OF KNOTS

All knots, after tying, should be dressed (the strands aligned and uncrossed) and compacted (all ends pulled down so the knot is compact). This ensures that the knot has its greatest holding power, while maintaining as much rope strength as possible.

Also, after being dressed, it is easier to identify knots and confirm that they are correctly tied.

KNOTS

Overhand Knot (for Rope and Webbing)

Applications:

♦ As a *foundation knot* for beginning other knots such as the ring bend (water knot).
♦ As a backup to secure other knots.

Figure 6-2, *A* through 6-2, *C* shows the tying of a simple overhand knot.

♦ **Do not mistake the overhand knot for a half hitch (a half hitch is shown for comparison in Figure 6-3).**
♦ **The overhand knot, when used as a backup knot, must be pulled down tightly and close to the knot it is backing up (as is shown in Figure 6-7, backing up a bowline).**

---

*Note: For clarity, many knots in this manual are not shown with backups. It should be assumed, however, that in each case they should have a backup.

The Figure 8 Family

The figure 8 family of knots will enable you to deal with many knot-tying needs in the high angle environment. High angle rope technicians increasingly prefer the figure 8 knots because:

♦ They tend to be secure, when tied correctly, and less likely to come apart under loading and flexing.
♦ It is easy to tell if they are tied correctly.
♦ They diminish rope strength less than some other knots.
♦ It is easy to remember how to tie them.

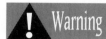

Figure 8 knots, as with all knots, should be dressed (the strands aligned and uncrossed) and compacted (all ends pulled down so the knot is compact). This ensures that the knot has its greatest holding power, while maintaining as much rope strength as possible.

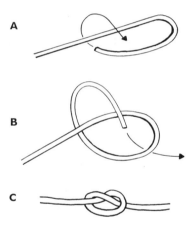

FIGURE 6-2
Tying a simple overhand knot.

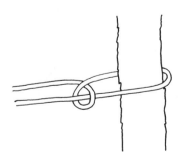

FIGURE 6-3
Half hitch.

Simple Figure 8 (for Rope)

Uses:

As a *stopper knot* for certain types of security, such as:

- Tied in the bottom end of a rope to prevent a person from rappelling off the end.
- To be tied in the top of a rope to prevent it from accidentally slipping through equipment.
- As a foundation knot for beginning the figure 8 follow through or the figure 8 bend (Figure 6-4).

Figure 8 on a Bight (for Rope)

Note that a *bight* is simply the loop formed when the rope is doubled back on itself. Creating a bight is the first step in tying this knot. You can do this in the middle of the rope, or at an end, as shown in Figure 6-5, *A*.

Uses:

As a secure loop in a rope for clipping into, for such things as:

- Safety lines.
- Persons being lowered.
- Litter and other rescue equipment.
- Anchor lines.

Optional Approach: Bowline Knot

Many authorities experienced in the high angle environment feel that the figure 8 family of knots is preferable to the bowline family for the following reasons:

- A figure 8 knot is more likely to be tied correctly.
- A figure 8 knot is more likely to be remembered.
- A figure 8 knot is easier to tell quickly if it is tied correctly.
- A figure 8 knot remains stable if loading on it comes from a direction different from what was intended.
- A figure 8 knot is more likely to remain tied after repeated loading and unloading.
- A figure 8 knot is less likely to invert and become untied when pulled across an obstruction, or when the trail of the knot is pulled.
- A figure 8 knot tends to weaken the rope less than a bowline.

> ⚠️ **Caution**
>
> **Be careful that you tie a figure 8 on a bight and not an overhand on a bight, which is illustrated in Figure 6-6.**

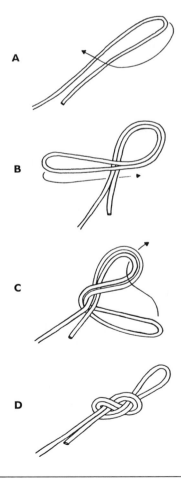

FIGURE 6-5

Tying a figure 8 on a bight.

> ⚠️ **Caution**
>
> **Do not confuse this knot with the simple overhand. Compare it with the overhand in Figures 6-2, A through 6-2, C and note the extra step in tying the simple figure 8. When you hold this knot up by either end of the rope, it should have the rough appearance of an "8."**

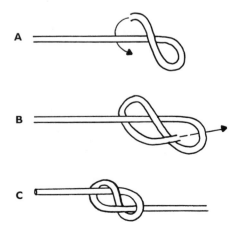

FIGURE 6-4

Tying a simple figure 8 knot.

However, due to the long tradition of using the bowline, there is often a passionate attachment to its use. A simple bowline is shown correctly tied, along with an overhand knot backup, in Figure 6-7.

If local policy dictates the use of a bowline for tying a loop in a rope, instead of a figure 8, then you should obtain instruction in the tying of a bowline from qualified personnel.

Figure 8 Follow Through

Use the figure 8 follow through to create a loop at the end of a rope in situations where a figure 8 on a bight cannot be tied (Figure 6-8). An example would be a

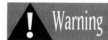

If you decide to use a bowline, make certain that it is tied correctly and also do the following:
- Make certain that the tail of the knot ("bitter end") is backed up with an overhand or other "keeper" knot.
- Avoid the use of a bowline on a moving rope. If the bowline snags, the knot may invert (changing the direction of the load on it) and fail.
- Do not load the tail of a bowline (it can also cause it to fail).

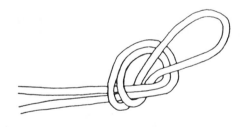

FIGURE 6-6
Overhand on bight.

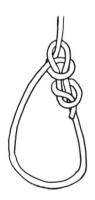

FIGURE 6-7
Simple bowline with overhand backup.

situation where you would want to anchor to a tall object, such as a tree, but a simple loop cannot be gotten *over the top*. Therefore a figure 8 follow through is tied *around it* (Box 6-1).

Figure 8 Bend (for Rope)

Note that the term **bend** as applied to knots refers to the joining of two ropes together (Box 6-2).
Uses:
For joining two ropes together:
- For connecting two pieces of rope.
- For creating a loop of rope by joining both ends of one rope together.

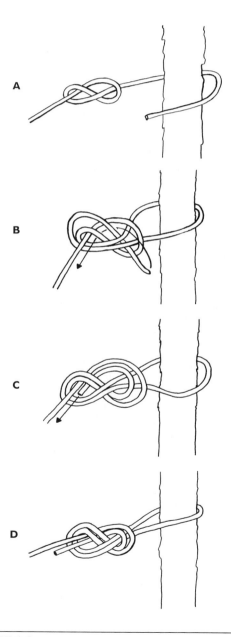

FIGURE 6-8
Tying a figure 8 follow-through knot.

Box 6-1 Suggestion for Use of Figure 8 Follow Through

1. Note that the figure 8 follow through always begins with the tying of a simple figure 8 knot as a foundation well back from the end of the rope.
2. After the simple figure 8 is tied, pass the end of the rope around the anchor point, then follow back through parallel to the first knot. Follow every contour of the first knot with both rope ends going *in the same direction.*
3. Do not confuse this knot with the figure 8 bend (Figure 6-9).

Box 6-2 Suggestion for Use of Figure 8 Bend

First try tying this knot using two ropes of different colors. This will make it easier to distinguish the different strands of rope.

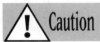 Caution

1. **Note that the figure 8 bend always begins with the step of tying a simple figure 8 knot as a foundation.**
2. **The next step is to exactly follow the contour of the first knot with the rope ends approaching from *opposite* directions.**

Optional Approach: Grapevine Knot

Another knot that can be used to securely join two rope ends to form a longer rope or to form a loop is the *grapevine knot* (also known as the *double fisherman's knot*). Although this knot is very secure, it may be more difficult to learn and to tell if it is tied correctly. The grapevine knot can be difficult to untie after it is loaded, particularly in softer lay ropes.

The grapevine knot should only be used for joining ropes of a similar diameter. It should not be used for webbing, for ropes of greatly unequal diameters, or for materials that may tend to untie or creep back through the bends of the knot (Box 6-3).

Ring Bend (Water Knot)

The ring bend knot is for webbing only and is also known as the *overhand bend.*
Uses:
   For tying webbing together:
   ◆ For joining two different pieces of webbing to form a longer piece.
   ◆ For tying the two ends of one piece of webbing together to form a loop (Box 6-4).

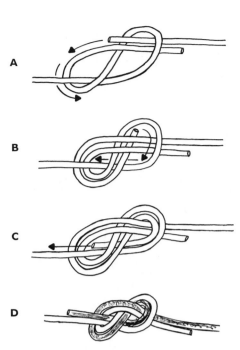

FIGURE 6-9
Tying a figure 8 bend knot.

Box 6-3 Suggestion for Use of Grapevine Knot

The tail of each rope, when tied correctly, should end up on the side of the knot opposite from the side it entered. The two turns from each half of the knot should lay flat against one another on one face of the knot and appear as a double X on the other face (Figure 6-10, D).

 Warning

The ring bend is to be used only for webbing. Do not use it for rope. Because of the flat nature of webbing, it tends to contour over itself. Rope does not have this quality and a water knot in rope may easily come out.

Figure 6-11, *A* through 6-11, *E* illustrate the tying of a ring bend (water knot) in webbing.

Double Overhand (for Rope)

Uses:
   For backing up other knots:
   ◆ The double overhand is essentially one half of a double fisherman's knot.
   ◆ Figures 6-12, *A* and 6-12, *B* illustrate the tying of a double overhand knot.

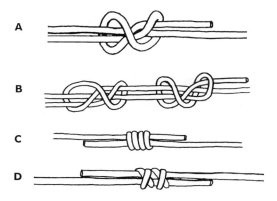

FIGURE 6-10

Tying a grapevine knot (also known as *double fisherman's knot*).

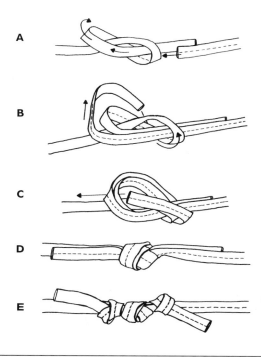

FIGURE 6-11

Tying a ring bend ("water knot") in webbing.

 Box 6-4 Suggestions for Tying a Ring Bend Knot

First try tying this knot using two pieces of webbing of different colors. This will make it easier to distinguish the different pieces of webbing as you tie the knot.

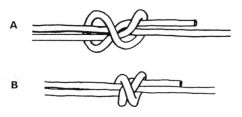

FIGURE 6-12

Tying a double overhand backup knot.

⚠ Warning

1. Always have at least two inches of webbing in the ends of ring bends *after they are tied and pulled tight*. Although webbing contours well in a ring bend, it tends to be slippery. For additional insurance, back up both sides of the knot with an overhand knot (see Figure 6-12, E) or sew loose ends down sufficiently to keep them from working through the knot.
2. A ring bend in webbing should be inspected frequently because over time it tends to work loose.
3. Be certain the webbing follows flat through the knot. A twist in the webbing inside the knot will allow the knot to slip at relatively low loads.

Evaluation Exercises

◆ COGNITIVE AND AFFECTIVE EXERCISES ◆

1. **Which of the following are uses for knots in the high angle environment?**
   A. Anchoring.
   B. Tying ropes and webbing together.
   C. Tying a person's seat harness directly to the rope.
   D. All of the above.
2. **Qualities of a good knot include all of the following,** *except:*
   A. It's easy to tie.
   B. It's easy to determine if tied correctly.
   C. It's hard to untie after loading.
   D. It has minimal effect on rope strength.
3. **Describe a use for each of the following:**
   a) Overhand knot.
   b) Simple figure 8.
   c) Figure 8 on a bight.
   d) Figure 8 follow through.
   e) Figure 8 bend.
   f) Ring bend ("water knot").
   g) Double overhand backup knot.
   h) Grapevine ("double fisherman's") knot.

▼ PSYCHOMOTOR EXERCISES ▼

4. Tie the following knots in a well-lighted room:
  a) Overhand.
  b) Simple figure 8.
  c) Figure 8 on a bight.
  d) Figure 8 follow through.
  e) Figure 8 bend.
  f) Ring bend "water knot."
  g) Double overhand backup knot.

5. Tie the following knots, while blind folded, or with your hands under a table:
  a) Overhand.
  b) Simple figure 8.
  c) Figure 8 on a bight.
  d) Figure 8 follow through.
  e) Figure 8 bend.
  f) Ring bend "water knot."
  g) Double overhand backup knot.

6. Put on your storm clothing, step into a cold shower with the lights off, and tie the following knots:
  a) Overhand.
  b) Simple figure 8.
  c) Figure 8 on a bight.
  d) Figure 8 follow through.
  e) Figure 8 bend.
  f) Ring bend "water knot."
  g) Double overhand backup knot.

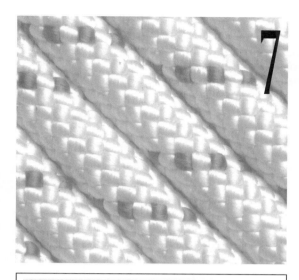

7 Anchoring

Key Terms ▼

Anchor (1) (n) A secure tie-in point for attaching a line. (2) (v) The act of attaching a line to an anchor.

Anchor Point A single secure connection for an anchor. An anchor point is used either alone or in combination with other anchor points to create an anchor system capable of sustaining the load on a rope rescue system.

Anchor System One or more anchor points rigged to provide a structurally significant connection for elements of a rope rescue system.

Artificial Anchors The use of specifically designed hardware to create anchors where good, natural anchors do not exist.

Backing Up The creation of a secondary or redundant system designed to provide added security and the creation of an additional independent anchor, or anchors, to sustain the high angle system should initial anchors fail. Backing up may be to the same anchor point if it is very solid, or to additional anchor points.

Back Tie Connector from a primary anchor to a second anchor that backs up the primary anchor.

Bombproof Jargon for an anchor or anchor system believed to be very secure.

Directional A technique for repositioning a rope at a more favorable angle than would exist by running the rope directly to the anchor.

Objectives _____ ▼

At the completion of this chapter, you should be able to:

1. Describe the purpose of anchoring.
2. Explain forces created on anchors and demonstrate ways to reduce or magnify these forces.
3. Given an anchor system example, estimate the forces on the anchor system.
4. Explain how to avoid overloading of an anchor system.
5. Given an example area, select anchor placement.
6. Explain the purpose of directionals.
7. Demonstrate how to set up a directional.
8. Select knots that are best employed in anchor systems.
9. Give examples of use of the tensionless hitch.
10. Use the following knots in an anchor system:
    ◆ Tensionless hitch.
    ◆ Figure 8 on a bight.
    ◆ Figure 8 follow through.
    ◆ Ring bend (water knot).
11. Cite examples of how rope and webbing are used in anchoring systems.
12. Identify what areas on a building would provide suitable and unsuitable anchor points.
13. Demonstrate secure anchor construction in a building.
14. Discuss what parts of a vehicle are suitable and unsuitable anchor points.
15. Demonstrate secure anchors in vehicles.
16. Demonstrate examples of when using multiple anchor points are needed.
17. Explain what angles on a multipoint anchoring system can create unacceptable forces.
18. Explain the concept of load-sharing anchors.
19. Correctly tie a load-sharing anchor using two anchor points.
20. Correctly tie a load-distributing anchor using a webbing loop on two anchor points.
21. Correctly construct a load distributing anchor system using three or more anchor points.
22. Explain the concept of a picket system.
23. Demonstrate the construction of a picket system.

ANCHORS AND THE HIGH ANGLE SYSTEM

Anchors are the means of securing the ropes and other elements of the high angle system to something solid. The place where the anchors are connected is the *anchor point.* Anchor points take a number of forms. They can be manmade, such as with structural beams, or natural anchors such as trees or rocks. Or they might be termed *artificial anchors* that people have placed in rock walls. On buildings, the most secure anchor points are structural parts such as integral beams and columns. In some situations, the only available anchor points may be on vehicles.

Anchoring is to the high angle system as a foundation is to a building. Without suitable and secure anchors, the remainder of the high angle system (ropes, hardware, and other gear) is in danger of failure, no matter how well you establish them. Just as a solid foundation is the primary concern before construction of a building you must have a suitable and secure *anchor system* before rigging the remainder of the system.

Anchor Points

The anchor point is the single secure connection for an anchor. The specific kind of anchor point will depend on the specific kind of high angle environment in which you are working.

Natural Anchors

The most commonly used natural anchors are trees and rocks around which webbing or rope can be wrapped. However, both have potential for failure. Before you use trees as anchors, you should examine them for potential rot. But even trees with sound wood may not be good anchors if their root systems are shallow or thin or if they are in wet soil. Boulders weighing tons can be pulled over by the stresses of anchor systems.

Anchors on Structures

In the industrial or urban setting, it will often be necessary to establish anchors on structures. You must do this carefully to make certain the anchor is structurally sound. On some modern buildings, it is often difficult to find any anchor points at all.

Some examples of deteriorated structures are:
- Corroded metals.
- Weathered stonework.
- Deteriorated mortar in brickwork.

Some examples of inherently weak structural features are:
- Vents constructed of sheet metal.
- Flashing.
- Gutters and downspouts.
- Brickwork without bulk, such as small chimneys.
- Fire hydrants.

When you rig anchors on buildings, choose anchor points that are inherently part of the building's structure or specifically constructed to support high loads.

Some examples include:
- Structural columns.
- Projections of structural beams.
- Supports for large machinery.
- Stairwell support beams.
- Brickwork with large bulk, such as corner walls.
- Anchors for window-cleaning equipment.

⚠ Warning

1. Do not confuse window cleaner eyebolts with guy wire hooks. Window cleaner eyebolts are substantial (usually ¾ inch), closed eyebolts in structural concrete. Guy wire hooks are used to stabilize items such as signs and antenna. They are not designed for life support.
2. Many window washer eyebolts are designed to be pulled vertically with cantilevered rigging. These may fail if pulled sideways. Always back up window washer eyebolts with other anchors.

Less Obvious Anchors

On some buildings, particularly those of recent construction, there may at first appear to be no anchor points. But after some practice at this type of problem, riggers may find some unexpected, but good, anchors.

Elevator and Machine Housings

Elevator and machine housings are generally very large compared with what is often expected as anchor points. But by taking a length of rope, running it around the housing several times, and tying the ends together with a figure 8 bend you may be able to create a secure anchor point for several lines.

Scuppers (Roof Drain Holes)

Many buildings have low parapets with drain holes set in them at roof level. By running rope or webbing through the drain hole and back over the top of the parapet, you can create an anchor point.

If possible, you should set the scupper on the side of the building opposite to the one over which you will run the main line. This will allow space on top of the building for rappellers to rig into the rope, and to set other rigging, such as lowering and raising systems.

The more substantial parapets are those constructed of reinforced concrete. If the parapet is constructed of brick or block, the riggers should be certain that several brick or block courses are involved and the mortar is in good condition. Even under the best of conditions for a brick or block parapet, it would be wise to rig with at least two anchor points. Be certain to pad all sharp edges.

Wall Sections between Windows and/or Doors

If a set of windows and/or doors are close enough together, then you can create a substantial anchor point by passing the anchor rope or webbing through an open window or door, around the intervening wall, and back through an adjacent window or door to tie it off. The anchor wall should be on the opposite side from where the main line will run out of the building. This will give more safe space for rappellers to rig into the rope, or to set rigging such as lowering and raising systems.

Stairwell Beams

Stairwell beams should be the structural beams. They are the open steel beams to which the stair risers are anchored.

Artificial Anchors

Artificial anchors are special types of hardware specifically designed for creating anchor points or "protection" where there are no natural anchors. Many artificial anchors are inserted into rocks or spaces in rock. They include such hardware as nuts, chocks, hexcentrics, and cams. For hardware to be safe and effective anchors, they need to be placed by a person who has a great deal of skill and practice in their use.

Among the artificial anchors, bolts are commonly used in rescue operations. But their placement is time consuming and they also require a great deal of practice and training for correct placement. They also create permanent damage to the rock, which is frowned on in managed areas such as parkland. (See Chapter 5, Basic High Angle Hardware, for more details on artificial anchors.)

Placement of Anchors

Whatever their nature, the placement of secure anchors depends very much on good judgment, which is developed though experience and practice. Although their specifics may vary from place to place, there are certain characteristics common to all anchors.

Strength of Anchors

Anchors must be able to sustain the greatest anticipated force on the high angle system as calculated through the *safety factor*. (See Chapter 3, Rope and Related Equipment, on how to calculate a safety factor.) Anchors that are so strong that they will withstand any force that the high angle system will deliver to them are said to be **bombproof.**

If the potential anchor point will not sustain the anticipated forces, then it must be abandoned for another more substantial one or teamed with one or more other anchor points (multiple anchors are described later in this chapter).

This ability of an anchor to withstand the necessary forces will depend on a number of factors, including:

◆ Condition of the anchor. For example, a live tree will usually withstand greater forces than a dead one.

◆ Structural nature of the anchor point. For example, a load-bearing structural column in a building will generally withstand greater forces than a handrail.

◆ Location of force on the anchor point. For example, a tree with the force pulling on it near the ground will generally withstand greater force than one with the stress higher up.

Direction of Pull on Anchor Point

Always consider the direction of pull that will be on the anchor point. Try to set anchors that will be in line with the direction of pull. Also consider what will happen if the direction of pull changes. Some anchors are rigged so that they are strong only when the pull comes from one direction. If the direction of pull changes, then the anchor could weaken or fail.

Positioning of Anchors

The position of an anchor will have an effect on the high angle activity. This is particularly true in rescue activity. Under the ideal conditions, the anchor should be close to and directly above the subject to be rescued. However, there would be circumstances where it might be preferable to have the anchor off to the side. Some examples are:

◆ Conditions where rocks or other dangerous objects might fall on the rescue subject or on the rescuers.
◆ Conditions between the anchor point and the rescue subject that could endanger rescuers or damage equipment such as rope.

Example. There is a flashover and fire from a window.

Example. The presence of a hostile or deranged person.

◆ Conditions where there are no suitable anchors directly above.

In any high angle activity, it is often desirable that segments of the high angle system, such as the belay rope, be off to the side to avoid rope cross or tangles. But if the primary anchor (the one bearing the greatest load) is off at an extreme angle, there could be problems for those people attempting to manage the rope work. They might, for example, have to make a wide swing on the rope (a *pendulum*) to reach their objective. However, there are some anchoring techniques that may solve such a problem.

Directionals

A *directional* is a technique for bringing a rope into a more favorable position or angle. There are numerous ways of creating directionals. You have to judge each method on its advantages and disadvantages specific to a given situation. As shown in Figure 7-1, there are two trees wide apart that could serve as strong anchors at the top of a cliff. But say, for example, that you want to use the rope to reach spot **X** on the ground that is between the trees:

1. If you anchor the rope to either one of the two trees, as it has been to the tree on the right in Figure 7-1, *A*, it would be difficult for you to reach spot **X** without a significant pendulum.
2. Now, say you add a secondary anchor, a directional, to the smaller tree on the left (Figure 7-1, *B*). In the end of this second rope, you tie a figure **8** on a bight knot and clip a locking carabiner into the figure **8**-knot. Finally, you clip this locking carabiner across the main anchor rope. Thus, the main rope is now at a better angle for you to reach **X**. One additional advantage with this approach is that the main rope runs freely through the carabiner so that as the exact position of the activity moves back and forth, the angle can change slightly.
3. A less desirable alternative would be to tie a figure **8** overhand knot in the main line and clip it directly into the carabiner that is on the directional (Figure 7-1, *C*). This would prevent the main line from sliding freely through the carabiner. This would also create a *multipoint anchor,*

but without the advantages of example (Figure 7-1, *B*). When the rope moved to one side or the other, it would create a great deal of loading on one anchor but very little loading on the other anchor.

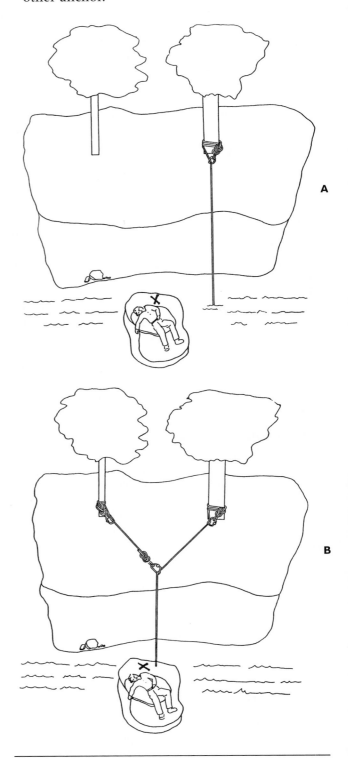

FIGURE 7-1

Setting a directional.

Location of Directionals

When you establish anchors and directionals you must keep in mind how safe and accessible their locations are for the high angle personnel who work with them. In Figure 7-1, for example, you could possibly make some improvements by changing the location of the anchors and directional. If there were anchor points, such as the trees, far enough back from the edge of the drop, then you could rig the anchor system and the directional on the top.

As a result:

1. Those people rigging the anchors and the directional would be in less danger of falling.
2. The rigging would be more accessible to the people and therefore would be more in their control.
3. With the rope running over the edge, not all the weight would be directly on the anchor; part of it would be taken by the edge of the drop. (The drawback would be possible abrasion on the rope.)

Backing Up Anchors

Anchor systems present a number of opportunities for failure, including:

◆ Uncertain strength of anchor points: Anchor-point failure is usually the most common cause of anchor system failure. You can rarely say for certain what kind of stress an anchor point will take.
◆ Failures in human judgment and experience: Knots may be tied incorrectly and carabiner gates may be left unlocked, for example.

◆ Equipment failures: Abrasion and cutting of rope and webbing and stressing of both hardware and software can occur.

Because of the potential for anchor system failure, and because the rest of the high angle system depends on anchors, it is good practice to back up anchors. *Backing up* is the creation of redundant anchors for safety. Two primary ways of backing up an anchor are:

1. Backing up to the same anchor point (Figure 7-2, *A*). Only do this when you are absolutely certain that the one anchor point can sustain any forces subjected to it by the high angle system (it is "bombproof"). This type of backup is done when there is the possibility of failure in other portions of the anchor system (carabiners, knots, slings, and so on).
2. Backing up to a separate anchor point (Figure 7-2, *B*). This requires a multiple anchor system. If the direction of loading will be shifting from side to side, you should make the multiple anchor system load sharing (explained later in this chapter).

Specifically the method of backing up the anchor system and the number of anchor points you will need depend on a number of variables:

◆ The condition of the anchor points. If there is the potential for failure of one of them, or of the equipment attached to it, then you need more than one anchor point.
◆ The nature of the high angle operation taking place. If there is a main line and a belay line, for example, then you should use separate anchor systems. If both the main line and the belay line originate from the same anchor point, then there is the danger of causing line tangles or damage to the rope from line cross (see Chapter 3, Rope and Related Equipment, on avoiding damage from rope cross).

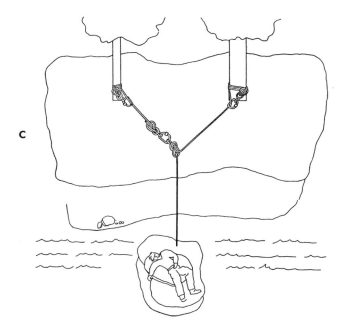

C

FIGURE 7-1—cont'd

Setting a directional.

> ⚠ **Warning**
>
> 1. Depending on the angle the primary anchor rope makes with the directional rope, there could be greater forces on the anchor system than if there were only a single anchor (see Figure 7-1, B). A directional is in effect creating a multiple anchor system. See the discussion later in this chapter on how multiple anchors create forces on the system depending on the angles the ropes create.
> 2. Remember, that should the directional fail, there will be a significant *pendulum*, the main line will drop, and the main line anchor will be shock loaded. In addition, the rope could be severely damaged or cut.

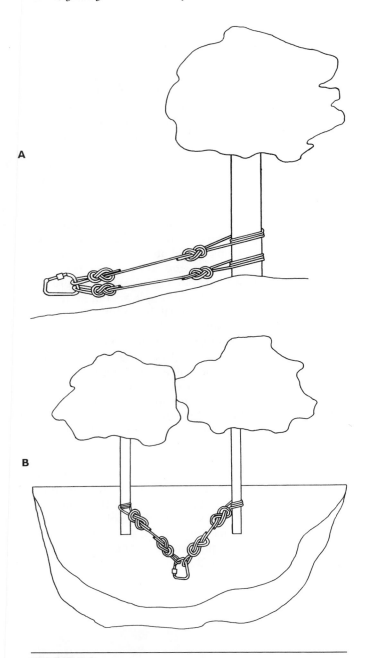

FIGURE 7-2
Backing up anchors.

The belay system would also have to be substantial enough to catch a fall, which means you need a substantial second anchor.

◆ The loads and stresses involved in the system: this will vary in intensity depending on the uses of the anchors:
1. Supporting only equipment.
2. Supporting the weight of only one person.
3. Directionals that create forces greater than the load ("load amplifiers").
4. Rescue lowering operations.
5. Hauling systems.

6. Highlines (a system of using a rope suspended between two points to move persons or equipment).

Materials for Anchors
Using Rope for Anchors

One of the simplest procedures in establishing an anchor is to connect the main line rope directly to the anchor point. In urgent situations, where time is critical, this may be the best solution. It also means a simpler anchor system, with less chance for failure than might be in a more complicated system.

However, if you rig the main line rope directly to the anchor point, it will reduce your flexibility and limit your ability to make modifications in the anchor system. These modifications may be necessary because of the changing conditions that can occur in rescue situations.

One potential solution is to use a separate piece of rope for the anchor system that is of the same strength or stronger than the main line and attach the main line to it:
1. Attach the anchor rope to the anchor point.
2. Tie a figure **8** on a bight knot in the ends of both ropes where they will meet.
3. Clip the figure **8** knots together with carabiners.

If a group involved in high angle activities has been established for some time, many of these rope pieces will become available. Often, when a main line rope has developed a small, bad section, that small section can be cut away, while the remaining pieces of the rope can be used as anchor lines.

Tieoffs for Anchor Ropes

One of the most attractive attachments for anchor ropes is the *tensionless* hitch (Box 7-1), also known as the *high strength tieoff*. It has advantages as an anchor knot for three reasons:
1. It is simple.
2. It reduces stress on rope and equipment.
3. It gives the flexibility to deal with changing conditions.

The tensionless hitch is wrapped around an object so that the friction of the wrap takes the load. With enough friction, all the force is applied to the object the rope is wrapped around. The end of the rope is tied off without any of the force of the load on the hitch itself, thus, the term, *tensionless hitch*. When the rope is tied correctly it is not weakened by a knot, so the rope maintains full strength. This assumes the object is bigger than 4 times the diameter of the rope (Box 7-2).

There is another knot that you can use in rope for anchoring. But it gives less flexibility for making changes than the tensionless hitch and may result in greater stress on the knot. However, where there will be lower loads on the anchor system, it may be preferable because it may be quicker to tie. This is the

Text cont'd on p. 74

Box 7-1 Procedure for Tying the Tensionless Hitch (High Strength Tieoff)

1. Take two wraps with the rope-around object being used as the anchor point (Figure 7-3). The number of wraps depends on the diameter of the anchor point and the coefficient of friction of the anchor point surface. A smaller diameter and slicker anchor point will require more wraps, but on any anchor point, there should be at least two. The objective is to have enough rope turns around the object so that the running end of the rope will have no tension on it. Instead, the tension is absorbed by the friction on the turns of rope around the object.
2. There should be no rope cross in the turns. If the anchor is above the load, the rope should spiral up with the running end at the top. This should be done in case the load has to be lowered slightly and in effect could be done by using the tree or vertical object as a lowering device.
3. Tie a figure 8 on a bight in the running end of the rope and clip a locking carabiner into the figure 8 knot.
4. Clip the carabiner across the standing end of the rope at the bottom of the spiral. The spiral should be adjusted (it's easier if two people are doing it) so that there is no slack in the spiral, yet no sharp angle where the carabiner is clipped across the standing end of the rope.

ALTERNATIVE APPROACH

If you do not have a carabiner, you can use a hitch or knot to replace the figure 8 knot and carabiner. Tie off the end in a way that prevents the rope from unwinding around the object and without placing any bends in the loaded section of the rope. The recommended method of figure 8 on a bight and a carabiner is more secure.

Box 7-2 Where the Tensionless Hitch may be Used

You can use the tensionless hitch on an anchor point around which you can wrap rope, which can withstand the stress of the forces in the system, and which will not damage the rope, such as on:

◆ Trees
◆ Columns
◆ Structural beams

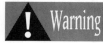 **Warning**

1. The tensionless hitch only works if there is adequate surface contact between the rope and the object. If the object is not shaped to allow this, choose another method of anchoring to it. For example an H-shaped beam will have rope contact in only four places. A tensionless hitch will not work here.
2. If the anchor point has sharp edges, as sometimes found on structural beams, then you should pad the rope appropriately. (See Chapter 4, Care and Use of Rope and Related Equipment.)

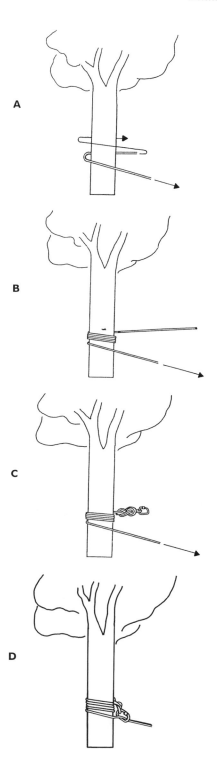

FIGURE 7-3
Tying tensionless hitch.

figure 8 follow-through knot. As with the tensionless hitch, it is used where a loop of rope cannot be laid over the top of an anchor point, such as a tree or column, but has to be tied around it. (See Chapter 6, Knots, for the procedure of tying a figure 8 follow through.)

If the vertical member to be used as an anchor point is short enough so that you can easily get a loop of rope over it, then you can tie a figure 8 on a bight in the end of the rope and place the loop over the anchor. (See Chapter 6, Knots, for the procedure of tying a figure 8 on a bight.)

Alternative Approach: Use of a Bowline. If local policy dictates the use of a bowline for tying a loop in a rope, such as for a simple anchor, then you must use a bowline in the place of a figure 8 follow through or a figure 8 on a bight. However, you should take the following precautions:

- Because the bowline is easily tied incorrectly, carefully inspect the bowline to be certain that it is tied correctly. Figure 6-8 in Chapter 6 shows a simple bowline correctly tied.
- Back up the bowline with a "keeper knot" such as the double overhand knot ("barrel knot").
- Before loading the bowline, pretension it to tighten it.
- See that the bowline is not subjected to loading from a direction different from the one intended.

Using Webbing for Anchors

Webbing is a convenient material for anchoring. Among some groups whose members have a background in climbing and mountaineering, the use of webbing has been common.

Advantage:
- Less expensive than rope.
- Fewer knots to learn.

Disadvantage:
- Cannot be tied into as many different knots as rope.
- Does not absorb shock loading as well as most ropes.

Webbing is convenient for making continuous loops known as runners or slings.

Presewn Slings. Properly sewn runners are often used as a quick and convenient means of setting anchors. The two advantages of the presewn slings are that they are quicker to use and there is less chance of tying the wrong knot when making a continuous loop. There are several brands of presewn slings that can be used for anchoring.

Presewn slings are available in a variety of webbing widths and lengths (Figure 7-4). Many of the slings are sewn with loops in both ends. When purchasing presewn slings, make certain they have adequate tensile strength for the safety factor you are using. Also, make certain you know how the manufacturer of the

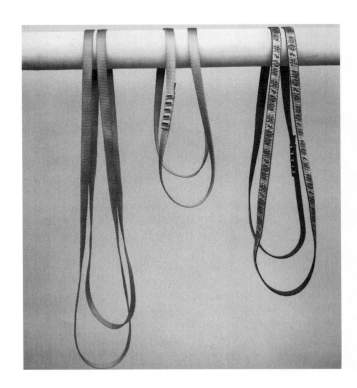

FIGURE 7-4
Presewn slings are available in various widths and lengths.

presewn slings tests them for strength. Anchor slings can have strength ratings based on being pulled end to end, pulled when rigged as a basket, or pulled when girded around an object. Before and after you use presewn webbing, always inspect it for wear on the stitching and the web material.

Anchor Straps. Anchor straps are heavy-duty webbing lengths with D rings sewn into each end. Anchor straps are commonly used in industrial and urban situations. Some anchor straps are made with a heavy-duty buckle to allow adjusting the strap to various lengths (Figure 7-5). Anchor straps, in addition to anchoring, can be used for other purposes such as litter bridles. Make certain anchor straps, as with other presewn slings, have adequate tensile strength for your system safety factor. In addition, make certain the manufacturer can provide you with specifications on how much loading it takes for the adjustable buckle to slip.

Creating Slings from Webbing Lengths. If you do not use sewn runners, then you can create a sling from a piece of webbing by tying it into a loop using a ring bend also known as a *water knot, overhand bend,* or *tape knot.* (See Chapter 6, Knots, for how to tie a ring bend.)

Placement of Webbing around Anchor Points. One secure method of placing the webbing around an anchor point is to tie it in a loop around the point using

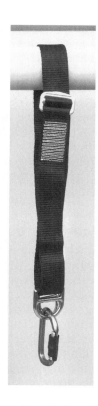

FIGURE 7-5
Anchor straps with heavy-duty buckles allow adjusting to various lengths.

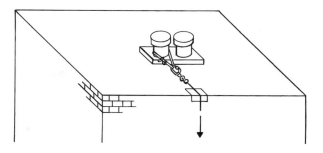

FIGURE 7-6
Tying webbing around anchor.

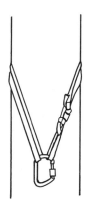

FIGURE 7-7
Wrapping webbing around anchor.

a ring bend as shown in Figure 7-6. If the object being used as the anchor point is very large, this procedure can be awkward and time consuming for one person.

An alternative is to first tie the runner. Next, wrap it around the anchor point and clip the two ends together with a carabiner as shown in Figure 7-7. However, such tied runners will require double the length of an untied length of webbing.

Keeping Anchors in Place

It is generally good practice to tie an anchor on a vertical member as low down as possible to reduce the stress on it.

However, if an anchor point is strong enough, there may be certain conditions where it would be an advantage to tie the anchor webbing higher up:

- ◆ It usually creates a better angle for a rappeller to get over the difficult edge of a drop.
- ◆ It might reduce rope abrasion on an edge.
- ◆ In rescue, it might improve conditions for lowering a stretcher over an edge.
- ◆ It could reduce the severe friction that is stressing a hauling system.

The problem is that a simple loop of webbing around a vertical member will tend to slip down on the member. One conventional method for holding

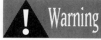

If you use tied webbing for slings, it is not wise to leave knots tied in webbing unless each runner is carefully inspected before being returned to the equipment cache and again inspected before being used. You should act to deal with the following problems:

- ◆ You may not know who tied the knot and what *kind* of knot it is.
- ◆ Knots in webbing may eventually work their way out.
- ◆ The knots may have been spot welded in webbing that has been shock loaded.

the webbing in place is to tie it around the anchor point in a girth hitch as shown in Figure 7-8, *A*. The drawback to this technique is the temptation to cinch the webbing back on itself as in Figure 7-8, *B*. This *should not* be done because it creates potentially dangerous stresses on the webbing.

One alternative to the girth hitch is to tie an interior loop in the webbing as shown in Figure 7-8, *C*. This, known as *wrap 1, pull 2*, will hold the webbing up on the anchor point and will not stress the webbing as will

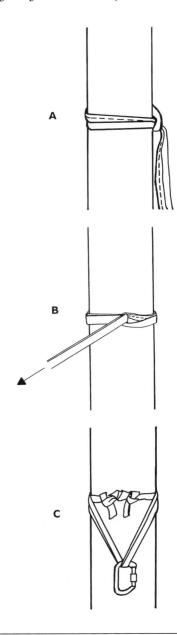

FIGURE 7-8

A and **B,** Girth hitch webbing. **C,** Wrap 2, pull 1 is preferable to the girth hitch.

a girth hitch. Note the location of the knot. It is on the interior loop, where there will be the least stress on it.

An even stronger anchor using webbing is a *wrap 3, pull 2*. In this system there are three wraps around the anchor, with two loops pulled out. Again, the knot is on the interior loop to maintain strength.

What to do when there are "No Anchors"

Extending Anchors

Although you sometimes may not find anchors nearby, you may be able to establish them by running lengths of rope, sometimes for a few hundred feet, to where there are anchors. *This should be done only with static rope. Attempting to extend anchors in such a manner with dynamic rope could potentially create a dangerous situation due to the large amount of stretch.* Even with static rope, there may be undesired stretch with only one line. Depending on the load, you can double, triple, or quadruple the lines to reduce the stretch.

One example of where extended anchors might work would be on the roof of a building where (absolutely, positively) no anchor points exist. Often, static rope can be run through the stairwell or through top-floor windows to lower floors where anchors do exist.

Using Vehicles for Anchors

A sort of "portable anchor" that is usually available is an *emergency vehicle*. However, there are some safety guidelines that you should follow when using vehicles for anchors:

◆ Begin by setting the parking brake.
◆ If automatic transmission, set in "park." If manual transmission, set in gear opposite to pull ("reverse" if pulling from the front).
◆ Forces created in a high angle system can move a vehicle with its brakes set, so chock wheels. If no chocks are available, use spare tire(s).
◆ Idiot proof your portable anchor by removing ignition key. Further disable starting system by pulling the coil wire.

There are portions of a vehicle that are structurally weak and should not be used:

1. Bumpers.
2. Tow hooks (these have often been subjected to intense and unrecorded stresses and contain the potential for failure).

Potential anchor points in a vehicle include structural parts, such as axles and cross members. But protect rope and webbing from oil and grease. As noted in Chapter 4, Care and Use of Rope and Related Equipment, rope and webbing must be protected from destructive substances such as battery acids, which are often found around vehicles.

Pickets

One alternative in a natural area where there are no anchors is the picket system. Although a picket system can work very well when properly rigged, it usually takes a great deal of time to properly establish it. In addition, not all soil types will hold pickets securely. Loose, sandy, or muddy soil, or snow may not hold well no matter how many pickets are used.

Most picket anchor systems consist of several rows of pickets. Figure 7-9 and Box 7-3 explain the construction of one row.

Multipoint Anchors

Multipoint anchors involve two or more anchor points. You use multiple anchors when one anchor

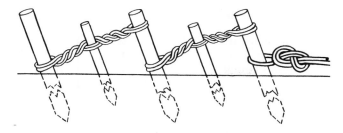

FIGURE 7-9
Establishing a picket system.

 Box 7-3 Establishing a Picket System

1. The pickets should have a minimum length of 5 feet, so that there will be a minimum of 3 feet in the ground and a maximum of 2 feet above ground.
2. Drive the pickets at an angle of 15 degrees away from the force to be anchored.
3. Connect the pickets in each row together by lashing from the top of the first picket (the one closest to the load) to the bottom of the next picket close to the ground. Continue in this manner until pickets in the row are lashed together.
4. Tension the lashings by twisting with a stick four to six turns. Drive this stick into the ground to secure it.
5. Construct the next rows of pickets as described above.
6. Connect the main line by clipping it to the front picket in each row with a *load sharing anchor* system as described above.

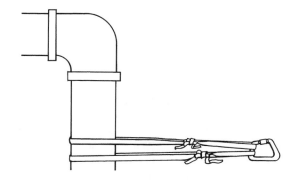

FIGURE 7-10
Backing up single anchor point.

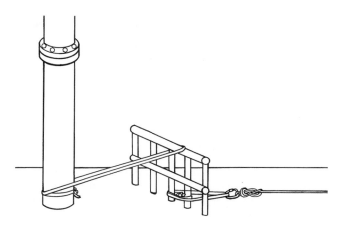

FIGURE 7-11
A back tie uses a connection to combine the two anchors.

point is insufficient to withstand the anticipated forces or when one anchor point is inconveniently placed.

Multiple Slings on Single Anchor Point

By adding additional attachments to an appropriate anchor point, you can help prevent the collapse of an anchor system due to the failure of a single item, such as webbing, carabiner, or improperly tied knots. Figure 7-10 shows the use of two slings of equal length on a single anchor point. This kind of system is used only where the single anchor point is absolutely secured ("bombproof"). There is *no insurance at all* in the additional webbing and carabiners if the anchor point fails.

Backing up Anchors

It is good practice to back up single anchors with a second anchor. This not only backs up the single anchor point but also gear such as anchor sling and carabiner. It also helps reduce the chance of failure due to human error such as badly tied knots and other rigging mistakes.

Backing up is essential when you encounter anchors that are in the right position but are not strong enough by themselves for a rescue load. In Figure 7-11 an anchor point is near the edge and in a good position but does not have the strength to take the load. You might consider this a *primary anchor.*

However, behind the primary anchor and directly in line with it is a second anchor. Its strength combined with the strength of the primary anchor will be enough to sustain the rescue load. This second anchor is called the *secondary anchor.*

To combine the two anchors run a rope or sling between the two anchors. This connector between the two anchors is known as **back tie.**

Two things must be kept in mind when employing a secondary anchor:

1. The secondary anchor must be *as strong* as the primary anchor.
2. The back tie must have no slack that would allow shock loading, which could cause both anchors to fail. One way to lessen the chance of shock loading is with a *pretensioned back tie.* (See volume II of this book, *Specialized and Advanced Techniques,* St. Louis, 1999, Mosby, for more information on pretensioned back tie.)

Load-Sharing Anchors

If anchor points are at all questionable, or inconveniently placed, then load-sharing anchors may be a solution. The simplest way to create a multiple anchor system for load sharing is to use two anchor ropes or slings of equal length. Run them from different anchor points and clip them together into a single point using one or two large locking carabiners (Figure 7-12). This point where you clip the two lines together with the carabiners is known as a ***master attachment point***. A master attachment point in load-sharing anchors is where the multiple lines come together at one point.

> ### ⚠ Warning
>
> A primary concern in rigging a load-sharing anchor is not to create too wide an angle between the legs of an anchor system. Ideally, this angle should not exceed 90 degrees and must never exceed 120 degrees. Beyond this point, the forces on each anchor will be greater than the total load itself.
>
> Remember, any angle in an anchor system will increase the loading on anchors and other elements of the system. Only when the angle between the legs of the anchor system is 0 degrees will each leg carry half the load. (See Figure 7-13 for diagrams of how angles affect the forces on anchor points and other elements of the system.)
>
> After you finish rigging the anchor system, check all the carabiners to make certain they will load correctly.

Load-Distributing Anchors

A major problem with a fixed, load-sharing anchor system as in Figure 7-14, *A* is that the stress on the anchor points will be equal only when the force from the main line pulls directly in the center of the angle. This is often not the case in high angle operations. Most of the time, the force will be pulling to one side or another, as in Figure 7-14, *B*. It can also be moving back and forth from one side to another. Obviously, if there is a possibility that either one of the anchor points cannot sustain these side-to-side forces, then the entire anchor system may fail.

One possible solution to this problem is to create a ***load distributing anchor system (LDA)***. When this type of system is correctly constructed and conditions are right, it can have some important advantages:

1. The forces on anchor points should remain distributed and shared by all anchor points, whatever the direction of pull.

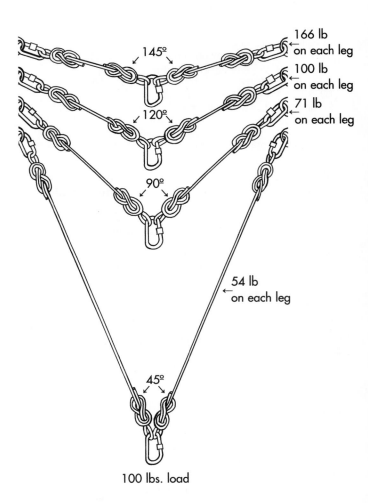

FIGURE 7-13

Relationship between anchor sling tension and a 100-lb load at different angles.

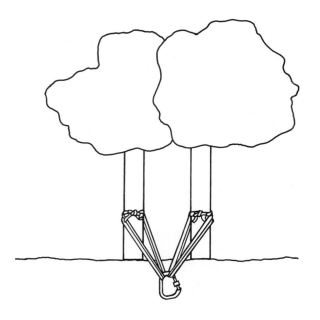

FIGURE 7-12

Load-sharing anchor.

2. Should any anchor point fail, the system should readjust to help redistribute loading on the remaining anchor point(s).

LDAs are sometimes called *self-equalizing anchors.* It is important to know that no anchor system can be made to be completely "self-equalizing:"

1. Because of the angles involved in rigging any LDA, there will be varying forces on the elements, so the LDA will never be completely equal.
2. In a shock-load situation, the redistribution of forces does not occur instantaneously. During this transition to redistribution, some elements of the LDA system will receive greater loads than others.

It is critical for all rescuers to realize that LDAs are not for casual use in rescue. Because of their complexity and potential for failure, use them only when there are no other options, such as load-sharing anchors or extending anchors.

Load-distributing anchors are the last choice when rescuers are faced with marginal anchors, and the only possibility of establishing anchorage is by making those marginal anchors work together. This situation would more likely be found by back-country rescuers having to use artificial anchors.

How well the system distributes the forces and survives the shock loading of one anchor point failing, depends on several factors:

◆ Keep the angles small, both to reduce magnification of forces on anchors and to help the system readjust to the new loading.
◆ Design the systems so that there will be as little drop as possible should any anchor fail. One way to do this is by keeping the anchor legs as small as possible.
◆ Avoid bulky rope or webbing and adjust the system so that knots are less likely to run through carabiners when the system readjusts.

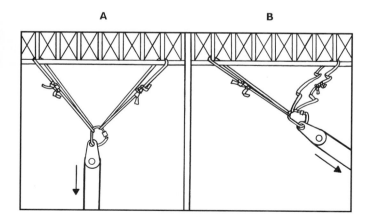

FIGURE 7-14
Forces on load-sharing anchors.

◆ Rope or webbing made of materials such as Kevlar or Spectra do not have the shock absorbing qualities of materials such as nylon. Only use Kevlar or Spectra in an anchor system if you include shock absorbing materials somewhere in the system.
◆ Make all of the anchor points in a load-distributing system as bombproof as possible.

A *Simple Two-Point, Load-Distributing Anchor System*

One of the simplest of the self-equalizing anchors involves two anchor points and uses a sling and a carabiner.

Creating a Simple Two-Point, Load-Distributing Anchor (Figure 7-15)
1. Configure a loop of webbing or rope in the shape of an **8**.
2. Clip a large locking carabiner across the inside loop.
3. Take each end of an outside loop and clip it into an anchor point.
4. Clip the carabiner on the inside loop into the main line. This will be the focal point for the anchor system.
5. Make certain that the angles made by the sling do not exceed the critical ones described in the Warning box on page 78.
6. Before loading this system, test it by hand. One at a time, simulate each one of the anchors failing to make certain that the system will catch the load.

Whatever the direction of the pull, the central carabiner should slip along the sling to equalize the forces. Should one anchor point fail, the webbing should set itself to pull on the other anchor point.

Tying a Load-Distributing Anchor System Using a Two-Loop Figure 8 (Figure 7-16)
1. Create a large loop by using a length of rope and tying the two ends together using a figure **8** bend (or double fisherman's knot).
2. For ease of operation, set the circle of rope on the ground or on the floor.
3. Place the knot at about 3 o'clock or 9 o'clock on the circle, so it remains out of the way.
4. Take a large bight of rope and flip it back inside the circle, about ⅔ of the way up.
5. The lower section of the circle is now doubled, so that there are four strands of rope.
6. Gather together these four strands of rope and tie a figure **8** knot with them.
7. At the top of the circle, there is now a large loop and a smaller loop inside. To reduce shock loading, keep the size of the large loop to a minimum, with a circumference of no more than 8 feet. At the bottom of the circle is a much smaller loop created by tying the figure **8** from the four strands.
8. Take the largest loop at the top of the circle and clip it into all the anchor points using a locking carabiner at each point.

9. Take the smaller loop at the bottom of the large loop. Using locking carabiners, clip this together to the larger loop between each anchor point.

10. Take the small loop below the knot created from the four strands. Clip this into the main line using one or two large locking carabiners. This will be the focal point for the anchor system.

11. If tied correctly, should any one point fail, the systems should redistribute the load among the remaining anchor points. The system should also distribute the load among all points whatever direction the load is coming from.

12. The riggers should inspect the system to make certain that it will indeed perform in this manner before the system is loaded by people. If there are any problems, such as a knot jamming, then the system must be adjusted so that it will work as intended.

⚠ Warning

Load-distributing anchor systems present the potential for dangerous shock loading as one anchor point pulls out and others take the load. Reduce potential shock loading by keeping angles small and slack to a minimum. Also:

◆ Try to keep anchor points close to one another. If this is not possible, it may be better to extend far-away anchor points with static rope to keep the load-sharing anchor's loop as small as possible.

◆ Keep outside angle to less than 90 degrees. Even better, limit angle to 60 degrees. The outside angle is measured from the two outer-most anchor points down to the master attachment point. This limits the forces on the remaining anchor points if one of the inside anchors fail in a LDA with three or more points.

◆ Rig load-distributing anchors with a minimum of slack in the system. Keep rope or webbing length at a minimum, approximately 8 feet or less, in the tied loop of a three-point system. Rig for a maximum of a 1 foot drop with the failure of an anchor point.

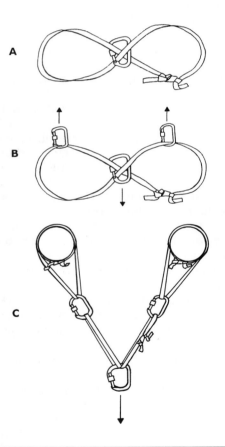

FIGURE 7-15
Simple self-equalizing anchor.

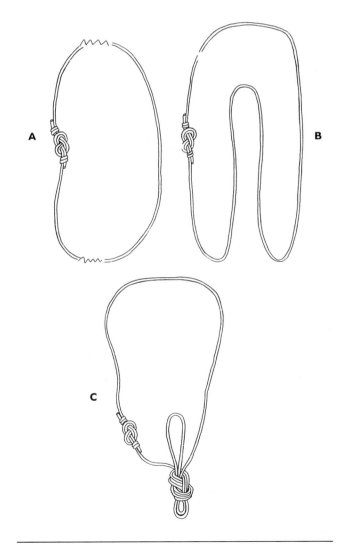

FIGURE 7-16
Complex self-equalizing anchor.

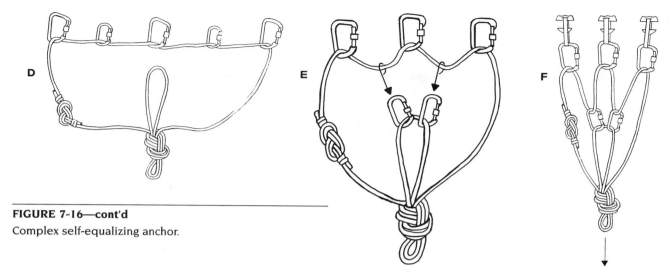

FIGURE 7-16—cont'd
Complex self-equalizing anchor.

Evaluation Exercises

◆ COGNITIVE AND AFFECTIVE EXERCISES ◆

1. Name three factors that affect the ability of an anchor point to withstand the forces of high angle activity.
2. Name three conditions where anchors should not be set directly above the high angle activity, but off to the side.
3. What is the purpose of a "directional" in an anchor system?
4. What would be the possible disadvantage in tying the main line directly into an anchor point?
5. What are three advantages in using the tensionless hitch or "high strength tieoff" in an anchor system?
6. In examining a tree for use as a potential anchor point, attention should be paid not only to the soundness of the wood but also to the nature of the _____ _____.
7. Why is it not prudent to leave knots tied in webbing (unless each runner is carefully inspected before use)?
8. How should webbing be tied to hold it in place on a vertical anchor point?
9. Name two typical reasons for anchor points on buildings being inadequate.
10. Name three potential anchor points on buildings that are an inherent part of the structure.
11. Describe parts of a vehicle that:
    a) Should not be used as anchor points.
    b) Might be used as anchor points.
12. Name two situations in which complex anchors are used.
13. Ideally, the angle between the legs of an anchor system should not be more than _____ degrees and never more than _____ degrees.
14. Name two ways to reduce the potential for shock loading when rigging LDAs.

▼ PSYCHOMOTOR EXERCISES ▼

15. Create a directional on an anchor system that was initially set at an inconvenient angle.
16. Set a tensionless hitch ("high strength tieoff") on a tree or column for a downward pull.
17. Do the following correctly:
    a) Tie a runner from webbing in a simple loop around a vertical anchor point.
    b) Tie a loop from a rope around the same anchor point.
18. Using an internal loop, set a runner tied from webbing around a tree or column so that it will not slip down.
19. Correctly set an anchor on a building using an anchor point that is an integral part of the structure. *Note:* if a training tower or similar structure is used, the student *will not* use any anchor points previously prepared, such as ring bolts.
20. Using webbing or rope on an anchor system with two anchor points, demonstrate the following:
    a) The angle that the two legs of the anchor *should not* exceed.
    b) The angle that the two legs *must not* exceed.
21. Correctly tie a load-sharing anchor using two anchor points.
22. Correctly tie a load-distributing anchor using a webbing loop on two anchor points.
23. Correctly set a load-distributing anchor system using three or more anchor points.

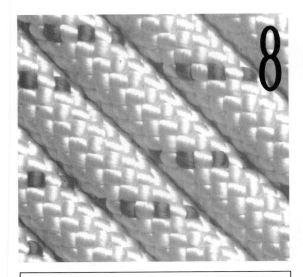

8 Belaying of One-Person Loads

Key Terms

Belay To protect against a fall by managing an unloaded rope (the belay rope) in a way that secures person or persons from falling in case their main line rope or support fails.

Belayer The one who performs the belay.

Belay Device A braking mechanism through which the belay rope is run. The belayer controls the device so that should the main line or support fail, the device holds the rope and secures person or persons on belay from falling.

Belay Line The line attached to person or persons that provides protection against fall or system failure.

Belay Plate A simple, metal plate containing one or more slots for rope and used to create rope friction with a carabiner. It is commonly used in belaying.

Lowering The controlled descent of persons and equipment using rope through a lowering device. A lowering rope goes one way: down. A lowering rope has weight on it throughout the lowering operation.

Munter Hitch A type of running knot that slips around a carabiner to create friction against itself. It is commonly used in belaying. Also known as *Italian hitch* or *half ring bend*.

◆ Prerequisites

Before attempting the activities described in this chapter, you must have demonstrated that you can properly:

1. Use and care for rope.
2. Use and care for other equipment employed in the high angle environment.
3. Tie correctly, and without hesitation, the eight knots described in Chapter 6.
4. Apply the principles of anchoring and rig a secure anchor.

Objectives

At the completion of this chapter, you should be able to:

1. Define belaying.
2. Distinguish between belay of one person and belay of a rescue load.
3. List the elements of a belay system.
4. Describe situations that might require a belay.
5. Repeat from memory and in sequence the belay voice communications.
6. Belay one person using a Munter hitch.
7. Belay one person using a one-person belay device.
8. Discuss why it is necessary to have both complete knowledge and thorough practice of belaying before attempting to belay a person in an actual high angle situation.

BELAYING

Belaying is a Serious Commitment

The word *belay* comes from the days of sailing vessels. On those ships, hefty belaying pins were set into the rails of the vessel. When sailors raised heavy objects, such as sails, they would attach a rope to the object and then take a turn of the rope around the belaying pin to prevent the line from slipping away from them.

In the high angle environment, the principle is the same except that the purpose of modern belaying is to keep a person from falling. The person is attached to a rope and the rope is managed in such a way, or belayed, to keep the person from falling far enough to be injured.

The ability to belay is a critical skill for anyone operating in the high angle environment. If you accept the assignment as a *belayer*, you have made a very serious commitment. It means that the well being, perhaps even the life, of the person at the end of the rope is in your hands. To say that you are able to belay when you cannot, or to allow your attention to lapse from the job of belaying, could possibly result in severe injury or death for the person at the end of the rope.

One-Person versus Rescue Belay

The techniques and equipment discussed in this chapter are designed for belaying one person. They should not be attempted with loads of more than one person. These larger loads are commonly known as *rescue loads*.

Many devices and techniques designed for one-person belay cannot reliably catch the load if it is more than one person's weight. See Chapter 12, Rescue Belaying, for information on belaying loads that involve more than one person.

The Belay System

The elements of a one-person belay system include the following (Figure 8-1):

♦ A person tied to the rope who is at risk of falling. (May be a person rappelling, ascending, or climbing, for example.)
♦ The rope attached to the person.
♦ A harness worn by the person and attached to the rope. The harness should be able to safely hold the person when caught by the rope, with the least amount of injury to the person.
♦ A *belay device.* It is in essence a braking mechanism. The rope is run through the belay device and controlled so that should the person being belayed fall, the belay device, under the control of the belayer, holds the rope.
♦ The belayer. He or she controls the belay device and the rope. The belayer's main duty is to brake the rope should the climber fall. But the belayer must also manage the rope so that excessive slack

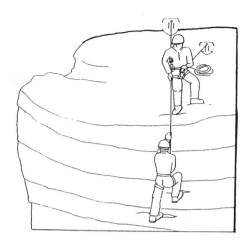

FIGURE 8-1
Elements of a belay system.

does not increase the shock load to the rope if the climber should fall.
♦ An anchor attached to the belay device. The anchor should be able to hold the highest shock load resulting from the fall of the person being belayed.

Situations Requiring a Belay

A belay may be called for any time there is "exposure" danger of falling. Some situations requiring a belay would be:

♦ When a person is rock climbing or mountaineering in hazardous terrain. Should the climber slip, a proper belay will be able to hold the climber.
♦ In a rescue situation where there is danger of falling. One example would be a *belay line* attached to a rescuer who is attempting to rescue a "jumper" from a bridge.
♦ When a person is crossing an area not generally dangerous, but there is a small area of exposure.
♦ When a person is unsure of himself or herself in attempting a new skill, such as rappelling for the first time.
♦ When a person's physical or mental capabilities are diminished, such as when he or she has been injured or is suffering from vertigo, exhaustion, or may be hypothermic.
♦ When environmental factors, such as potential rock falls or areas slick with ice, increase the danger of falling.
♦ When one or more persons are being lowered by rope, such as in a rescue.
♦ When one or more persons are being raised by rope, such as in a rescue.

Judgements about When to Belay

There will be times when the need for a belay is not completely clear cut. Some examples are:
♦ A person who is very experienced in the high angle environment is rappelling or ascending.

He or she may feel that a belay would only be a hindrance.

- ◆ When a belay might cause a greater problem than not having one. An example would be a situation in which there are already several rope lines involved. An additional line from a belay could cause an entanglement.
- ◆ In free drops where the load may spin. A belay line could entangle the main line and stop everything.

Judgments about these situations have to be made locally by those people who are experienced and well trained. If you are not sure, then it is probably best to belay (Box 8-1).

Belay Failure and Hand Protection

There have been many accidents due to belayer failure. These are often caused by one, or a combination, of two factors:

1. The belayer having a momentary lapse of attention just as the person on the rope fell.
2. The belayer not automatically performing the correct actions due to lack of adequate training in belaying.

One basic principle about human nature is this: *In a sudden emergency, humans respond with what is instinctive.* Such emergency situations could relate to driving experience during the threat of a vehicle accident or to weapons training in a law enforcement confrontation.

Belaying is a similar activity in that it must be thoroughly learned under realistic conditions and followed by constant practice until it becomes instinctive. Otherwise, the belayer may fail to take the correct action when the sudden emergency occurs. Such failure could result in severe injury or death.

It is not enough to have *intellectually* learned belaying. That is, it is not enough to have read about belaying, to have watched it, or even to have practiced the hand positions.

You must have combined both the *mental* and *physical* experience of the actual belay situation (Box 8-2).

Belay Practice System

Figure 8-2 shows an overall view of a belay practice system for one person (see Chapter 12 for belaying a rescue load). It consists of the following elements:

- ◆ A weight or a dummy of at least 200 lb to simulate the weight of a falling person (see the Suggestion box on p. 86).
- ◆ A method of raising the weights. A winch may be the easiest and most convenient way of doing this. However, a mechanical advantage hauling system can be used for raising the practice weights (Figure 8-3).
- ◆ A belay "station" where a belayer is located.
- ◆ An instructor's station.
- ◆ The instructor has a rope that triggers the weight's fall. The triggering mechanism can be created from a seatbelt buckle, a parachute harness release, or a military helicopter harness release (Figure 8-4 and Box 8-3).

Such a belay practice system that simulates the forces of a falling climber is essential to the instruction of belaying. This system is very simple and inexpensive to construct. Details on the system for hauling the weight and on the triggering mechanism are shown in Figures 8-3 and 8-4.

Belaying Signals

When you are belaying, it is essential that you use the standard voice signals (also called *commands* or *calls*). Otherwise, even momentary confusion could cause an accident.

In climbing and mountaineering, there are a group of voice signals that have been standard in belaying

---

Box 8-1 A Belay is not the Same as Lowering

Belays and **lowerings** (see Chapter 15, High Angle Lowering) involve different techniques, different equipment, and are for different purposes (although they may be used together). Do *not confuse the two.*

A BELAY

A belay is a safety to catch persons should they fall. A belay rope can be run either way (up or down) while it is being used for a belay. A belay rope does not have weight on it unless there is a fall on it or "tension" is called for in special cases. The belay rope, depending on the activity, may be maintained with some slack in it. A belay uses specialized equipment such as a **belay plate** or special knots such as the **Munter hitch.**

A LOWERING

A lowering is the controlled lowering of persons and equipment using rope through a lowering device and hardware such as the large ring of a figure 8 descender or a brake bar rack (both of which should not be used for a belay). A lowering rope goes one way: down. A lowering rope has weight on it throughout the lowering operation.

However, should a fall occur, a good belay system should have the ability to lower the load a short distance to where it can be stabilized.

Box 8-2 Hand Protection

In belaying, the belayer must wear gloves to protect his or her hands from rope friction. This must be done for two reasons:

1. To protect the hands from possibly severe rope burns from a running rope.
2. To prevent the potential pain caused by grasping a running rope and enables the belayer to hold the rope firmly and stop the fall of the person on the rope.

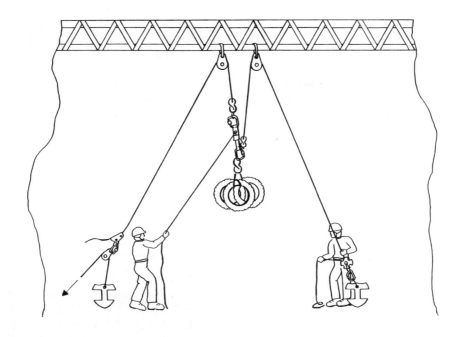

FIGURE 8-2
Overall view: belay practice system.

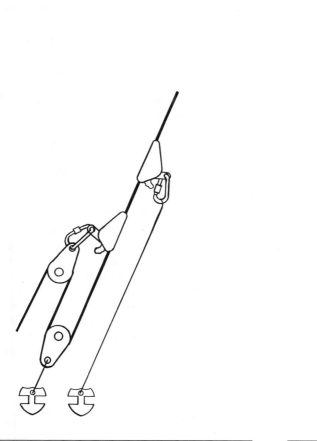

FIGURE 8-3
Hauling: belay practice system.

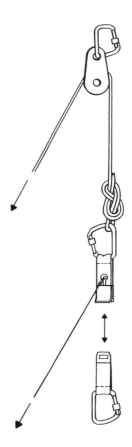

FIGURE 8-4
Trigger: belay practice system.

Suggestion

Discarded truck tires work well as the weight for a belay practice system. They are inexpensive and tend not to cause damage to concrete and asphalt floors when they drop.

Box 8-3 Belay Practice System Procedure

---

1. The belayer and the instructor take their stations.
2. An assistant begins to haul the weight up.
3. The student belayer "belays" the raise by keeping slack out of the rope.
4. At some point, without warning, the instructor pulls the line that triggers the fall of the weight.
5. The student belayer attempts to arrest the fall of the weight.

---

for years. These same calls work well in both the work and rescue environment.

They take place as an exchange of voice signals between a climber (or rappeller) and the belayer to ensure that both are ready for any possibility.

The standard belay signals in sequence are as follows:

Climber	Belayer	Phrase Meaning
1. "On belay?"		*A question: "I am about to climb (or rappel), are you ready to catch me if I fall?"*
2.	"Belay on."	*A statement: "I am ready to catch you if you fall."*
3. "Climbing" (or: "rappelling").		*"I am starting to climb" (or: "to rappel").*
4.	"Climb" (or "rappel").	*"Go ahead."*

Once a climber is in place where he or she no longer needs the belay, then the climber initiates an exchange to end the belay:

5. "Off belay."		*"I am in a secure place now. I no longer need the belay."*
6.	"Belay off."	*"I am no longer belaying you."*

There are some additional signals that can help communication between climber and belayer during the belay cycle. One of these is in response to a situation where the belayer is holding the rope too tightly:

Climber	Phrase Meaning
"Slack."	*"There is too much tension on the rope; I cannot move as well as I would like."*

(This requires no verbal response from the belayer, only the action of letting an appropriate amount of slack into the rope.)

⚠ Warning

When the weight falls and the belay catches, the belay rope will come taut with great force. To avoid injury, the belayer, and others around the belayer, must take the following precautions:

◆ Be aware of the position the rope and belay device will take when it catches and stay out of its path. Otherwise, the impact of the rope and/or belay device can cause serious injury.
◆ Keep fingers, hair, and clothing free of the rope near the belay device. Otherwise, these could be swept into the belay device possible causing injury and impeding the belay.

⚠ Warning

As with all belay techniques, the Munter hitch belay must be practiced on level ground and with a weight or dummy drop before attempting it with a person in the high angle environment. This practice must be under the guidance of a qualified instructor.

The other situation is the opposite. There is too much slack in the rope. It may be that the climber is at a particularly tricky point and he or she needs the support of the rope to make a move.

Climber	Phrase Meaning
"Tension."	*"Hold the rope tightly for a bit; this might be a difficult move."*

(Requires no verbal response, only the action of taking slack out of the rope.)

Consistency of Communications

It is important that once these voice communications have been agreed upon, there must be no change in them without prior agreement. Otherwise, there could be some confusion in communication. If this occurs, even briefly, it can be dangerous.

It is also important that all people involved discuss and clarify their understanding of the signals, even if they know one another and have worked together before. Slight variations in interpretation can cause accidents.

Make Yourself Heard

For the belay voice communications to work, they must be heard by those involved. Do not be timid when you use them. Wind, falling water, machinery, or other conditions can interfere with voice communications being heard. The belay communications will

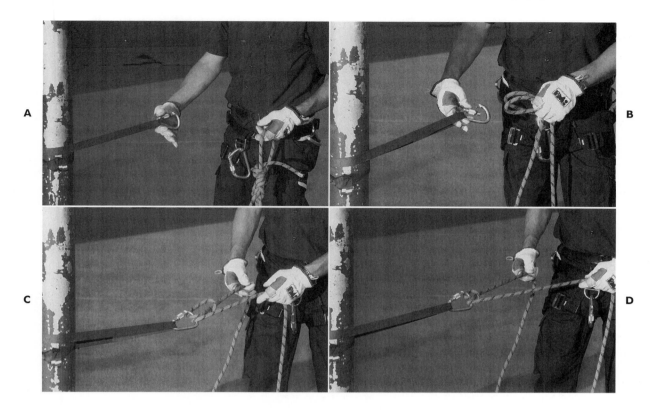

FIGURE 8-5
Setting belay/level ground.

take at least shouting, perhaps yelling, to be effective. If the required response to a command is not received, repeat it *louder.*

BELAYING TECHNIQUES

There are a number of belaying techniques used for the high angle environment. They all work essentially the same way: they create a braking action on the rope to prevent the person at the end of the rope from falling far enough to be injured.

We will examine two of these techniques in detail. These techniques are among those considered to be simple to learn, easy to use, and pose less of a danger to the belayer and the person on the rope.

The Munter Hitch

The carabiner used with the Munter hitch (also known as the *Italian hitch*) must be a carabiner designed for use with the Munter hitch, or an HMS carabiner. The HMS carabiners are designed for use with the Munter hitch. The gentle curves in these pear-shaped carabiners allow the Munter hitch to move freely back and forth through the carabiner when the direction of the belay is reversed. A narrow

carabiner or even a large D carabiner can cause jamming of the Munter hitch.

Procedure for Belaying One Person with the Munter Hitch

Setting the Belay on Level Ground (Figure 8-5).

1. Tie a piece of webbing or rope sling into a secure anchor (see Chapter 7, Anchoring).
2. Clip a large locking carabiner into the anchor sling.
3. Tie a Munter hitch near the end of the rope where the person being belayed will be. Although there are several ways of tying a Munter hitch, Figure 8-7 on p. 89 shows a simple, easy-to-remember way of doing it.
4. Clip the HMS carabiner across the portion of the Munter hitch that has two sections of rope parallel to one another. Lock the carabiner.
5. It is important to remember that the Munter hitch "runs" in both directions.

This means that if the person on the rope is moving away from you, the loop in the bight will be on the side of the carabiner toward the climber. If you are pulling up rope (the climber is moving toward you), the loop will be on the side of the carabiner facing you.

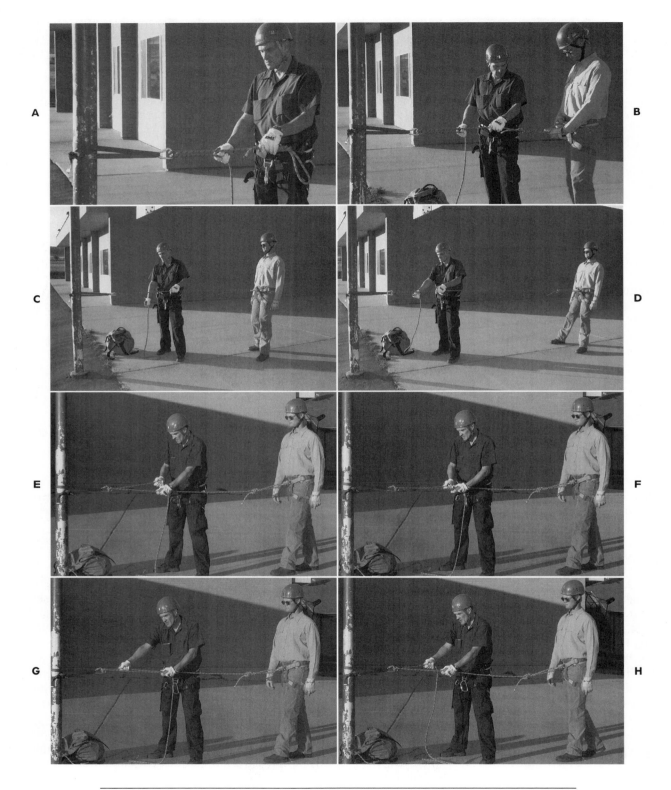

FIGURE 8-6
Practicing Munter hitch on level ground.

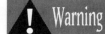

When anchoring yourself as a belayer, never place yourself into the system. That is, do not belay with a device clipped to the front of the harness and the anchor clipped to the back of your harness. Should the climber fall and the system shock load, you could be severely injured, possibly with a fractured pelvis. You could be disabled or suffer life-threatening injury.

Practicing the Munter Hitch Belay on Level Ground (Figure 8-6)

1. Face the carabiner. Take the rope on the side of the carabiner away from the climber in your dominant hand (the right hand for right-handed people). This is your *braking hand. You must not take this hand off the rope when the person is "on belay" unless the belay is tied off.*
2. Take the rope on the side of the carabiner near the climber in your weaker hand (the left hand for right-handed people). This is your *guide hand.* You will use it to help manipulate the rope. The guide hand needs no more force than what the forefinger, index finger, and thumb can provide to manipulate the rope. The guide hand does not provide braking force.
3. Now, have a partner wearing a seat harness clip into the end of the rope.
4. Remove slack in the rope between the carabiner and the climber by pulling it out with the brake hand.
5. Begin the belay voice communications. The person on the rope says, "on belay." If the belayer is ready, he or she says, "belay on."
6. Have the person on the rope begin slowly walking backwards. With the guide hand, pull the rope out from the carabiner and feed it to the climber. Allow the "climber" to set the rate of rope run. As your brake hand approaches within a foot of the carabiner, slide it back *while still holding the rope. Never take the brake hand off the rope.*
7. Now, to give a feel of the control you have, hold the rope firmly with the brake hand, stopping the person on the rope from going farther.
8. In an area where he or she will not slip, have the "climber" firmly plant his or her feet on the ground and lean back from the rope. Hold the rope firmly with the brake hand.
9. To get a feel of the control, slowly let a few inches of rope out with the "climber" leaning against the rope.

Reversing Direction
10. Now have the partner walk slowly toward you. The problem now is to take in rope while keeping the person safely on belay.

For maximum friction (maximum control) when using the Munter hitch, keep the braking side of the rope close to the rope going to the load. That is, keep the angle of the rope as small as possible to provide maximum friction.

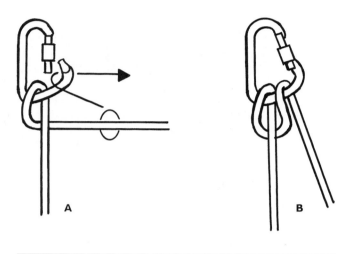

FIGURE 8-7
Tying the Munter hitch.

11. Have your brake hand on the rope about 1 foot from the carabiner.
12. Place your guide hand about 3 feet from the carabiner and on the rope.
13. As slack comes into the rope, pull it out by pulling with the brake hand. Also pull the rope with your guide hand to reduce friction on the Munter hitch and help ease the rope through the carabiner.

Note that reversing the Munter hitch can sometimes take a bit of effort. There can be difficulty getting the hitch to pop back through the carabiner and reverse direction. It is easiest to do this when the Munter Hitch is in the middle of the rounded portion of the carabiner.

Just as your guide hand approaches your brake hand, grasp both sides of the rope with your guide hand. *Do not cross hands.*

14. Holding both lines in place with the guide hand, move your brake hand up the rope toward the carabiner *without taking it off the rope.*
15. Continue the procedure until the person on the rope reaches your position.
16. Exchange the voice signals that conclude the belaying cycle. *(Person on rope: "off belay." Belayer: "belay off.")*

The moving of hand positions on the rope is one of the most critical operations in belaying. Remember: the person at the end of the rope may fall *any time* while you are belaying. If you do not have your brake hand on the rope at all times, ready to grasp it in an instant, you may drop the person and cause severe injury or death.

When the weight falls, and the belay catches, the belay rope will come taut with great force. To avoid injury, the belayer, and others around the belayer, must take the following precautions:

◆ Be aware of the position the rope and belay device will take when it catches and stay out of its path. Otherwise, the impact of the rope and/or belay device can cause serious injury.

◆ Keep fingers, hair, and clothing free of the rope near the belay device. Otherwise, these could be swept into the belay device possibly causing injury and impeding the belay.

◆ One-person belay devices are designed for catching one-person loads and may not be the most appropriate device for catching rescue loads.

Belay Practice with a One-Person Weight and Dummy

Now practice belaying with a Munter hitch using the belay practice system with one-person dummy or weight as shown in Figure 8-2. Do a procedure first with the weight falling as it is being raised and then with it falling as it is being lowered.

In an actual belay situation, you would, if possible, keep the "climber" in view. But for practice, you will face away from the weight and dummy so you cannot visually anticipate the fall. This will sharpen your skills at catching an unexpected fall.

As each fall of the dummy and weight comes onto your rope, and you catch it, lower it to the ground using the Munter hitch.

Using a One-Person Belay Device

Another method of belaying is the use of a one-person belay device. There are several different devices designed for one-person belay. Figure 8-8 shows various designs of one-person belay devices. Many traditional belay devices use a variation of the belay plate design. The plate, combined with a carabiner, creates

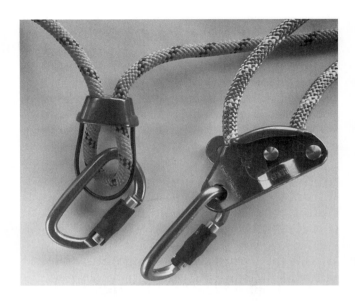

FIGURE 8-8
Various belay devices.

rope friction on the device so the belayer can control the belay line. Some plate-type belay devices have two slots of the same size. They are designed for belaying both with single- and double-rope system. Some plates have two slots for different sizes. They are designed for people who might be using an 11 mm rope on one occasion and a 9 mm rope another time.

Belay plate devices are designed only for use with kernmantle ropes (either static or dynamic). *They are not designed to be used with laid ropes.*

Another design of personal belay devices uses a toothless camming device. The camming action squeezes and stops the rope running to the person being belayed. One example of a camming action belay device is the GriGri (Petzl, France).

For this practice session, use the ATC (Black Diamond, USA). The ATC is a variation of the belay plate design and uses friction to create control of the rope. This friction is created when the carabiner presses the belay rope against the plate section of the ATC. This happens when the belayer brakes the rope with the control hand and spreads the two sides of the rope apart. This causes the rope to pull the carabiner against the plate, creating friction.

Belaying with the ATC
Rigging the One-Person Belay Device (ATC) (Figure 8-9)

1. Tie a webbing or rope sling into a secure anchor (see Chapter 7, Anchoring).
2. Clip a locking carabiner into the end of the loop.
3. Take a bight of rope near the end of the rope where the person to be belayed will be.

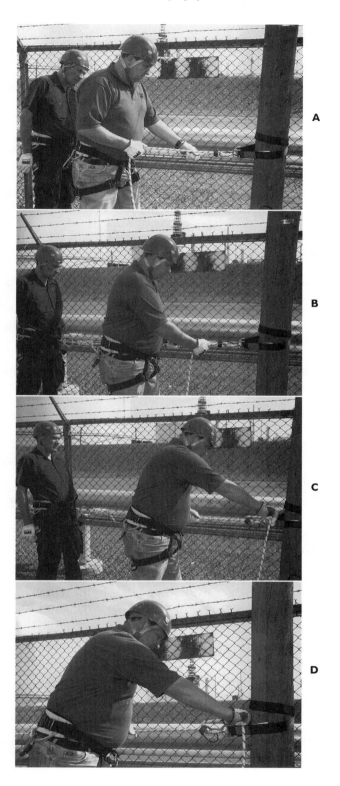

! Warning

Belaying with a one-person belay device must be practiced on level ground and with a weight or dummy drop before attempting it with a person in the high angle environment. This practice must be under the guidance of a qualified instructor.

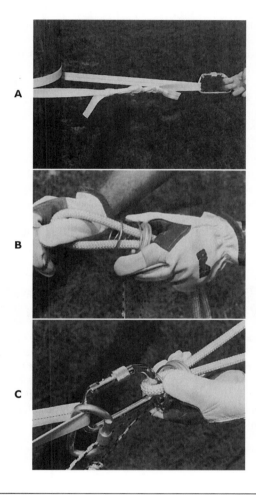

FIGURE 8-9
Rigging the belay plate.

4. Push a few inches of the bight through the hole in the smaller end of the tapered plate of the ATC.
5. Clip both the loop of the rope and the ATC's wire cable through the locking carabiner.

Practicing the Belay on Level Ground (Figure 8-10)

1. Face the belay device. Take the rope that is on the side of the belay plate away from the "climber" in your dominant hand (the right hand for right-handed people). This is your *brak-*

FIGURE 8-10
Belay plate/level ground.

ing hand. You must not take this hand off the rope when the person is "on belay" and the belay is not tied off.

2. Take the rope on the side of the brake device that is nearest the climber in your weaker hand (the left hand for right-handed people). This is your *guide hand.* You will use it to help manipulate the rope.

3. To stop the rope from running out, pull back on the rope with the brake hand so that the angle of the rope strands is at an approximate angle of 180 degrees. Keep the guide hand in position to help maintain control of the rope. Note that this forces the plate portion of the belay device against the carabiner, causing friction on the rope. To maintain the braking action, hold the rope tight with your brake hand.

4. Now, have a partner wearing a seat harness clip into the end of the rope.

5. Remove slack in the rope between the belay device and the climber by holding the rope strands at a small angle and pulling the slack out with the brake hand.

6. Begin the belay voice communication. *(Person on the rope: "on belay." If the belayer is ready, he or she says, "belay on.")*

7. Have the person attached to the rope begin slowly walking backwards.

8. Feed rope into the belay device with the brake hand and pull it with the guide hand. Maintain just enough slack so it is noticeable and allows the climber freedom of movement.

9. Now, initiate a braking action. Pull back on the rope with the brake hand so that the angle of the rope strands is at an approximate angle of 180 degrees. Keep the guide hand in position to help maintain control of the rope.

10. In an area where the climber will not slip, have the climber firmly plant his or her feet on the ground and lean back from the rope. Hold the rope firmly with the brake hand.

11. Stop feeding rope through with the brake hand. The device should lock, holding the climber in place.

12. To get a feel of control, slowly let out a few inches of rope with the "climber" leaning against the rope. Do this by bringing the two sides of the rope toward one another and by moving your brake hand toward the belay device.

Reversing Direction

13. Now have the partner walk slowly toward you. The problem now is to take in rope while keeping the person safely on belay. To practice control of rope tension, do not allow the rope between the climber and the belay device to touch the ground.

14. Have your brake hand on the rope about 1 foot from the belay device.

15. Place your guide hand about 3 feet from the brake plate.

16. As slack appears in the rope, pull the slack out by pulling the rope with the brake hand. Your guide hand can help move rope toward the brake plate.

17. Just as your guide hand approaches your brake hand, grasp both sides of the rope with your guide hand.

18. Holding both lines taut with the guide hand, move your brake hand quickly up the rope toward the brake plate *without taking the hand off the rope.*

19. Continue the procedure until the person on the rope reaches your position.

20. Exchange the voice signals that conclude the belay cycle. *(Person on rope: "off belay." Belayer: "belay off.")*

Practice with a Belay Weight and Dummy

Now practice belaying with the ATC using a belay weight or dummy as shown in Figure 8-2. Do a procedure first with the weight or dummy falling as it is being raised and then with the weight or dummy falling as it is being lowered. In each case, as the weight comes onto your belay line, lower it to the ground with the brake plate.

⚠ Warning

The moving of hand positions on the rope is one of the most critical operations in belaying. Remember: the person at the end of the rope may fall *any time* while you are belaying. If you do not have your brake hand on the rope at all times, ready to grasp it in an instant, you may drop the person and cause severe injury or death.

⚠ Warning

When the weight falls and the belay catches, the belay rope will come taut with great force. To avoid injury, the belayer, and others around the belayer, must take the following precautions:

◆ Be aware of the position the rope and belay device will take when it catches and stay out of its path. Otherwise, the impact of the rope and/or belay device can cause serious injury.

◆ Keep fingers, hair, and clothing free of the rope near the belay device. Otherwise, these could be swept into the belay device, possibly causing injury and impeding the belay.

In an actual belay situation, you would try to keep the "climber" in view as you belay him or her. But for practice, you will face away from the weight and dummy so you cannot visually anticipate the fall. This will sharpen your skills at catching an unexpected fall.

Belay Plates in Figure 8 Descenders

Some figure 8 descenders are designed with a belay plate either in the small ring or between the two rings. However, you should use 8 belay plates with caution for the following reasons:

- ◆ The slot in the figure 8 may not be the correct size for the rope you are using.
- ◆ Some figure 8s have slots that are not well-designed for use as a belay plate.
- ◆ A figure 8 is not as well balanced as some devices and may not be as easy to use.

ADDITIONAL CAUTIONS FOR BELAYERS
Belay Direction

The main elements of the belay system, the anchor, belay device, and climber must be in as direct a line as possible, so the instant the climber falls, the force will come directly onto the belay device and the anchor. If these elements are not in a direct line, any or all of the following could happen:

- ◆ The belay device could fail to work properly.
- ◆ The belayer could be thrown off position.
- ◆ The anchor could fail.
- ◆ The system could be shock loaded.

Also, the belay rope must not be around or against the belayer or any other person. They could be injured by the rope's suddenly coming taut.

Maintaining Proper Slack in the Belay Rope

It is critical that the belayer maintain a proper amount of slack in the belay rope. If the rope is too taut, it can interfere with the climber (if there is a climber on the rope) or with the brakeman (if the belay is a safety for a separate lowering system). Good judgment on belay rope slack is another skill that develops with practice at belaying. There should be at least some *visible* slack in the rope but not so much slack that there would be intense shock loading of the rope during a fall.

Securing the Belayer

If the belayer is near a place where he or she could fall, he or she must be secured via a safety line to an anchor.

If possible, connect your safety line to an anchor separate from the belay. This would help ensure that you, as the belayer, are not endangered by a climber's fall and that whatever happens, you remain in a stable situation to continue the belay or otherwise assist the climber.

Bottom Belay (Only for Rappelling)

A bottom belay is a pull on the rappel rope from the bottom (Figure 8-11). A common use of the bottom belay is to assist a rappeller who is in danger of losing control. It is, in essence, a substitute for the rappeller's control hand. This pull from the bottom increases friction on the rappeller's descender.

A bottom belay is not a substitute for the belays previously described. It should be used when a top belay is not available and in an emergency. Bottom belays have the following drawbacks:

- ◆ The rope can easily slip out of the grip of the person at the bottom.
- ◆ The belayer can only exert as much pressure as his or her body weight. This is often sufficient if the belayer is directly below the rappeller and the rappeller has not gained too much momentum out of control. But it is often not effective if applied from an angle.
- ◆ A bottom belay is not effective with all rappel devices.
- ◆ A person doing a bottom belay is in danger of being hit by objects, such as rocks, being dislodged by the person or rope above.
- ◆ A bottom belay does not provide backup for the failure of the main line rope, anchor, or rappel device, but only for an out-of-control rappel.

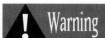

Warning

Do *not* use the figure 8 descender as a belay device with the rope wrapped in the large ring as for rappelling or lowering. This large ring is not designed with enough friction to stop a rope that is shock loaded from a fall.

Warning

When anchoring yourself as a belayer, never place yourself into the system. That is, do not belay with a device clipped to the front of the harness and the anchor clipped to the back of your harness. Should the climber fall, and the system shock load, you could be severely injured, possibly with a fractured pelvis. You could be disabled or suffer life-threatening injury.

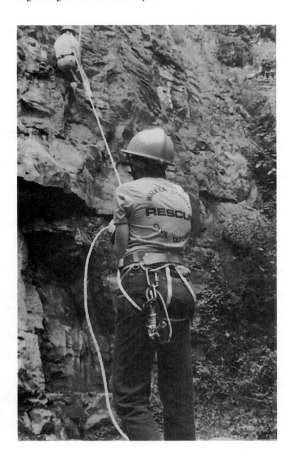

FIGURE 8-11
Bottom belay.

⚠ Warning

When the weight falls, and the belay catches, the belay rope will come taut with great force. To avoid injury, the belayer, and others around the belayer, must take the following precautions:

- Be aware of the position the rope and belay device will take when it catches and stay out of its path. Otherwise, the impact of the rope and/or belay device can cause serious injury.
- Keep fingers, hair, and clothing free of the rope near the belay device. Otherwise, these could be swept into the belay device, possibly causing injury and impeding the belay.

Body Belays

One additional technique for belaying is known as the *body belay*. With this technique, the belayer creates friction by running the rope around his or her body, usually around the waist. Except in emergen-

cies, the technique is not recommended for the following reasons:

- It is not as easy to stop a fall as with a belay device.
- It can injure the belayer.
- The belayer's ability to hold a fall is only as high as his or her pain threshold.
- If the belayer is at the top of a drop, it can pull him or her over.
- It can entangle the belayer in the rope. If the climber falls, it may entrap the belayer and put him or her into a position where he or she is unable to assist the climber.

Evaluation Exercises

◆ COGNITIVE AND AFFECTIVE EXERCISES ◆

1. List the six elements of a belay system.
2. Describe six situations that might require a belay.
3. Describe how a belay differs from a lowering in the following:
   a) Purpose
   b) Technique
   c) Equipment
4. With you playing the role of a belayer and another person playing the role of a climber, recite from memory the cycle of belay voice communications. Reverse roles.
5. List three reasons why belay plates on figure 8 descenders may pose problems.
6. List the conditions in which a bottom belay should be used.

▼ PSYCHOMOTOR EXERCISES ▼

7. On flat ground, rig a Munter hitch belay system. Using a partner tied into the rope, have him or her walk away from you in a belay cycle.
8. Repeat the above with the partner approaching you.
9. Repeat numbers 7 and 8 using a personal belay device.
10. Using a belay dummy and weight fall, rig a Munter hitch belay and simulate a situation where a climber falls as the rope is being let out.
11. Using a belay dummy and weight fall, rig a Munter hitch belay and simulate a situation where a climber falls as a rope is being taken in.
12. Using a belay dummy and weight fall, repeat numbers 10 and 11 using a one-person belay device.

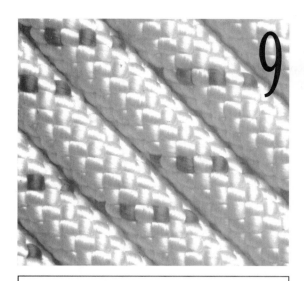

9 Rappelling

Key Terms

Arm Rappel ("Guide's Rappel") A type of rappel in which the rope wraps around both outstretched arms and across the person's back. The technique is sometimes used in sloping terrain. It does not give enough control for vertical situations.

Body Rappel (Dulfersitz Rappel) A type of rappel that uses the body as friction by running the rope through the legs, across one hip, over the opposite shoulder, and to a braking hand. Because of the discomfort involved and the potential injury to body parts, the technique has largely been supplanted by other techniques.

Brake Bar Rack A rappel device that consists of a series of short metal bars fixed to, and sliding along, a U-shaped metal rack with an eye at one end for attachment.

Brake Hand The hand, usually the dominant one, that grasps the rope to help control the speed of descent during a rappel.

Carabiner Wrap A rappel technique that uses several rope wraps around a seat harness carabiner to create friction and control the descent. It is generally not considered a safe and secure technique for rappelling.

Descender A rappel device that creates friction by a rope running through it and is attached to a rappeller to control descent on a rope. Most descenders can also be used as a fixed brake lowering device.

◆ Prerequisites

Before attempting the activities described in this chapter, you must have demonstrated that you can properly:

1. Use and care for rope.
2. Use and care for other equipment employed in the high angle environment.
3. Tie correctly, and without hesitation, those knots necessary for effective and safe work in the vertical environment (see Chapter 6, Knots, for examples).
4. Apply the principles of anchoring and rig a secure anchor.
5. Apply the principles of belaying and safely and confidently belay another person using either a Munter hitch or personal belay device.

Objectives ▼

At the completion of this chapter, you should be able to:

1. Describe the purposes of rappelling.
2. Describe the necessity for maintaining control during a rappel.
3. Discuss the principles behind the body rappel, along with its dangers and limitations.
4. Discuss the principles behind the arm rappel, along with its dangers and limitations.
5. Set a secure anchor for rappelling.
6. Safely belay a person who is rappelling and interact with a person belaying you while you are rappelling.
7. Discuss the principles behind rappelling with figure 8 descenders.
8. Describe the advantages and disadvantages of using a figure 8 with ears.
9. Safely and under control, rappel with a figure 8 descender and be able to securely lock off the device while on rope and then return to a rappel.
10. Discuss the principles behind the use of a brake bar rack.
11. Safely and under control, rappel with a brake bar rack, securely lock off the device while on rope, and then return to a rappel.
12. Discuss the principles behind self-belay techniques.

Key Terms—cont'd

▼

Dulfersitz Rappel See Body Rappel.

Figure 8 Descender A commonly used descender made roughly in the shape of an 8.

Guide Hand The hand, usually not the dominant one, which cradles the rope to help in balancing the rappeller.

Locking Off The technique of jamming a rope into a descender or tying off securely so that the rappeller can stop the descent and operate hands free of the rope.

Munter Hitch Rappel A limited use rappel technique using a Munter hitch attached to the seat harness carabiner.

Rappelling The controlled descent of a rope using the friction of the rope against one's body or through a descender.

RAPPELLING

Rappelling is controlled descent on a rope by using the friction of the rope against one's body or through a descender. It is a necessary skill for a person to operate safely in the vertical environment. The learning of safe and controlled rappelling skills is a step toward developing vertical competency. Rappelling, to the inexperienced, may appear to be a spectacular art. However, just to be able to rappel does not necessarily mean that a person is skilled and knowledgeable in the vertical environment. Rappelling is not the ultimate goal for a high angle technician. It is just one personal skill to be used in combination *with other* skills for activities in the vertical environment. Rappelling, for example, may be the means of travel in a controlled descent of a vertical face. It may be used in combination with other essential vertical skills for performing a rescue.

Importance of Control

One important sign of a person's competence in rappelling is *control*. Evidence of control includes:

◆ Being able to control the descent with minimum physical effort.
◆ Rappelling in a controlled manner so that the rope is not damaged by heat buildup in the rappel device, and anchors are not damaged by shock loading.
◆ Being able to stop the rappel any time.
◆ Being able to tie off securely and operate hands free of the rope and rappel device.
◆ Being able to operate in any body position including upside down.

How Rappelling Works

Any technique for rappelling uses friction with the rope to slow the rate of descent. Both the *body rappel* and the *arm rappel* use friction of the rope on the body to slow the descent. This friction and the resulting heat and discomfort can make these techniques unpleasant to use. Because of this discomfort (and because of the potential dangers associated with them) these techniques are no longer widely used.

Most modern techniques use *rappel devices* or *descenders*. They are attached to the rappeller, usually by means of a seat harness carabiner. The rope runs through the device to create friction, so the heat and discomfort go into the device and not the rappeller's body. Also, a well-designed rappel device offers more control of the descent than a body rappel.

With most rappel devices, the rate of descent is controlled by pulling down on the portion of the rope that is below the device. This increases friction by increasing rope tension and pressure on metal parts of the device. The rappeller usually does this controlling action with the dominant hand (usually the right hand for a right-handed person). This hand is known as the *brake hand.*

The rappeller's other hand cradles the rope above the device or (with some descenders) cradles the device itself. *This hand does not support body weight by grasping the rope.* In most rappel devices, this hand is known as the *guide hand* and helps to balance the rappeller. In some rappel devices, it may also help in controlling the descender.

Types of Rappels
Arm Rappel

Figure 9-1 shows the *arm rappel,* which is sometimes used for short distances on low angle slopes.

The user sets up the rappel by having his or her upper back to the anchored rope while facing uphill. The rappeller then wraps both extended arms around the rope. The friction, and rate of descent, is controlled by varying handgrips.

! Warning

It is essential that, from the beginning, anyone learning to rappel maintain absolute control of the descent. Among the ways of ensuring this control are:

◆ Avoiding rapid, bouncing rappels that can lead to loss of control, damaged rope, overloaded anchors, and injuries.
◆ Using a top belay.
◆ Learning under the guidance of a qualified and experienced instructor.

The arm rappel is *only* for use on short, low-angle slopes. It does not produce enough friction to adequately control full body weight in a completely vertical situation. Because of the potential of rope abrasion injuries on arms and hands, it must be used only when wearing long-sleeved shirts and gloves.

Make certain that your rope is long enough so you end up in a safe zone at the end of the rope.

The body rappel must be practiced on a low-angle slope before it is attempted on a steep slope. The body rappel should not be used in general practice but only in case of emergency, when no hardware is available to use as a rappel device.

The body rappel technique presents two potential dangers:

1. The rope could become unwrapped from the leg. As a result, the rappeller would lose friction with the rope and possibly fall free to the ground. This is a particular danger on a vertical face.
2. Rope abrasion and pressure can injure body parts, particularly the crotch and shoulder. Thick padding in these areas in recommended.

Body Rappel ("Dulfersitz")

Figure 9-2, *A* through 9-2, *C* illustrates a procedure for wrapping the rope for a body rappel.

1. The rappeller straddles an anchored rope facing the anchor.
2. He or she brings the strand of rope that is below him or her around one hip (the side with the dominant arm).
3. He or she then brings the rope across the chest and over the opposite shoulder.
4. He or she now brings the rope down across the back to the braking hand (the dominant hand),

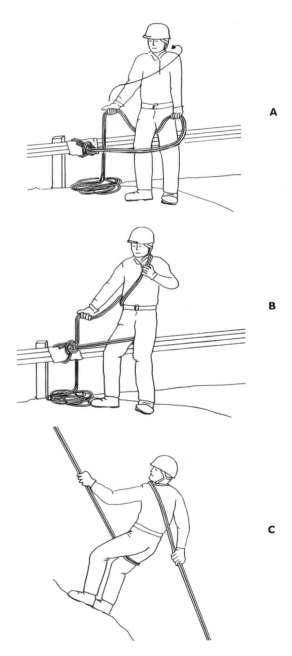

FIGURE 9-2

Body rappel.

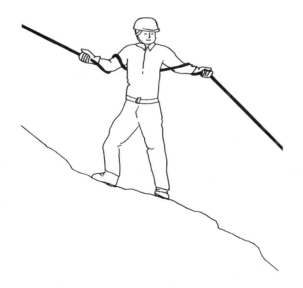

FIGURE 9-1

Arm rappel.

which is on the same side as the hip where the rope runs.

5. Control of the descent is maintained by (dominant) hand strength and by bringing the rope across the torso with the brake hand.

As mentioned earlier, one of the dangers of the body rappel is on high angle rappels where the rope can become unwrapped from the leg. Therefore the wrapped leg must be kept lower than the unwrapped leg and the upper body.

The body rappel technique will result in large amounts of pain and may have the undesirable effect of causing the rappeller to let go to relieve the pain.

MECHANICAL RAPPEL DEVICES
Figure 8s

One design of a conventional *figure 8 descender* is shown in Figure 9-3. (For more details on materials and the various designs, see Chapter 5, Basic High Angle Hardware.) The larger ring of the figure 8 may be rounded or squared off, depending on the specific design. The larger ring is the portion of the descender that creates friction on the rope, while the smaller ring attaches to a seat harness carabiner.

Most conventional figure 8 descenders are found in smaller sizes. Because they are compact and lightweight, smaller figure 8s are often used by climbers and other individuals involved in recreational activities.

Although the conventional figure 8 is a strong device for rappelling, it has significant drawbacks in some situations (Box 9-1).

Box 9-1 Drawback of Figure 8 Devices

◆ You cannot use the smaller version with larger diameter rope.
◆ You may find it difficult to use the smaller figure 8 descender "double wrapped" ("double wrapping" of a figure 8 descender is explained on page 107).
◆ When you are rappelling with the conventional figure 8, it is possible for the rope wraps to slip up and around the larger ring to form a girth hitch (Figure 9-4).

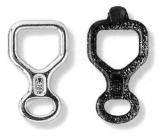

FIGURE 9-3
Regular figure 8 descender.

The Girth Hitch Problem

Accidental girth hitching of the figure 8 ring tends to occur in two circumstances:

1. When you attempt to ease over a difficult edge or ledge, and the edge catches a wrap of rope on the bottom of the figure 8. The weight of the rappeller forces the wrap over the top of the ring and into a girth hitch. To help prevent this from happening, lace the rope onto the descender by first bringing the bight of rope into the large ring from the top, as shown in Figure 9-5.

2. When you cause momentary slack in the rope, such as rappelling over ledges or uneven faces, or in bouncing rappels. These situations cause a momentary slack in the rope wrap, allowing it to slip over the large ring.

The girth hitching of the figure 8 immediately stops the rappel and prevents you from descending further. You will begin to move again only when you can re-

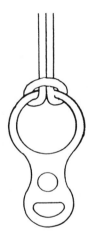

FIGURE 9-4
Figure 8 descender with girth hitch.

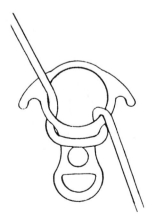

FIGURE 9-5
Lacing rope into figure 8 from top.

move your weight from the girth hitch long enough to slide it back over the large ring. Unless you possess the appropriate skills and equipment, this is a difficult and hazardous position to escape. If you have good upper-body strength, you might be able to forcefully extricate yourself from this situation by lifting your weight from the figure **8**. But it would be easier and usually safer for you to set an ascender or Prusik knot on the rope above the figure **8** and step into an attached sling. (See page 135 in Chapter 10, Ascending, for possible ways of extricating yourself from this kind of situation.)

The best solution to the girth hitch problem on a figure **8** ascender is to prevent it from happening. One method of prevention is to use a figure **8** with ears (Figure 9-6). The "ears," which are protrusions on the larger ring, primarily serve to prevent the rope from slipping over the larger ring to form a girth hitch. But the ears also serve other functions, such as helping to contour the rope around the ring and holding the rope in place when it is locked off.

Consequently, unless space and weight are strong considerations, the figure **8** with ears is preferable for most rappellers.

Procedure for Using the Figure 8 with Ears
Using the Figure 8 with Ears on Level Ground (Figure 9-7)

1. Don a sewn, manufactured seat harness with thigh supports and a front tie-in point.

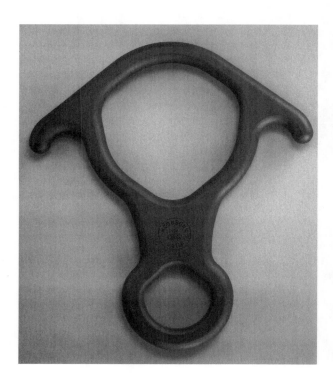

FIGURE 9-6
Figure 8 descender with ears.

2. Clip a large locking carabiner or a screw link into the seat harness tie-in point. If the carabiner or screw link is in a vertical plane after being clipped on, make certain that the gate is toward your body. (This is to help prevent friction against a vertical face from opening the gate.)
3. Establish a secure anchor point.
4. Firmly attach a main-line rappel rope to the anchor point.
5. Take a figure **8** with ears in your guide hand (Figure 9-7, *A*).
6. Face the anchor with the rope running past you on the brake hand side.
7. On the rappel main line near the anchor, take a bight of rope in your brake hand. Push it through the large ring of the figure **8** descender *from the top* (Figure 9-7, *B*).
8. Bring the bight of rope around the end of the small rung of the figure **8** descender and across the waist of the rappel device. Pull the rope snugly around the figure **8** descender by pulling on the strand of rope that is on the side of the descender away from the anchor (running end). If the figure **8** descender will be in a horizontal plane when it is clipped into your seat harness, the rope should run across the *top* of the waist of the figure **8** descender. If the figure **8** descender will be in a vertical plane once it is clipped into your seat harness, the rope should lay across the side of the descender that is near your brake hand (Figure 9-7, *C*).*
9. Clip the small ring of the figure **8** descender into your seat harness carabiner. Lock the carabiner (Figure 9-7, *D*).
10. Take the running part of the rope (that is on the lower side of the figure **8** descender) in your

> ⚠ **Warning**
>
> 1. The learning and practice of rappelling techniques must be under the guidance of a qualified instructor.
> 2. Rappelling techniques must be practiced first on level ground and then on short and moderate slopes before using them on a steep face.
> 3. Everyone practicing rappel techniques on a steep face or any other area where a severe fall is possible must use a top belay.

*Note that when you have to slide over a difficult edge to rappel, you could get the figure **8** descender caught on the edge. If the rope is on the side of the descender away from the edge, you will be less likely to jam on the edge. Also, if you are using a conventional figure **8** descender and you keep the rope on the side away from the edge, the edge is not as likely to push the rope up over the larger ring to form a girth hitch.

dominant hand (the right hand on right-handed people). This is your *brake hand.* When you are rappelling and the descender is not *securely* tied off, you must *never take your brake hand off the rope.*

11. With your less-dominant hand (the left hand for right-handed people), lightly cradle the rope above the figure 8 descender. This is your *guide hand.* This hand is *not* for supporting your weight but to help balance yourself. *You must not*

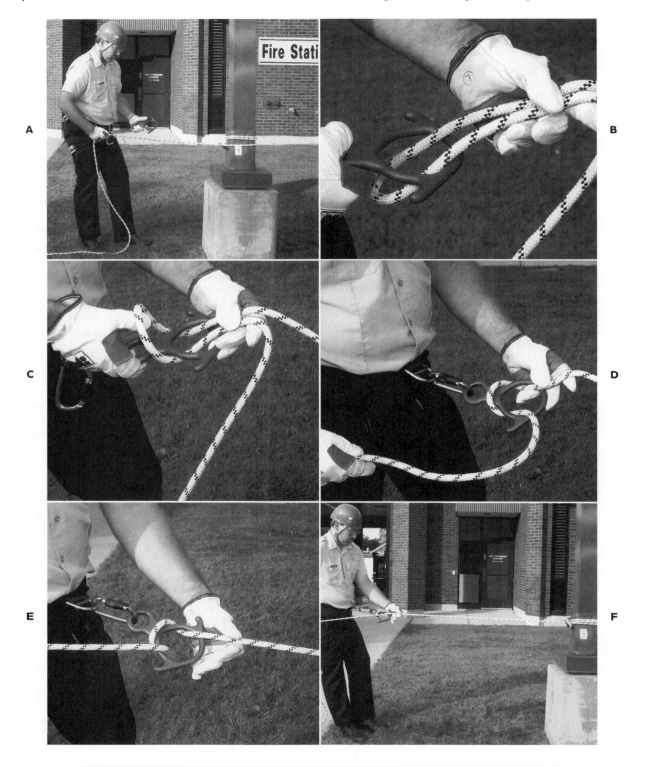

FIGURE 9-7

Using figure 8 on level ground.

support your weight with the guide hand, or it could throw you off balance when you try to rappel.

12. Now, by pulling down on the rope with your brake hand, pull the slack out of the rope between the figure **8** descender and the anchor. If this is difficult, you can help the process with your guide hand (Figure 9-7, *E*).

13. Grasp the rope below the figure **8** descender with your brake hand and pull it taut against your hip with your hand about 6 inches below your hip. This is the best position to assume that will provide extra stopping power by using the friction of the rope against your hip. However, you should not constantly keep the rope against your hip because it may abrade your seat harness webbing. So, while keeping the rope taut with your brake hand, swing the rope out about 2 feet from your hip at an angle that is comfortable for your arm.

    Now is the time for a safety check. Have your instructor check the rigging, carabiners, your descender, gloves, and so on.

14. Lean back away from the anchor so that the rope between the figure **8** descender, and the anchor becomes taut. Always remove the rope slack between your descender and the anchor before beginning a rappel.

15. As you lean back against the rope, begin to walk backwards, letting the rope slowly slip through the figure **8** descender with the brake hand and holding your guide hand lightly on the rope above the rappel device. As you let the rope slip through your brake hand, keep the same distance on the rope between your hand and the figure **8** descender (Figure 9-7, *F*).

Locking Off (Figure 9-8)

16. Gripping the rope with the brake hand, allow rope to slide through the descender until the brake hand is about 1 foot from the rappel device (Figure 9-8, *A*).

17. Now, *hold the rope taut with the brake hand.* In a continuous, smooth motion, use your brake hand to pull the rope in an arc from the rappel position, straight out in front of you. Pass the brake side of the rope below the main line and then to where the rope and your hand are 180 degrees from the rappel position (Figure 9-8, *B*).*

18. *Maintain a firm grip on the rope with your brake hand.* With the brake hand, take the strand of rope the hand is holding and pull it down far-

ther toward you to trap it between the strand of rope that goes to the anchor and the large ring of the figure **8** descender (Figure 9-8, *C*).

   *The braking side of the rope must be firmly trapped between the rope that goes out of the descender to the anchor and the large ring of the figure **8**. For this to happen, there must be tension on the rope between the figure **8** descender and the anchor.*

Unlocking

19. Take the rope *firmly in your brake hand.* In a smooth, continuous motion, pull the rope first straight toward the anchor and in an arc back to the rappel position. You will hear a slight "pop" and feel a slight bump as the rope unlocks from the rappel device. *Keep the rope firmly in your brake hand.* Continue rappelling as before.

Rappelling with the Figure 8 Descender on a Slope (Figure 9-9)

1. Establish a secure anchor point at the top of a short slope of about 45 degrees (if a slope is not available, then use a stairway). Attach the rappel rope securely to the anchor point.

2. Establish an anchor point for a belay. Attach an anchor sling securely into the anchor point. Clip a large locking carabiner into the end of the anchor sling.

3. Have a belayer take position. If a Munter hitch is being used for belay, have the belayer create the hitch in the belay rope and clip it into the belay carabiner. If the belayer is using a personal belay device, attach it to the rope and clip it into the belay anchor carabiner. Be sure the carabiner gate is locked.*

4. Clip into the belay rope. Initiate the belay cycle with the belay voice communications. *(Rappeller: "on belay?" Belayer: "belay on." [Figure 9-9, A]).*

5. At a secure point where you are not in danger of falling, follow steps 5 to 14, beginning on page 99, to lace the figure **8** descender onto the rope (Figure 9-9, *B* and *C*). *Do a safety check on all equipment and rigging. In particular, inspect carabiners for sideloaded gates and unlocked gates and anchor slings in need of adjustment. Make certain that loose clothing is tucked in, hair is not in danger of being caught, and the helmet chin strap is secure.*

---

*Note that this may be a little difficult to do while standing on flat ground. Once you are suspended by the rope on a steep slope or on a vertical face, this movement is much less awkward to perform. This has to do with the angle of the rope and anchor in relation to the figure **8** and the rappeller.

---

*Note to keep a proper distance between the belay anchor rope and the main-line rappel rope. As noted elsewhere in this book, it is good practice to keep rope strands (such as the belay line and the main-line rappel rope) apart to prevent tangling and damaging the rope from heat fusion as a result of rope cross. However, the distance between the rappel line and belay anchors should not be too great. If there were a great distance between the anchors and the main-line rappel anchor failed, but the belay caught, there would be a possibility of a *pendulum fall* (a sudden swing on the line that could result in an injury to the rappeller or damage to the rope).

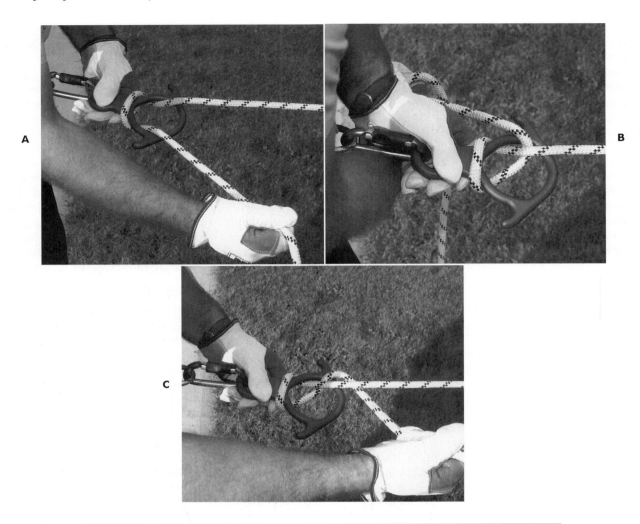

FIGURE 9-8
Locking off figure 8 descender.

6. Begin to back down the slope, controlling your descent with the brake hand and following the steps outlined in 15 through 18 on page 101. Keep the following principles in mind (Figure 9-9, *D*):
   ◆ Keep your body generally perpendicular to the slope.
   ◆ Keep your feet apart, about the width of your shoulders.
   ◆ Keep your knees relaxed and slightly flexed.
   ◆ Take slow and deliberate steps backwards.
   ◆ Keep your body slightly turned in the direction of the brake hand, looking down slope to select a path of travel.
   ◆ Use your guide hand for balance. *Do not support your weight with the guide hand.*
   ◆ *Never take the brake hand off the rope unless the belay device is securely locked off.*
7. When part way down the slope, stop the rappel and lock off the figure 8 descender using the principles described in steps 16 through 19 on page 101 (Figure 9-9, *E and F*).

> ⚠ **Warning**
>
> 1. The learning and practice of rappelling techniques must be under the guidance of a qualified instructor.
> 2. Rappelling techniques must be practiced first on level ground and then on short and moderate slopes before using them on a steep face.
> 3. All personnel learning rappel techniques on a steep face or any other area where a severe fall could result, must use a top belay.

8. Unlock and continue the rappel to the end of the slope (Figure 9-9).
9. Conclude the belay cycle with the belay voice communications. *(Rappeller: "off belay." Belayer: "belay off.")*

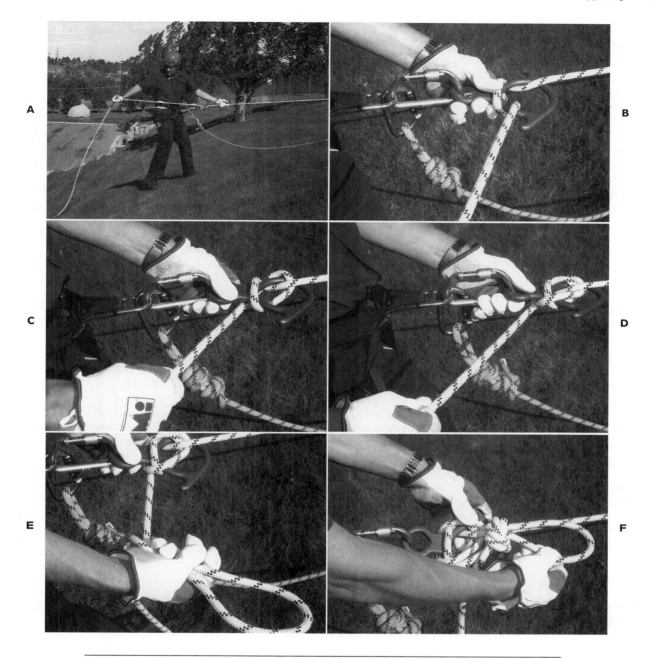

FIGURE 9-9
Using figure 8 on slope.

Rappelling Down a Vertical Face with Figure 8 Descender (Figure 9-10)

1. Choose a short vertical face (approximately 20 feet) where the top breaks over gradually into a steep face. On the first try, do not choose a face with a sharp edge.
2. Establish a secure anchor (as described in Chapter 7) at a safe distance from the edge. If possible, have the anchor point high above the edge. This will assist any rappeller going over the edge. Attach the main-line rappel rope securely to the anchor point.

3. Establish a separate anchor for a belay at a safe distance from the edge. Attach a sling securely to the anchor point. The anchor point and sling should be established so that when the belayer takes position, he or she has a good field of view of the top and face but is not in danger of falling over the edge. In the end of the sling, clip a large locking carabiner.
4. Have a belayer take position to belay. If there is danger of falling, have the belayer secure himself or herself to a safety line. If a Munter hitch is being used for belay, have the belayer tie the

Munter hitch into the belay rope and clip it into the belay carabiner. If the belayer is using a personal belay device, attach it to the rope and clip it into the belay anchor carabiner.

5. Clip into the belay rope with a knot or locking carabiner. Initiate the belay cycle with the belay voice communications. (*Rappeller: "on belay."* Belayer: *"belay on."* [Figure 9-10, *A*]).

6. At a secure point, where you are in no danger of falling, follow steps 7 through 14 on page 99 for attaching the figure 8 descender to the rope (Figure 9-10, *B, C,* and *D*).

7. Make certain that the slack is out of the rope between the figure 8 descender and the anchor. Do a safety check on all connectors such as carabiners, on the seat harness, on the anchor, and other rigging. Make certain that no loose clothing or hair is going to be sucked into the descender. Make certain your helmet is secure.

8. Slowly begin backing to the edge. Keep the following principles in mind:
   ◆ *Keep the body generally perpendicular to the slope.* This means that you will have to deliberately lean out as the slope becomes vertical. At first, this may seem an unnatural stance. But this position is necessary to keep your feet from slipping out from under you (Figure 9-10, *E* and *F*).
   ◆ Keep the feet apart about shoulder width for balance. This will help you from being pulled over to one side.
   ◆ Keep the knees relaxed and slightly flexed.
   ◆ Take slow and deliberate steps backwards.
   ◆ Keep the body slightly turned in the direction of the brake hand, looking down slope to pick a path for your descent.
   ◆ Use the guide hand for balance. *Do not support your weight with your guide hand.*
   ◆ Never take the brake hand off the rope unless you are *securely* locked off.

The belay, as it is normally used, is for the safety of the rappeller. *It is not* to be used by the belayer to control the rate of descent of the rappeller nor to share the load when the rappeller is in a controlled descent. For students to learn proper control of a rappel device, they must be controlling their full weight with no control coming from the belayer. Therefore it is important that the belay line have a small amount of slack as the rappeller descends.

Only if the rappeller loses control or requests assistance (such as "tension") does the belayer control the rappeller's weight and/or rate of descent.

9. As you move over the edge, more of your weight will be held by the rope. This means you need greater effort for control with the brake hand. As the rope is weighted, you may feel pulled in a direction right or left. Step slightly in that direction until you feel a better balance (Figure 9-10, *G*).

10. If you slip, fall over, or even turn upside down, *keep calm. Hold tight with your brake hand until you*

orient yourself. Then, slowly, place your feet against the face and rebalance yourself.

11. When you are midway down the face, stop the rappel and lock off. On a vertical face, with your weight on the rope and descender, you will find it more difficult to trap the rope between the main line and the large ring of the figure 8 descender. But hold the brake line steady and pull it across and down with deliberate force until it is securely trapped (Figure 9-10, *H* and *I*).

A More Secure Lock off for the Figure 8 Descender

In certain vertical situations a more secure lock off for the figure 8 descender may be desirable. Such situations include when the rappellers may have to be locked off for long periods of time, when they have to do a great deal of moving about in one position to manipulate equipment or a rescue subject, or any other circumstance where they feel they need greater security.

Figure 9-11 illustrates and Box 9-2 describes one technique for more securely *locking off* a large figure 8 descender.

To unlock, untie the overhand knot and unwrap the brake side of the rope from around the figure 8. *Always keep the rope firmly in your brake hand with no slack in the rope between your brake hand and the figure 8.*

12. Unlock. Untie the overhand knot. You will find it will be more difficult to pull the brake side if the rope is out of its trap between the large ring and the standing part of the rope, because in a vertical situation your full weight is involved. But *grasp the rope tightly* and pull it slowly away from you until you feel the slight jolt indicating that it has come unlocked. (You may have to use both hands to pull the rope out of its locked position.)

Box 9-2 Locking off a Large Figure 8 Descender

1. Trap the brake side of the rope between the line going to the anchor and the large ring on the descender.
2. Pull the brake side of the rope firmly down toward the seat harness carabiner, across the surface of the figure 8, and around *behind* the ears. *Do not bring the rope through the large ring of the figure 8.* It should be between the line going to the anchor and the large ring and above the line first locked off. Make certain that the rope lies firmly around the device and there is no slack.
3. Bring the brake side of the rope down and around the figure 8 again as in Figure 9-11, *C*, and then behind one ear, but do not place it between the line going to the anchor and the large ring. Instead, form a large bight of rope from the brake side of the rope.
4. Bring the bight up parallel with the rope going to the anchor.
5. Tie an overhand knot with the bight onto the rope going to the anchor.
6. Be certain that the overhand knot is contoured well and there is no slack in the knot.

Maintain tension on the rope with your brake hand. *Never take your brake hand off the rope.*

13. Rappel to the bottom and complete the belay cycle (Box 9-3). *(Rappeller: "off belay." Belayer: "belay off.")*

Gaining Extra Friction from the Figure 8 Descender

One advantages of the figure 8 with ears is the ease of creating increased friction and therefore greater control of the descent. This is because those figure 8 descenders that have ears are larger devices with greater surface area to create friction. Also, the ears help to contour the rope and hold it in place.

Double Wrapping a Figure 8 Descender (Figure 9-12)

Double wrapping a figure 8 descender cannot be done once the rappeller is on rope. It must be done before attaching the figure 8 descender to the seat harness carabiner.

1. Face the anchor with the rappel rope running past you on your brake hand side.

2. At the place on the rappel rope where you want to attach yourself for the rappel, take a bight of rope in your brake hand. Push it through the large ring of the figure 8, downward through the top (if the ascender will be in a horizontal plane) or from the side with the brake hand (if the descender will be in a vertical plane).

Box 9-3 Getting off the Rope

With any rappel device, it is easier to get off rope if you have a small amount of slack in the rappel rope to work with. A quick trick to gain this slack is to keep your weight on the rope and rappel device as your feet touch the bottom and do a deep-knee bend before stopping your rappel. As you return to standing straight up, you will have a foot or so of slack in the rappel rope that will help you in unlacing the rappel device.

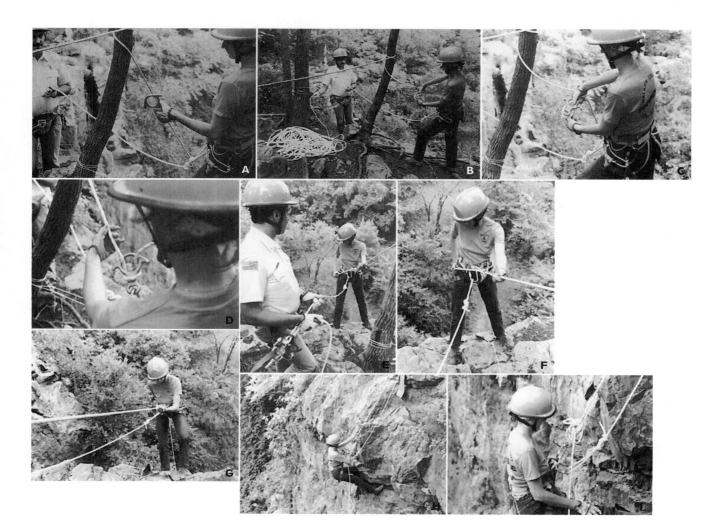

FIGURE 9-10
Using figure 8 on vertical.

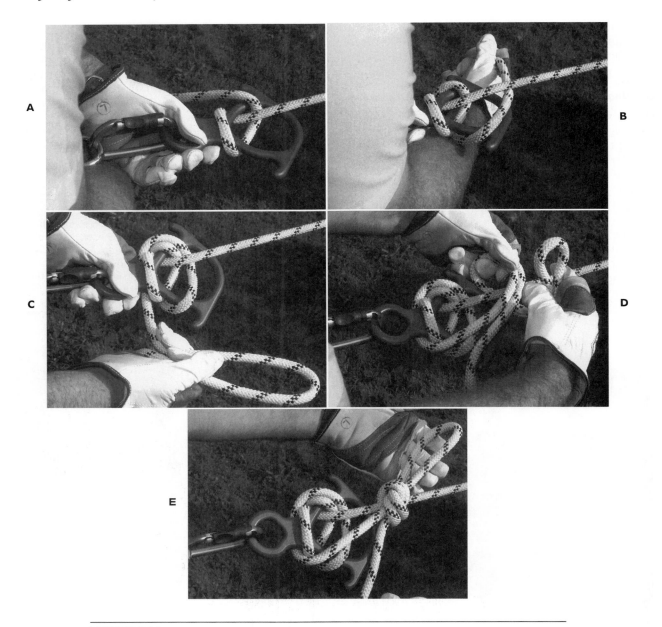

FIGURE 9-11
Secure lock-off for figure 8.

3. Bring the bight of rope around the small ring of the figure **8** and over the waist of the device.
4. Push the bight of rope through the large ring again, between the two strands already there. If you need more rope, pull on the bight.
5. Now bring the center of the bight back over the waist and pull the rope strands snug.
6. Attach the figure **8** descender to your seat harness carabiner and lock the carabiner.

Rappelling with a Double-Wrapped Figure 8 Descender. Although a double-wrapped figure **8** descender can give a rappeller added control through greater friction, it does require some increased attention to technique.

The double-wrapped figure **8** descender works smoother with the brake hand out to the side as shown in Figure 9-13. This position will help to guide the rope into the figure **8** descender. If the hand is closer to the body, the following may occur:

1. The strand of rope running around the figure **8** descender on the brake-hand side may begin to cross itself.
2. There is no danger in this, but the increased friction will slow the rate of descent. The descent may also feel a little rougher.
3. To uncross the strands, simply bring the brake hand back away from the body. You will feel a slight bump as the rope strands uncross.

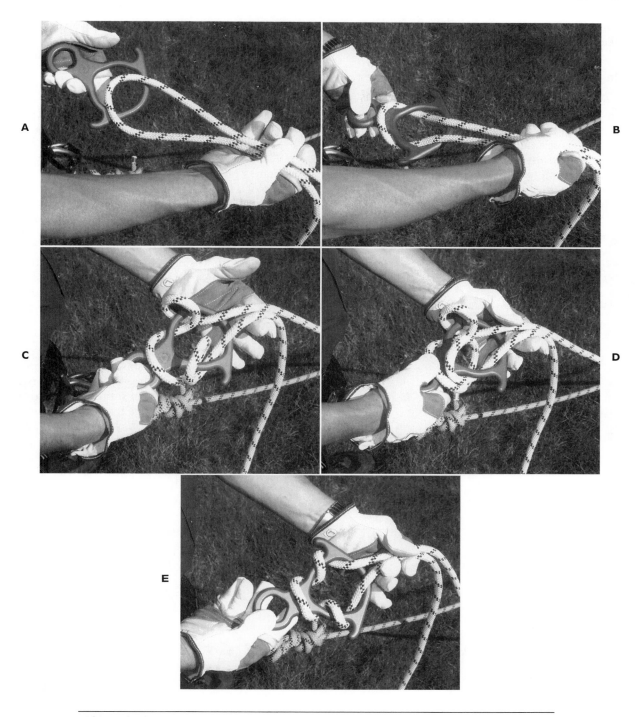

FIGURE 9-12
Double wrapping the figure 8.

GAINING EXTRA FRICTION WHEN ON RAPPEL

A rappel should only be done when the rappeller has friction and, therefore, control to spare. If during the rappel there is not enough friction, there are techniques to create additional control.

Increasing Friction with the Body

One technique for increasing friction in the body is to bring the rope sharply against the thigh as shown in Figure 9-14. It is not a good rappel technique to continually have to do this because:

◆ The rope may run across seat-harness webbing and damage it.

◆ This leaves no extra friction to spare in case it is needed.

Gaining Extra Control with Spare Carabiner

There may be situations where you may need more friction than the figure 8 descender may offer. Some of these would be:

◆ When using a new or wet rope.
◆ Rappelling with extra equipment.
◆ Doing an emergency rescue ("pickoff") of another person.

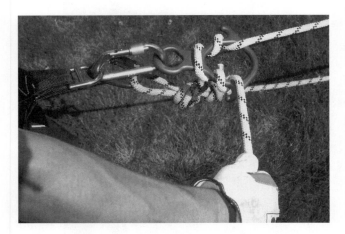

FIGURE 9-13
Hand position with double wrapped 8.

Figure 9-15 shows the sequence of using a spare carabiner to gain extra friction:

1. Add a second locking carabiner to your seat harness tie-in point. Always place the extra carabiner on the side the rope comes out of the figure 8 (usually your brake-hand side).
2. (If you are locked off) unlock the second carabiner and clip the rope into the carabiner. Lock the carabiner.
3. Firmly grasp the brake side of the rope where it comes out of the second carabiner.
4. Unlock the figure 8.
5. Control with the brake hand using the second carabiner by pulling upward, instead of downward as you would do if you did not have the spare carabiner.
6. To lock off, raise the rope across toward the guide hand and lock off in the normal way.

RAPPEL STANCE

When most people are learning to rappel, they feel uncomfortable backing over a sharp edge while standing. However, for most circumstances, this is the most effective stance for rappelling. When rappellers are intimidated by a difficult edge, some may try to "sneaky Pete" their way over the edge by rolling over it on their side or stomach. If this action can be avoided, it should not be done for the following reasons:

◆ The friction of your body against the edge can unlock the carabiner, causing it to disconnect from your seat harness.

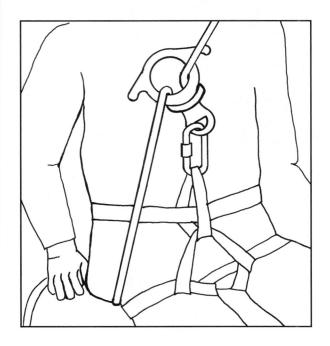

FIGURE 9-14
Gaining hip friction on rappel.

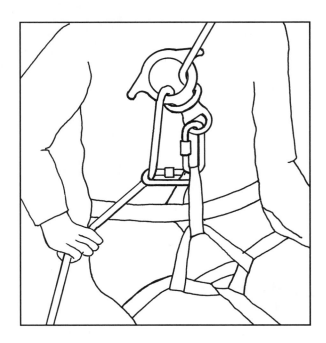

FIGURE 9-15
Gaining friction with extra carabiner.

◆ This method can easily trap feet or hands between the rappel rope and the edge.
◆ It can damage equipment, such as carabiners and seat harnesses, which get snagged on the edge.
◆ On cliffs, this method will brush rocks and other debris over the side and endanger those people who are below.

The preferred stance is on both feet (or alternatively, on both knees). On particularly difficult edges, there are variations that can help in getting over.

GETTING OVER THE EDGE

Usually, the most difficult part of a rappel is getting over the edge. This often has to do with apprehension. But there is often the physical challenge of getting over the edge of a wall or cliff. There are several techniques that you can use to help get started over the edge. *Do not attempt any of the following for the first time without a top belay.*

Variation # 1: The Butt Thrust (Figure 9-16)

1. Face the anchor. Back up, slowly letting slack through your descender until you are standing with the balls of your feet on the edge.
2. Imagine that something is pushing you at your waist, so that your butt is slowly being thrust back out over the drop and opposite the anchor. *Keep your feet in place.* This should get the weight off your toes and onto the insteps of your feet against the face of the wall (this serves to have your weight pressing against the wall).
3. As this is happening, the rope should be coming downward to meet the edge of the drop. When the rope does reach the edge, it will create greater stability for you by making a three-legged tripod (the rope on the edge plus your two feet kept a shoulder's width apart).

4. If you need to help this process of getting the rope down to the edge, you can quickly shuffle your feet down the face of the wall. Taking small steps increases your stability.

Variation #2: Knees (Figure 9-17)

1. Walk back to the edge with slack out of the rope.
2. Get down on your knees at the edge of the drop.
3. Lean back, getting your butt back away from the edge.
4. Slide over the edge on your knees. Your toes will hit the wall and you will stabilize as the rope comes down on the edge. Continue to rappel backwards, with your feet a shoulder width against the wall and your torso parallel to the face.

Clearing the Descender

It is very important that as you clear the edge on a rappel, the descender also clears and does not catch on the edge. Otherwise, the descender may become jammed and you will be stranded in a precarious position.

Therefore when you're backing over the edge in a rappel, *always observe the position of the descender and make certain that it is going to clear the edge.*

Effect of Rope Angle on Rappelling

One factor that will significantly affect the degree of difficulty in rappelling over an edge is the angle the rope makes from the rappeller to the anchor point (Figure 9-18). This will range from the most difficult for a horizontal angle (the anchor on the same level or lower than the rappeller) to the easiest for a vertical

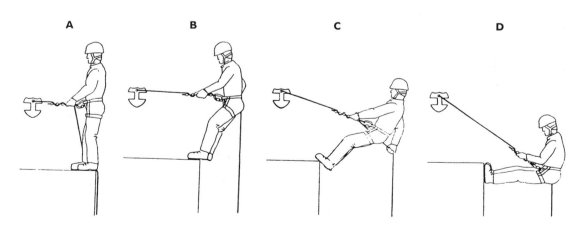

FIGURE 9-16
Butt thrust.

A   B   C   D

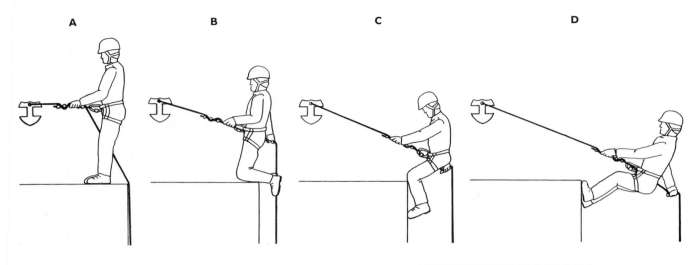

FIGURE 9-17

Knees over edge rappel.

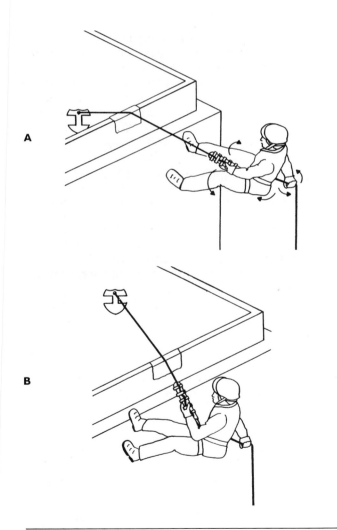

FIGURE 9-18

Effect of rope angle on rappel. **A,** Lower anchor point.

B, High anchor point.

angle (the anchor above the rappeller). It is rare that a vertical angle will be found. Most of the time it will be a compromise: getting the rope angle as high up as possible while maintaining a safe and secure anchor point.

Undercut Edges

Undercut edges are those where the edge is overhung so far back that your legs cannot reach the wall as you start your rappel over the edge. Undercut edges present the rappeller with a special problem. It requires an advanced technique, to be attempted only after you have developed full confidence and skill to control the descender.

Rappelling from an undercut edge is similar to rappelling from a helicopter skid. The procedure involves maintaining your feet on the edge, while lowering the rest of the body until your head is well below the feet and the edge of the overhang. Only after you are certain that the rappel device and your torso are far enough below the edge to clear it, do you step off the edge. *This often results in a forward pendulum.* Your feet must absorb the shock of the forward motion against the vertical face (if there is one).

The Brake Bar Rack

The *brake bar rack* descender offers several advantages and disadvantages for rappelling.

Advantages:

- ◆ It offers greater friction; therefore greater control than most descenders.
- ◆ It provides the ability to change friction once you have begun to rappel.
- ◆ Its variable friction provides the ability to more comfortably rappel longer drops than most descenders.

> ## Suggestion
>
> There is one technique of getting over the edge that can avoid the dropping over and pendulum and potential shock loading of the rappel system. This involves hanging an anchored, separate rope loop, sling, or daisy chain over the edge to use as a step.
>
> Before starting over the edge, always rig in your descender and take any rope slack out of it. This will help you in weighting the rope as quickly and smoothly as possible.

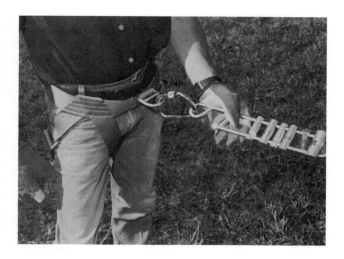

FIGURE 9-19
Brake bar rack on harness.

Disadvantages:

♦ The brake bar rack is somewhat more complex than descenders such as the figure 8, so it takes a bit longer to put it on the rope, and it is somewhat bulkier and heavier.

Rappelling with the Brake Bar Descender

See Appendix C for guidelines on attaching the bars to the rack. For more specific details on the brake bar rack itself, see Chapter 5, Basic High Angle Hardware.

Attaching the Rack to Yourself

1. Decide on how many bars to begin the rappel with. When learning to use the brake bar rack, always begin a rappel with all six bars engaged. As you become more experienced, you will learn how many bars are needed according to specific situations. Figure 9-19 shows the brake bar rack in position on a seat harness ready to be put on the rope (this figure shows the rack in position for a right-handed person).
2. If your seat harness carabiner is in a horizontal plane, attach the rack to it with the short leg of the rack down. If you have a seat harness carabiner in a vertical position, then have the short leg of the rack toward the brake hand (the right hand on a right-handed person).

Attaching the Brake Bar Rack to the Rope (Figure 9-20)

3. Establish a secure anchor point.
4. Attach the rappel rope securely to the anchor point.
5. Clip the rack into your seat harness carabiner and lock the carabiner (with the gate toward your body).
6. Stand facing the anchor with the rappel rope on your brake-hand side.
7. Hold the rack out in front of you in your guide hand.
8. Disengage all bars except the top one on the rack. Do this by sliding them one at a time toward the bottom of the rack (towards the eye). Squeeze the two legs of the rack together with one hand and, with the other hand, flip back each bar.
9. Pick up the rope with your brake hand. Guide the rope between the two legs of the rack and across the top bar. *Do not pass the rope between the top bar and the bend of the rack* (Figure 9-21). *This will pinch the rope, make the descent harder to control, and cause excessive wear on the rack.*
10. Reach down below the rack, grab the rope, and pull it across the top bar away from you (toward the anchor), pulling the slack out of it (Figure 9-20, *A*).
11. With the other hand, clip in the second bar at the bottom of the rack and slide it up to trap the rope between it and the top bar (Figure 9-20, *B*).
12. Now bring the free end of the rope back across the second bar, pulling it toward the anchor so that the second bar is snugged in by the force of the rope pulling against it. Note that the rope must be on the side of the bar opposite the notch to hold the bar in place on the rack frame (Figure 9-20, *C*).
13. Repeat the process with the remainder of the bars, until all six are clipped in (Figure 9-20, *D* and *E*).
14. In an area with good footing, so that you will not slide down, lean back against the rope. The preferred position for the brake hand is for it to be below the rack and off to the side. This position for the brake hand is similar to other rappel devices (Figure 9-20, *F*).
15. The difference is in the position for the guide hand. Instead of being on the rope above the device, as with other descenders, the guide hand should be resting on the bars of the rack, holding the bar ends between the thumb and fingertips.

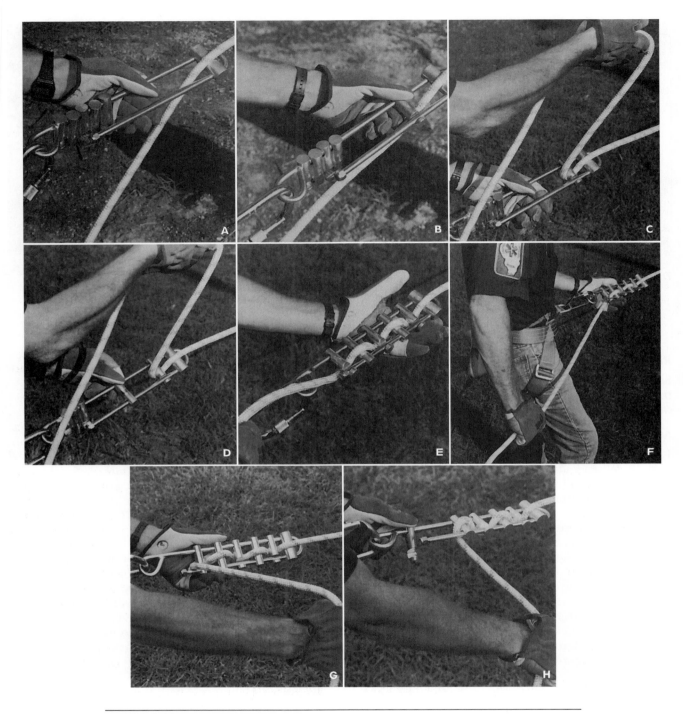

FIGURE 9-20
Attaching rope to rack.

16. Take your brake hand and pull the rope away from you (using the anchor). If they are laced correctly, this should pull all of the bars together toward the top of the rack. This is known as the *quick-stop* position when you are rappelling (Figure 9-20, *G*).

17. Now bring the rope back to the normal rappel position.

18. With your guide hand, grasp the bottom bar on either side of the rack and push it (along with the other bars) toward the top of the rack. This is the "stop" position for the guide hand. By jamming the bars together in this manner, toward the top of the rack, you increase the friction on the rope and add another element of control.

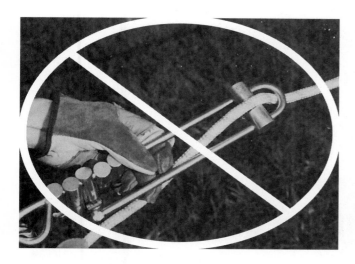

FIGURE 9-21
Incorrect lacing of brake bar rack.

19. Using the guide hand, pull the bars, one by one, back toward you. As you are doing this, ease your grip on the rope with the brake hand. This is increasing the "go" mode of the rack by reducing the friction between the bars and the rope. As you are leaning back against the rope, you may feel the rope begin to move a bit through the rack and through the brake hand.

20. If you have not moved, disengage the bottom bar. Do this by first swinging the rope with the brake hand in an arc to the opposite side of the rack to uncover the bottom bar (Figure 9-20, *H*). Then squeeze the two legs of the rack together at the open end of the rack that is near you. Unclip the bottom bar. Let it slide down the rack toward the eye and out of the way. Now spread the remaining bars apart along the length of the rack. This is lessening the friction even more.

21. If you still have not moved, remove the fifth bar (which is now on the bottom) in the same manner that you disengaged the sixth bar. Spread the remaining bars along the length of the rack.

22. Now, reverse the process by clipping bars back in to gain friction. Do this by using your guide hand to squeeze the legs of the rack together and clip the bars in one at a time at the bottom and lacing the rope back between them. This is the same process you used when you initially laced up the rack on the rope.

Tying Off (*Figure 9-22*)

23. Lean back against the rack so that the rope between the rack and the anchor is taut. Start the tie-off process by taking the rope with your brake hand and pulling it away from you, to the top of the rack and toward the anchor (Figure 9-22, *A*).

24. With the brake hand, pull the rope over to the side of the rack by your guide hand so that the rope runs across the top bar and is pinched between the curve of the rack and the section of the rope going to the anchor (Figure 9-22, *B*).

25. Bring the rope back toward you, pulling it taut so that it locks all the bars together. Bring the rope through the two legs of the rack and across the bottom bar.

26. Pull the rope away from you, toward the anchor, in the same path you did before. Pull it firmly so that all the rope sections are taut and the bars locked together (Figure 9-22, *C*).

27. The rack should now be locked in a "stop" position. With your brake hand extended parallel with the strand that runs to the anchor, hold the rope out away from you. At the point the trailing end of the rope crosses your brake hand, form a large bight in the rope using the assistance of your guide hand (Figure 9-22, *D*).

28. Treating this bight as one rope, use it to tie an overhand knot in the line that is going to the anchor. Cinch the overhand knot firmly against the top bar of the rack. *There must be no slack in the rope running over the bar nor space between the bars.* The rack is now locked off (Figure 9-22, *E* and *F*).

Unlocking

29. When unlocking, *always keep a firm grip on the rope and allow no slack in the brake end of the rope.* To unlock, reverse the locking process. To untie the overhand knot, pull slowly toward you on the brake end of the rope, holding your guide hand at the center of the bight of rope so that it comes out slowly.

30. With your brake hand firmly on the rope, pull the brake end of the rope in a 180-degree arc until it is straight out in front of you.

31. Now, still grasping the rope firmly with the brake hand, pull the rope straight out towards the side by the guide hand, then through a 180-degree arc and back to the normal rappel position.

32. Place the guide hand back in its normal position of cradling the bars. If you have not begun to move again, pull the bars apart with the guide hand until the decrease in friction allows you to rappel again.

Getting Off Rope

33. Getting the rack off the rope reverses the process of putting it on. You may leave the rack attached to your seat harness carabiner while doing this. With your brake hand, pull the rope back in the direction of the anchor so that it uncovers the bottom bar completely.

34. Using your guide hand, squeeze the legs of the rack together and unclip the bottom bar. Let the bar slide to the bottom of the rack.

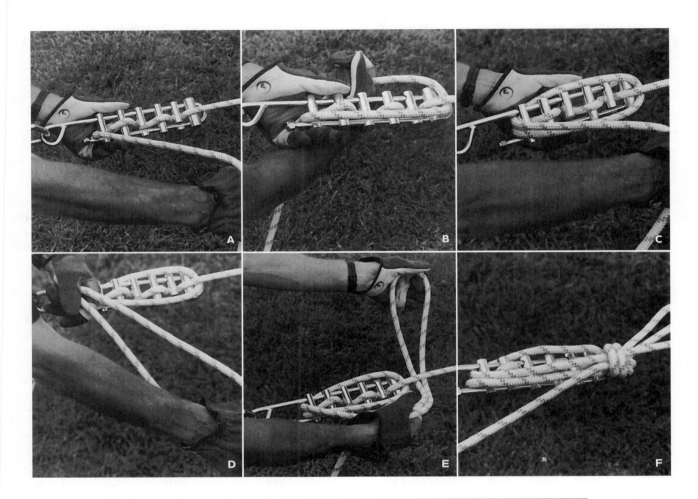

FIGURE 9-22
Tying off brake bar rack.

35. With the brake hand, move the rope back through the leg of the rack, uncovering the next bar up and pulling the rope back toward the anchor. Unclip the next bar up with the guide hand. Continue this procedure until all bars are disengaged.

Rappelling with the Brake Bar Rack on a Slope (*Figure 9-23*)

1. Establish a secure anchor point at the top of a short slope of about 45 degrees. (If a slope is not available, then use a stairway.) Securely attach the main line rappel rope to the anchor point.
2. Establish an anchor point for a belay. Attach a sling securely to the belay anchor point. Clip a large, locking carabiner into the end of the anchor sling.
3. Have a belayer take position. If a Munter hitch is being used for belay, have the belayer tie it in the belay rope and clip the Munter hitch into the belay carabiner. If the belayer is using a personal belay device, attach it to the rope and clip it into the belay anchor carabiner.
4. Clip the rappeller into the belay rope. Initiate the belay cycle with the belay voice communications (*Rappeller: "on belay." Belayer: "belay on."* [Figure 9-23, *A, B,* and *C*]).
5. In a secure position, where you are not in danger of falling, follow steps 5 through 15 on p. 111 to lace the rope onto the rack. Be certain that there is no slack between the rack and the anchor (Figure 9-23, *D*).*
6. Begin backing down the slope, controlling your descent with your brake hand and, if necessary, with the guide hand on the bars. If you are unable to move, use the guide hand to pull the bars down toward you, as in step 20 on p. 113 (Figure 9-23, *E*).
7. If, after spreading the bars along the length of the rack, you still have not moved, disengage bars as described in steps 21 and 22 on p. 113. But *never have less than four bars on the rack.*
8. Rappel until you are about midway down the slope. With your brake hand, do a "quick stop" as described in step 16 on p.112.
9. Rappel a short distance farther. Now, using your guide hand on the bars, attempt to stop yourself as described in step 18 on p. 112.
10. Relax your guide hand and tie off the rack as described in steps 24 through 29 on p. 113.

---

*Have the instructor do a *safety check.* Among the other critical elements in the belay system, make certain that the bars are secured correctly. Check all connectors such as carabiners to make certain they are locked and in position of function. Be certain the seat harness is buckled correctly and the anchors are secure. Be sure that no loose clothing or hair will be drawn into the rappel device. Be certain that the helmet is secure.

Rappelling with the Brake Bar Rack down a Vertical Face (*Figure 9-24*)

1. Choose a short vertical face (approximately 20 feet) where the top breaks over gradually into a steep face. On the first rappel, do not choose a face with a sharp edge.
2. Establish a secure anchor point safely back from the edge. If possible, have the anchor point high up. This will help the rappeller in going over the edge. Attach the main line rappel rope securely to the anchor point.
3. Establish a separate anchor point for a belay. Securely attach a sling to the belay anchor point. The anchor point and sling should be established so that when the belayer is in position of operation, he or she has a good field of view of the top and face but is not in danger of falling over the edge. Clip a large-locking carabiner into the end of the belay anchor sling.
4. Have the belayer tie into a safety line and take position. If a Munter hitch is being used for belay, have the belayer tie a Munter hitch in the belay carabiner. If the belayer is using a personal belay device, attach it to the rope and clip the rope into the belay carabiner.
5. The rappeller clips into the belay rope. Initiate the belay cycle with the initial belay voice communications (*Rappeller: "on belay?" Belayer: "belay on."* [9-24, *A*]).
6. In a secure position, where you are in no danger of falling, follow steps 5 through 15 on. p. 111 to lace the rope onto the rack. Be certain that there is no slack between the rack and the anchor.
7. Begin backing to the edge. Because you are on top, there is a great deal of friction in the rack but little weight to pull the rope through. Consequently, you may have to feed the rope through the rack by letting slack with the brake hand. And you may have to reduce friction with your guide hand by spreading the bars apart or perhaps disengaging one or two bars. *But remember: as soon as you start over the edge, your full weight will come onto the rack and you may need the friction. So be prepared to reengage the bars with your guide hand and to establish control with your brake hand* (Figure 9-24, *C*).
8. As you go over the edge, keep the following principles in mind:
   ◆ Keep the body generally perpendicular to the wall. This means that you will have to deliberately lean out as the wall becomes vertical. This may seem unnatural at first, but it is necessary to keep your feet from slipping out from under you.
   ◆ Keep the feet a shoulder's width apart for balance. This will help prevent you from being pulled over to one side.
   ◆ Keep the knees relaxed and slightly flexed.
   ◆ Keep the body slightly turned in the direction of the brake hand, looking down slope, picking a path.

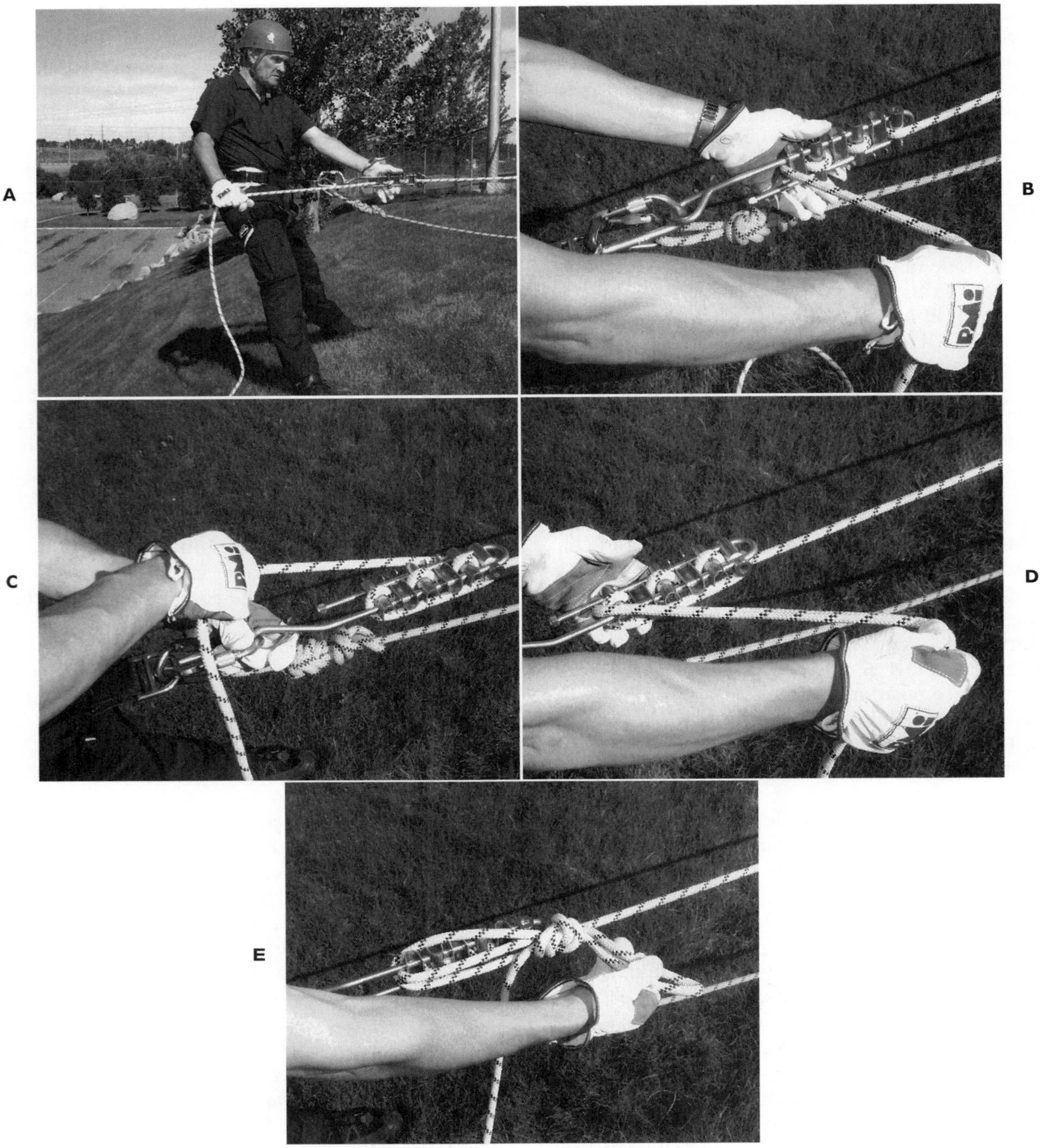

FIGURE 9-23

Using brake bar rack on vertical.

♦ Use the guide hand for balance and for control of the bars. *Do not support your weight with it.*

♦ *Never take the brake hand off the rope unless you are securely locked off* (Figure 9-24, *D*).

9. After you are over the edge, rappel a few feet, then bring the brake side of the rope up in a "quick stop" by pushing it away from you toward the anchor (Figure 9-24, *E*).

10. Tie off the rack so you can be hands free of the rope (Figure 9-24, *F* and *G*).

11. Unlock and rappel a few feet farther.

12. Attempt to stop your descent with the guide hand by jamming the bars up together.

13. Pull the bars apart and rappel to the bottom.

14. Complete the belay cycle with the appropriate voice commands. *(Rappeller: "off belay." Belayer: "belay off.")*

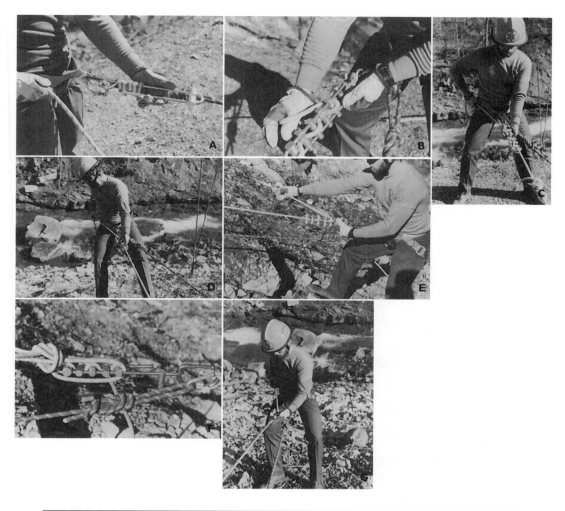

FIGURE 9-24
Using brake bar rack on slope.

⚠ Warning

One of the major concerns in going over the edge with a rack is the possibility of catching the device on the edge. This is possible with any rappel device. But, because of the rack's length, you need to be particularly cautious about catching it on the edge. If you do catch the rack on the edge, any of the following things might happen:

1. You could jam the rack on the edge, preventing the rope from running through the device, thereby stranding yourself in that position.
2. The pressure of your body weight could bend the rack, causing it to malfunction in the future.

The solution to these problems is to avoid edge catch. As you go over the edge, make certain that you lean out enough and push back with your feet before you step down so that the rappel device clears the edge before the rope lays across the edge (Figure 9-25).

15. Remove the rack from the rope.
16. Immediately move away from the "drop zone" to lessen your chances of being hit by falling objects and to clear the rope for others.

EMERGENCY DESCENT SYSTEMS

There may be emergency situations when a rappel is necessary, but the person has no descender with him or her. There are possible solutions to this problem.

One solution might be the *body rappel,* described earlier in this chapter. But, as noted, it has some distinct disadvantages and dangers.

One system used in the past is the ***crabiner wrap***. This consists of wrapping a seat harness carabiner with several turns of the rappel rope to create friction. However, *the carabiner wrap rappel is not considered a satisfactory and safe technique* for rappelling for the following reasons:

♦ If the rope wraps are not correctly put onto the carabiner, they can spiral out of the carabiner gate, resulting in a free fall.

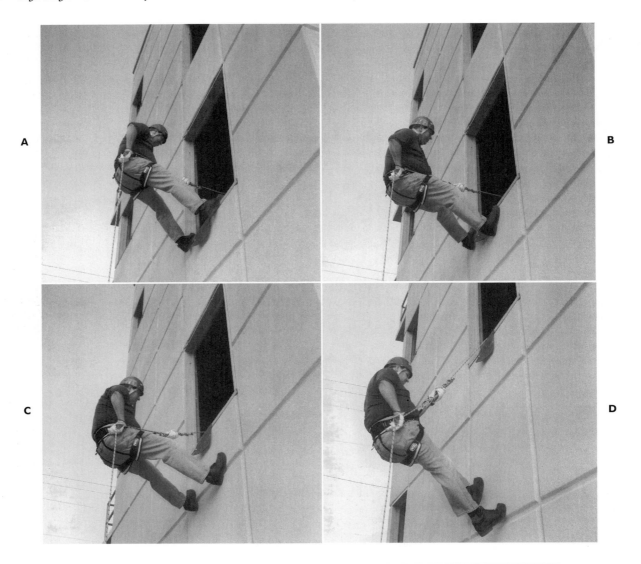

FIGURE 9-25
Clearing rack from edge.

◆ The wraps can bear on the carabiner gate and break it. One alternative to the carabiner wrap might be the ***Munter hitch rappel*** (see Chapter 6, Knots, Figure 8-7 in Chapter 8, Belaying, and Figure 9-26).

Self-Belay Techniques

Where the belay of a rappeller by another person is not possible or practical, self-belay techniques may be possible. Most self-belay techniques are based on the use of some type of rope-grab device on the main rappel line *above* the descenders. Usually the rappeller is attached to the device via a short sling to a chest harness. The self-belay mechanism is triggered by a definitive action by the rappeller, such as leaning over backwards.

One example of a self-belay device is the *spelean shunt* as shown in Figure 9-27. The spelean shunt

consists simply of a Gibbs cam, an oval carabiner, and a short piece of webbing or rope that attaches to a chest harness.

One disadvantage of the spelean shunt is that it can catch and set at times when not desired. This often happens when the rappel is not completely free.

Regulations of the Federal Occupational Health and Safety Administration (OSHA) require that in a workplace environment, such as in high angle window cleaning, there be the use of a "secondary safety system." This could be, for example, self-training rope grab on a belay or safety line.

Using a Prusik "Safety" in Rappelling

One traditional means of rappelling safely has been the use of what is called a *Prusik safety*, which uses a sling with a Prusik knot on the rope and connected to the rappeller's harness (see Chapter 10, Ascend-

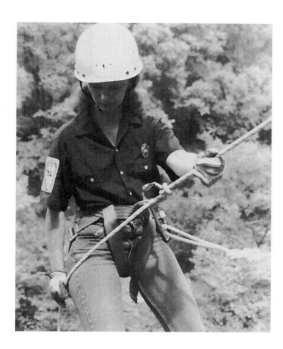

FIGURE 9-26
Munter hitch rappel.

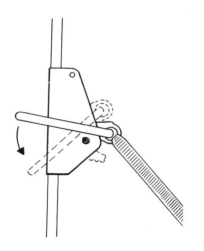

FIGURE 9-27
Spelean shunt.

ing, for further information on the Prusik knot). The theory is that should the rappeller get out of control, the Prusik knot can be used to tighten on the main rope to stop the fall. However, there are pitfalls a rappeller must avoid or the "safety" may not work at all.

In a panic, the falling rappeller may grab for the Prusik knot itself, which does not close it but opens it up. The result is a free fall, until the rappeller hits bottom. This usually occurs when the user pulls down on the top of the Prusik instead of letting go. There are

! **Warning**

The Munter hitch rappel, as with all other rappel techniques, must be practiced on level ground, on a moderate slope with a rappel, and on a short drop with a rappel.

Because the Munter hitch rappel wears the rope, twists the rope, and wears the carabiner, it is a limited-use technique.

! **Warning**

Self-belay techniques are *not* completely automatic safeties but require some positive action by the rappeller. Remember: *in an emergency, one reacts with an instinctive action.* Whether one responds with the correct action in a self-belay emergency may depend on how well trained and disciplined he or she is to do so.

some precautions that can help the Prusik safety work as designed:

- Practice the use of it at a safe height so that your emergency actions become automatic.
- Make certain that the Prusik is tight enough and properly dressed so that it will catch when it is supposed to.
- Place the Prusik safety *under* the belay device. However, this means that you must make the sling short enough that it will not jam into the belay device.

Protecting the Rappel Rope That Is Below You

In most cases, the rappel rope is simply dropped down the vertical face where the rappeller is about to travel. There are, however, circumstances where this might not be desirable:

- In tactical operations where there is a hostile person below you who could grab the rope (and thereby control you).
- Where there is a very frightened and unpredictable person below you.
- Where unstable rocks could be knocked loose by the rope and fall on people below.
- Preventing the rope below you from being damaged and cut from falling debris and rock.
- Where the rope could become tangled or jammed and you could not retrieve it.

In these cases, it might be desirable for the rappeller to keep the rope with him or her. One way of doing this is to attach the rope bag to the rappeller as shown in Figure 9-28. Among the ways of attaching the bag are:

- If it is very light, then the bag may be attached to a seat-harness equipment sling.

Whenever you use a self-belay device, such as the Spelean shunt, you must be certain that the sling connecting the device to the person is not too long. Otherwise, it could put the device out of reach on the rope above you. The result would be that the device could lock itself out of reach and you could be stranded on the rope.

Suggestion

One way of managing a Prusik safety under the belay device is to attach the Prusik sling to the harness leg loop instead of to the belay loop. If the Prusik sling is attached to the harness belay loop, it may be impossible to make the sling short enough not to catch in the rappel device. If it is attached to the leg loop, there is minimal force, as though the Prusik is acting as a "hand."

⚠ **Warning**

1. It is difficult to accurately estimate the length of a rope when it is in a bag. So there is the danger that when rappelling from a bagged rope, you could rappel off the end of the rope. Always either tie a stopper knot in the bottom end of a bagged rope or tie the rope end to the bag to prevent rappelling off the end of the line. (See the section on Preventing a Rappel off the End of a Rope on pages 120–121)

2. Rappelling with a bag attached to your body requires special care to avoid rope tangles that could jam in your descender. You must also be very cautious that the bag does not jam in your descender. This is a particular problem when rappelling from helicopters where a jammed rappel device could leave you stranded on the rope hanging from the helicopter and could lead to severe injury or death.

♦ If the bag is heavy, then it may be attached with a carabiner directly into the bottom of the descender.
♦ Special design rope bags have straps that attach to the lower leg.

EXTRICATING JAMMED RAPPEL DEVICES

Rappel devices are notorious for snagging loose material to become jammed and, perhaps, strand the rap-

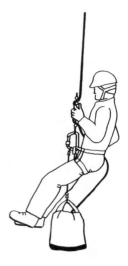

FIGURE 9-28
Rappelling with bagged rope.

peller in a very difficult and painful position that might require a rescue. Among the possibilities are:
♦ "Tee" shirts and other loose clothing.
♦ Hair.
♦ Body parts, such as loose flesh on an underarm.
The best solution to this problem is, of course, prevention:
♦ Tuck in shirt tails and other loose clothing.
♦ Keep hair trimmed or tied back and tucked into helmets.
♦ Keep flabby body sections (underarms, stomachs, and so on) away from rappel devices.

Techniques for Extrication

Avoid using knives. It is very difficult to use a knife in such situations without damaging the rope or cutting it completely. If you are trying to cut jammed material from a descender, you are probably under pressure, physically unbalanced, and, possibly, also in pain. So it is extremely difficult for you to cut away the offending material without also touching the rope with the knife.

Another problem in using a knife involves hair jammed in a descender. Remember that hair is usually attached to scalp. An attempt to cut hair out of a descender could also inflict a significant scalp wound.

One way out of such a situation is to take your weight off the descender with the use of an ascender or Prusik knot above the descender. See Chapter 10, Ascending, for a description of this technique.

Preventing a Rappel off the End of a Rope

There is the potential in some situations of rappelling off the end of a rope. This usually occurs when you cannot see the bottom of the drop before you begin the rappel. As you near the bottom end of the rope, you may not be paying attention or you may lose control. One form of insurance against rappelling off the end of a rope is to use a "stopper knot." One way to do this is to tie a figure 8 knot in the bottom end of the rappel line (or tie the knot in both strands, if rappelling on a doubled rope).

An even better knot is a figure 8 on a bight, which forms a loop. This gives you something to stand in while you figure out what to do next.

Evaluation Exercises

◆ COGNITIVE AND AFFECTIVE EXERCISES ◆

1. List five characteristics of controlled rappelling.
2. Why are the body rappel and arm rappel uncomfortable to use?
3. The rate of descent in rappelling is controlled by the _____ hand.
4. The _____ hand helps to balance the rappeller but does not support weight.
5. The arm rappel should only be used for what situations?
6. What two dangers are posed by using the body rappel?
7. What are the two main drawbacks in using the conventional figure 8 descender?
8. What is one way of getting out of the girth hitch occurrence with the conventional figure 8?
9. What is one way of preventing the girth hitch occurrence?
10. What is one way of lacing up a figure 8 descender that will help prevent it from jamming if caught on an edge?
11. Why should you keep a proper distance between a rappel line anchor and a belay anchor?
12. What is the danger in having too great a distance between a rappel line anchor and a belay anchor?
13. Name seven principles to keep in mind when rappelling down a vertical face.
14. What is one technique for gaining extra friction from a figure 8 descender?
15. What can occur when rappelling on a figure 8 with the brake hand too close to the body?
16. Describe the preferred stance for rappelling.
17. Describe the effect of the angle the rope makes from the rappeller to the anchor point.
18. Why is it important that a rappeller not catch the rappel device on the edge of a drop?
19. Name three advantages and three disadvantages of the brake bar rack.
20. In lacing the rope onto the brake bar rack, one *(should) (should not)* pass the rope between the top bar and the bend of the rack.
21. What is different about the position for the guide hand when using a brake bar rack in contrast to other rappel devices?
22. What is the minimum number of bars that one should use on a brake bar rack?
23. What are two reasons that the carabiner wrap rappel is not considered a satisfactory and safe technique?
24. When using a self-belay device, why should one not get the connecting sling too long?
25. What should you do to the bottom of your rope to prevent rappelling off the end?

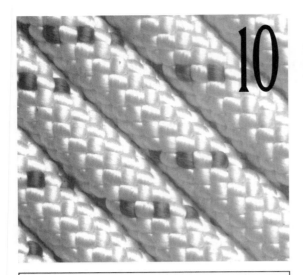

10 Basic Ascending Techniques

◆ *Prerequisites*

Before attempting the activities described in this chapter, you must have demonstrated that you can properly:

1. Use and care for rope.
2. Use and care for other equipment employed in the high angle environment.
3. Tie correctly, and without hesitation, the eight knots described in Chapter 6.
4. Apply the principles of anchoring and rig a safe and secure anchor.
5. Apply the principles of belaying and safely and confidently belay another person using either a Munter hitch or personal belay device.
6. Apply the principles of rappelling: rappel safely, confidently, and under control; tie off the rappel device to operate hands free of the rope and then return to a safe and controlled rappel.

Objectives ▼

At the completion of this chapter, you should be able to:

1. Describe the purposes of ascending and the principles behind it.
2. Select equipment for an ascending system.
3. Tie and use a Prusik hitch.
4. Safely and efficiently use personal ascenders.
5. Ascend a fixed rope safely and efficiently using an ascending system created from three ascenders.
6. Define what is meant by "changing over" from ascending to rappelling, or from rappelling to ascending, and what is involved in these procedures.
7. Safely and efficiently change over from ascending to rappelling.
8. Safely and efficiently change over from rappelling to ascending.
9. Describe what is meant by an ascending "system" and what criteria are necessary for ascending systems that are safe and efficient.
10. Describe the need for and use of the procedure known as "tying off short."
11. "Tie off short" when ascending.
12. Describe how ascenders can be used to extricate yourself from a jammed rappel device or other similar emergencies.

Key Terms ▼

Ascenders Rope grab devices used by individuals to ascend a fixed rope or, with specific types of ascenders, used in the creation of hauling systems. There are basically two categories of ascenders: (1) *personal ascenders*, which are normally used for no more than one person's body weight and (2) *general-use ascenders*, which are used both as personal ascenders and in hauling systems for progress capture devices and as rope grabs.

Ascending A means of traveling up a fixed rope with the use of either mechanical devices or friction hitches attached with slings to the user's body.

Ascender Sling Attachments of webbing or rope that connect a person to his or her ascenders.

Changeover To transfer from an ascending mode to a rappelling mode or from a rappelling mode to an ascending mode.

Chicken Loop A safety loop that fits around the ankle to secure the ascender sling and prevent the foot from slipping out of the sling should an upper connection fail and the person ascending fall backwards.

General-Use Ascenders Mechanical rope grab devices that operate primarily by the force of a cam action wedging the rope against the inside of their shell. They are designed to slide in one direction on a rope and are used for both personal ascenders and in hauling systems for progress capture devices and as rope grabs.

THE PURPOSE OF ASCENDING

Ascending a rope is, in essence, the opposite of rappelling. It is the use of mechanical devices or friction hitches to safely and efficiently ascend a fixed rope. *Ascending* is a further development of competency in the vertical environment. To only be able to rappel means that you can only travel one way on the rope: down. But to be able to both competently rappel *and* ascend means that you have developed the freedom to travel both down and up the rope.

To further develop competency and enhance skills at rappelling and ascending, you must also be able to safely transfer between rappelling and ascending while on rope. This procedure is known as *changeover.* If you are skilled at changeover, you have the ability to both make the transition from rappelling to ascending and from ascending to rappelling.

To be able to both ascend and make changeover safely and efficiently requires a mix of equipment and the simultaneous use of skills. This means that you must have an absolute knowledge of the equipment and an instinctive use of the skills. These only come through practice of the necessary techniques.

Along with the development of ascending and changeover skills and a thorough knowledge of the equipment involved comes the ability to extricate yourself from certain difficult situations. You may, for example, use these skills to extricate yourself from a jammed rappel device without the potentially dangerous use of knives.

HOW ASCENDING IS ACCOMPLISHED

Ascending is accomplished through the use of rope grab devices, called *ascenders.* When ascenders are properly used and secured to the rope, they can be made to slide in only one direction: up.

Types of Ascenders
Friction Hitches

There are several kinds of friction hitches, but the type most commonly used is the *Prusik hitch.*

Mechanical Ascenders

Mechanical ascenders work by an offset camming action that presses against the rope to keep the device from sliding down the line. They are further subdivided into two types: general-use ascenders and personal ascenders.

General-use Ascenders. *General-use ascenders* grip the rope primarily by squeezing it against the inside of the ascender shell. The two best known brands currently on the U.S. market are the Gibbs and the Rescucender.

Personal Ascenders. *Personal ascenders* work primarily by gripping the rope with teeth on a cam and also pressing the rope inside the shell of the device. There are several brands of personal ascenders available, including CMI, Petzl, Jumar, and SRT.

In all cases, ascenders are attached to the user's body by *slings,* which are connectors made either of webbing or of rope. These slings may be connected through various combinations to seat harnesses, chest harnesses, and feet.

The actual ascending process works by an alternating action of the user. While resting his or her weight on the first ascender as it grips the rope, the person keeps weight off the second ascender and moves it up the rope. He or she then shifts weight to the second ascender and takes weight off the first ascender as he or she moves it up the rope. The person moves up the rope, by repeating this cycle.

In most ascending activities, *at least two* ascenders are required. Three ascenders increase the margin of safety.

THE BASICS: A PRUSIK HITCH

Friction hitches were the first type of rope grab devices used in ascending. For the most part, they have been replaced in ascending by mechanical devices. But the knowledge of how to tie and use a friction hitch is still important. If you know how, you can improvise a friction hitch with rope or cord when you do not have mechanical ascenders. On numerous occasions, the ability to improvise a friction hitch has saved lives by helping people extricate themselves from difficult situations. Friction hitches have also helped people perform a self-rescue after the failure of a mechanical ascender. In addition, friction hitches are used in rigging for some rope rescue systems. Although there are a number of different friction hitches, the one most commonly used is the *Prusik hitch.*

Selecting Material for a Prusik Hitch

Diameter

The Prusik hitch will operate more efficiently if the rope it is made from is a smaller diameter than the main line rope to which it is attached. A rule to start with is to have the Prusik cord diameter between ⅔ to ¾ the diameter of the main line rope. This usually works out to 8 mm Prusik cord to be used on 11 mm (⁷⁄₁₆ inch) rope, or 9 mm Prusik cord for 12.5 mm (½ inch) rope.

Be careful to avoid extremes. The Prusik cord must be strong enough to support the intended load, with a proper safety margin. But it should not be so large that it is hard to get the hitch to "set."

Stretch

The Prusik material should not be stretchy, otherwise it will be difficult to loosen once it is "set" on the rope.

Construction

Construction of ropes is a compromise among the following:

◆ A softer braid construction grips better but will be more difficult to loosen and move up the rope and will wear out faster.
◆ Harder braid ropes are easier to loosen and move up the rope but do not grip as well.

Creating a Prusik Loop

To create a *Prusik loop,* make a continuous loop from an approximately 6-foot length of rope that you have chosen for the loop material. Do this by tying the two ends together with a grapevine ("double fisherman's") knot.

Attaching the Prusik Loop to a Rope (Figure 10-1)

1. Securely anchor a main line static kernmantle rope vertically so that it will support a person. There should be some means of letting slack into the rope while it still supports a person. (This is

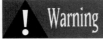

Warning

Materials used for Prusik hitches wear quickly and should be inspected before each use.

so that the person practicing with a single Prusik hitch can be let back to the ground when he or she gets up as far as possible.) One possibility is to use the ascending practice system described on page 130.
2. Wear a sewn, manufactured seat harness with leg and thigh supports. Clip a locking carabiner into the seat harness' front attachment point.
3. Stretch the Prusik loop out between two hands with the connecting knot about midpoint.
4. At about eye level begin to place the loop on the rope by forming a Prusik hitch. Do this by holding the loop against the rope on the side of the rope near you. Have a smaller portion of the loop (about 6 inches) off to the right of the rope (Figure 10-1, *A*).
5. Bring the larger side of the loop around the main line rope toward you and pull it through the smaller side of the loop. Be sure that the figure 8 bend (or grapevine knot) passes well through and that the coils formed around the main rope are even (Figure 10-1, *B* and *C*).
6. Bring the larger side of the loop through the same path again as before. Make certain that the coils of the Prusik hitch around the main rope are even and parallel (Figure 10-1, *D*).
7. Tighten the Prusik hitch around the main rope. Do this by doing the following: (1) with one hand, pull the end of the Prusik loop away from the main rope; (2) at the same time, with the other hand, grasp the knot by placing the fingers on the coils of the hitch on the side away from you, with the thumb on the bar portion of the hitch on the side next to you. Grasp the hitch with the thumb and pull the bar tight against the rope (Figure 10-1, *E* and *F*).

Weighting the Prusik Hitch

8. Clip your seat harness carabiner into the end of the Prusik loop. Lock the carabiner (Figure 10-1, *G*).
9. Now sit down so that the Prusik hitch sets on the rope and the loop supports your weight. If the hitch begins to slide, set it further by holding it in your hand and pressing it closed using the thumb as in step #7 above.
10. Stand up on the floor and take your weight off the hitch.
11. Slide the hitch 6 inches up the rope. Unset the hitch by grasping it with your hand as before. But this time pull the bar on the hitch with your thumb *away* from the main rope so that it breaks the hitch loose. As you do this, move the hitch up the rope with your hand around it. Be certain that you have taken your weight off the Prusik sling.
12. After you slide the hitch up the desired length, reset it as you did before. Sit down with the hitch supporting your body weight (Figure 10-1, *H*).

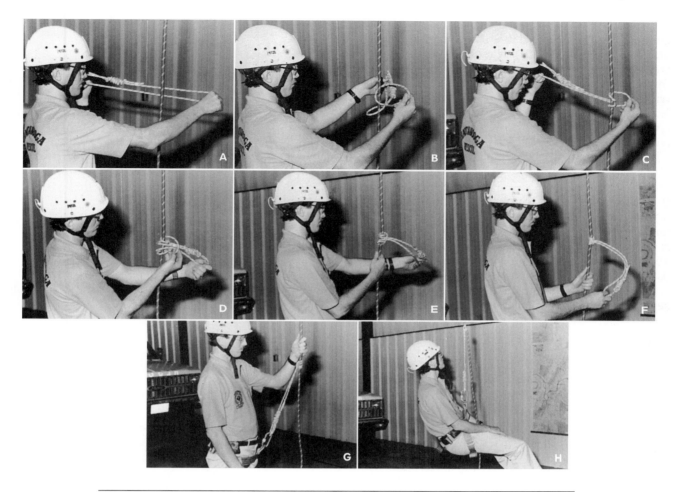

FIGURE 10-1
Attaching Prusik loop to rope.

13. Repeat this process until you cannot slide the hitch any farther up.
14. If you cannot get back down, have someone allow slack into the rope so you have your weight off the hitch. Remove the hitch from the rope.

You have now examined the basics of using a Prusik hitch. Because you have used only one hitch, your movement was obviously limited. In the actual practice of ascending with Prusik hitches, you would not shift your weight to the ground in order to raise the Prusik hitch. Instead, you would shift your weight to another Prusik hitch, which you would also be advancing up the rope.

Other Uses for the Prusik Loop

As mentioned in Chapter 1, The High Angle Environment, it is a good idea to carry with you a couple of Prusik loops that can be used quickly for unforeseen needs. If, for example, your descent device became jammed while rappelling, then you could use a Prusik on the line above the device to get your weight off

> ### ⚠ Warning
>
> Never press down on the top of a Prusik or other friction hitch, unless you want it to slide down. In a life-support situation, a downward pressure could release the hitch, causing a fall, which could result in severe injury or death.

and unjam the rappel device. See page 120 for specific details on using an ascender to unjam a rappel device. A Prusik might also be used as a self-belay on safety lines at the edge of a drop.

Greater Holding Power: The Three-Wrap Prusik

The two-wrap Prusik hitch, described earlier, will be adequate for most personal-use vertical applications. However, for greater holding power, such as where the rope is made slippery by mud or ice or where greater weight is involved, the three-wrap Prusik may be desired (Figure 10-2). The three-wrap Prusik is created by running the Prusik sling one more time through the loop. This is known as "adding another wrap."

Although the three-wrap Prusik hitch offers the potential of greater holding power, it may be more difficult to manipulate than the two-wrap Prusik hitch.

PERSONAL ASCENDERS

In personal ascending, most people now use mechanical ascenders. They tend to be easier, more efficient, and more convenient to use than hitches. One type of mechanical ascender is the *personal ascender*. Figure 10-3 shows a typical personal ascender with a handle. Although some models may not have the parts exactly as shown here, they all work in essentially the same manner.

Parts of the Personal Ascender

The Frame (A)

The frame is what the parts are attached to and what mostly determines the ascender strength. The frame may be fabricated from extruded, stamped, or plate aluminum or, in some cases, from cast aluminum.

The Handle (B)

The handle may be an integral part of the frame or it may be attached to the frame with rivets or bolts. In some designs, the handle is molded to fit the contour of the hand and can be comfortably used with gloves or mittens. Not all personal ascenders have handles. Those without handles are usually designed for direct attachment to the user's body without the use of the hands.

The Safety Lever (C)

When the safety lever is in the locked position, it prevents full downward movement of the cam. This is designed to help prevent the ascender from accidentally coming off the rope. (However, see the Warning box on p. 127.)

The Nose (D)

The nose forms the inside channel into which the cam pushes the rope so that the ascender stays on the rope.

Tie-In Points

Tie-in points are usually an integral part of the frame and are used to fasten a sling that is attached to the user. Most ascenders have tie-in points at the bottom, so that the ascender can support a person below him or her. Some ascenders also have an additional tie-in point at the top. These are used in certain ascending systems where the ascender is pulled along as the user advances up the rope.

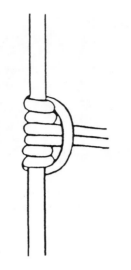

FIGURE 10-2
Three-wrap Prusik.

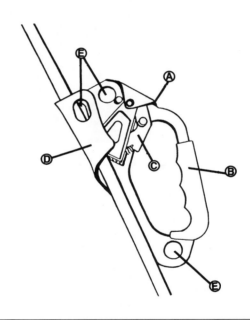

FIGURE 10-3
Typical personal ascender (right hand).

Right- and Left-Handed Ascenders

Most ascenders with handles are manufactured in right- or left-handed models. Some manufacturers color code the ascender so you can tell the difference. However, you can tell the difference between a right- or left-handed model by doing the following:

◆ Turn the ascender so that the opening for the rope between the nose and the cam is facing you.
◆ The left-handed model will have its handle to your left. The right-handed model will have its handle to your right.

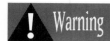

Warning

Personal ascenders *can and do fail when misused*. The most common modes of failure include the following:

FRAME BREAKAGE

Ascender frames constructed of cast aluminum can crack or break when subjected to the high stress of being dropped. Cast aluminum frames can crack under their paint so there is no outward sign of damage. Previously owned ascenders of any type may have been subjected to stresses that could result in failure. For this reason, a previously-owned ascender should not be used unless its complete history is known.

ROPE DAMAGE

Rope damage occurs when the ascender pulls on the rope with such force that the teeth of the cam tears the rope sheath. Sheath tearing has been known to occur with as little force as 800 lb on the ascender and rope. For this reason, ascenders with toothed cams should never be used in situations where more than one person's body weight is involved. One example of where toothed cams, such as found on personal ascenders, should not be used is in rescue hauling systems.

ROPE SLIPPING OUT OF AN ASCENDER

Personal ascenders are designed to operate most efficiently and safely on vertical ropes and when moved in a direct line with the rope. Personal ascenders have been known to slip off the rope when they have been pulled away from the rope or torqued on the rope. This could happen when using personal ascenders on a rope that is not completely vertical but at an angle, such as ascending a sloping highline or traversing rope along a ledge.

If there is a chance that the ascender might be operated in this kind of situation, which they were not designed for, then a safety carabiner should be clipped across the ascender and the rope as shown in Figure 10-4. This may not prevent the ascender from slipping from the rope, but the sling will remain connected to the rope via the carabiner.

Ascender Slings

Ascenders, to be used safely and efficiently, must be attached to the user's body with connections known as *slings*. These slings may be made either of webbing or of rope. Many people prefer rope for the following reasons:

◆ An appropriate design of rope may abrade less easily than webbing.
◆ Rope will operate better than webbing if the sling has to go through a roller device, such as is used in certain ascending systems.

If you decide to construct **ascender slings** from rope, you may be able to use line that is a smaller diameter

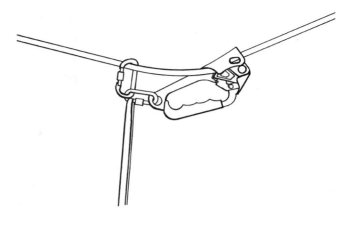

FIGURE 10-4
Clipping carabiner across ascender and rope.

than what is normally used for the main line rope. A sling made of $3/8$- or $5/16$-inch rope might be appropriate as long as it has an adequate safety factor.

Most experienced ascender users prefer slings constructed of static rope. Static rope tends to stretch less than dynamic rope, thereby transferring the energy involved in ascending directly to the ascenders, rather than absorbing it.

The actual length of the slings will depend on factors such as the proportion of your body and the type of ascending system you use. These factors are explored later in this chapter.

Tying the Slings to the Ascender

Because of the different designs for ascender tie-in points, the actual method of connecting the slings to the ascender will vary depending on the individual brand and design. See the manufacturer's instructions for specific information.

In connecting the sling to an ascender, remember that a sharp bend in a rope will diminish the strength of the rope (see Chapter 3, Rope and Related Equipment, on the 4:1 rule). If the tie-in point of an ascender is wide enough, then the sling may be tied directly into it using a figure **8** follow-through knot. If the tie-in point is narrow so that it will create too sharp a bend in the rope, then the rope should be first clipped into a carabiner or snap link. The carabiner or snap link is then clipped directly into the carabiner tie-in point.

A figure **8** on a bight knot is tied in the end of the rope sling to be attached to the person. If the sling is to go into a seat harness, then the knot is connected to the carabiner, which is clipped into the seat harness' front tie-in point. If the sling is to go to a foot, then a large loop in the figure **8** knot will be needed. This should be large enough to slip through a **chicken loop** and onto a boot. (More on this in the section on Ascending Systems on p. 129.)

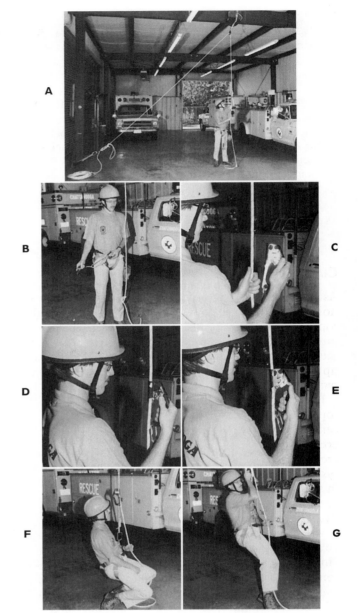

FIGURE 10-5
Using a personal ascender.

⚠ Warning

Some people warn against clipping a carabiner or snap link directly into an ascender with a cast aluminum frame. It is thought that under a severe impact, the carabiner or snap link might cause the cast aluminum frame to crack.

Using a Personal Ascender (Figure 10-5)

1. For this exercise, you will need only one personal ascender with a handle. It may be either right- or left-handed, depending on which feels more comfortable.
2. Using rope, create an ascender sling. For this exercise, the total length after tying should only be about 2 feet. Attach the sling to a lower tie-in hole of the ascender either directly or with a carabiner following the guidelines outlined previously. Tie a figure **8** on a bight loop in the end of the rope sling that is to attach to the person.
3. Wear a sewn, manufactured seat harness with leg and thigh supports. Clip a locking carabiner into the seat harness tie-in point.
4. Clip the seat harness into the loop of the ascender. Lock the carabiner.

Attaching the Ascender onto the Rope

5. Securely anchor a main line, static, kernmantle rope vertically so that it will support a person's weight with an adequate safety factor. As in the exercise with the Prusik hitch, there must be a means for the person on the rope of getting back down once he or she has pushed the ascender up as far as it will go (Figure 10-5, *A* and *B*).
6. Take the ascender in one hand and press the safety lever so that the cam swings down and open. The literature that comes with the ascender should provide specific instructions for triggering the safety lever. The triggering is usually done with the thumb of the hand that is holding the ascender. With some ascenders, this triggering can be done as the hand grasps the handle. With other ascenders, the hand must be grasping the entire ascender, with the handle against the palm and the index and middle finger around the nose (Figure 10-5, *C* and *D*).
7. Place the ascender on the rope at about eye level with the nose up. Do this by holding the cam down with the trigger. Place the ascender so that the main line rope runs in the channel of the nose. Release the cam so that it presses the rope into the channel of the nose and the ascender remains on the rope. Release the safety lever, making sure it now locks the cam on the rope.

When you are ascending, never touch the safety lever unless you intend the ascender to come off the rope (Figure 10-5, *E*).

8. Sit down so that the sling comes taut and the ascender supports your weight on the rope. (If the rope stretch is such that you end up on the ground, reset the ascender up the rope so that you are being supported [Figure 10-5, *F*]).
9. Now, stand up so that your weight is off the sling and push the ascender up a foot. Sit down again (Figure 10-5, *G*).

Backing the Ascender down the Rope

10. Stand up so that your weight is completely off the ascender. While grasping the upper part of the ascender around the nose, take your thumb and move the cam down while slightly lifting the ascender. *Do not touch the safety lever.* Move the ascender down a foot and release the cam so that it reengages the rope. Sit down again on the ascender until it supports your weight.

You have now examined the basics of using a personal ascender. Because you used only one ascender, your movement obviously was limited. In the actual practice of using ascenders, you would not shift your weight to the ground in order to raise the ascender. Instead, you would shift your weight to another ascender, which you would also be moving up the rope.

CREATING AN ASCENDING "SYSTEM"

As seen from the previous exercise, one ascender can hold you on the rope. But to effectively move up the rope, you need two or more ascenders. When two or more ascenders, whether they be friction hitches or mechanical ascenders, are worked together to travel up a rope, the arrangement is known as an ascending *system*.

Dozens of different ascending systems are used in rope work. They differ in terms of what kinds of ascenders they use, what combinations the ascenders are attached to the body, what parts of the body they are attached to, and in other ways. Each ascending system may offer advantages in safety, in ease of use, in speed of movement, and in ease of movement. No one ascending system includes all these advantages. Every system has at least one drawback.

When you are beginning to work with ascending, you should initially seek ascending systems that combine safety and ease of use. Some characteristics of ascending systems that contribute to safety and ease of use are:

♦ The system should require more use of your legs and feet and less use of your arms and hands. Your legs and feet are stronger and have greater stamina than your hands and arms.

♦ The system should hold you upright on the rope with your body weight over the legs. This requires less arm strength, encourages use of the legs, and contributes to safety.

♦ The system should be able to support you in a sitting position while you are on the rope. Ascending is a tiring activity, and short periods of rest while sitting are essential.

♦ The system should have attachments to the seat harness (and in some cases to a chest harness). Some systems have attachments only to the feet and depend on arm and body strength to hold the user upright. These systems are sometimes called *death rigs*.

It is important that whatever system you use, it be fine tuned to your body height and build. A well-

tuned system makes rope ascending no more work than climbing a ladder. A poorly fitted, untuned system will quickly exhaust even the most physically fit person (Box 10-1).

Tying off Short

Tying off short is the safety procedure of tying directly into the main rope to ensure an additional attachment. It is used in certain situations during ascending when there are less than three points of attachment on the rope. Examples include:

♦ When a person is using only two ascenders and he or she must take one of the ascenders from the rope for a procedure such as moving past a knot or going over an edge of a cliff or building.

♦ When, for any reason, there are less than three ascenders on the rope.

To tie off short, do the following (Figure 10-6):
1. Reach down below the lowest ascender to the slack rope hanging below you (Figure 10-6, *A*).
2. Take a large bight of that rope and pull it up.
3. Tie a figure 8 on a bight in the bight.
4. Clip the figure 8 on a bight into a spare carabiner that is clipped into the seat harness (Figure 10-6, *B* and *C*).
5. Make your move past the obstacle (Figure 10-6, *D*).
6. When finished with this safety, unclip the figure 8 on a bight from the carabiner, untie the knot, and allow the rope to drop back down below you (Figure 10-6, *E* and *F*).

If it happens that you are ascending with only two ascenders, you can create a continuous safety by tying off short:
1. Tie off short as soon as you have ascended high enough so that a fall would injure you.
2. Leave the figure 8 on a bight knot clipped into your seat harness carabiner as you continue to ascend.
3. Ascend until you create enough slack in the rope so it no longer offers adequate protection from a fall (this distance is usually around 10 feet, or one story).
4. Tie a second knot closer to you and place it in the carabiner above the first knot.

Box 10-1 Maintaining Three Points of Attachment in Ascending

A commonly accepted safety guide in ascending is the "three points of attachment" rule. This means that when the user is moving one ascender, the person is attached to the rope by two devices. In many ascending systems, such as the ones shown in this chapter, three ascenders are used on the rope. When using only two ascenders, it may be necessary to "tie off short" to maintain a margin of safety (see the next section).

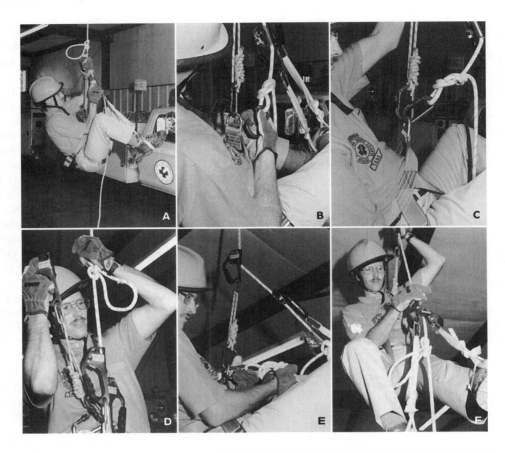

FIGURE 10-6
Tying off short.

5. Take the first knot out of the carabiner, close the carabiner, untie the old knot, and drop the slack out of the main line rope.
6. Repeat this procedure until you have finished the climb.

Chicken Loops

One feature that should be used when using ascenders that are attached to the foot is called the *chicken loop* (Figure 10-7). In ascending systems where feet are used, ascenders are often attached to the feet via foot stirrups. These stirrups are often simple loops of webbing or rope sling. In addition, chicken loops should be used around the ankles to serve the following purposes:

♦ It helps prevent the feet from slipping out of the stirrups while the user is ascending.
♦ Should the person ascending lose all upper-body attachments and fall over backwards, the chicken loops help keep the feet in the stirrups to prevent a fall to the ground.

Chicken loops are constructed of webbing (1 inch or larger) and stitched, or securely tied, into a loop that is larger than the ankle but smaller than the boot.

The chicken loop must be able to hold a person's weight without failing.

Ascending with Example Systems

The following portions of this chapter will explore ascending techniques with some example systems. These systems may be used with Prusik hitches (or other comparable friction hitches), general-use ascenders, or personal ascenders. However, in these examples, the systems will be described in use with personal ascenders because they are more easily manipulated when learning ascending techniques.

An Ascending Practice System

Because ascending is a new and unique activity for most people, an *ascending practice system* can be very helpful in learning the technique in a safe environment.

This system consists of the following elements (Figure 10-8):

1. A main line, static kernmantle rope on which the practice takes place. The rope runs over a directional pulley that is securely attached to a beam in

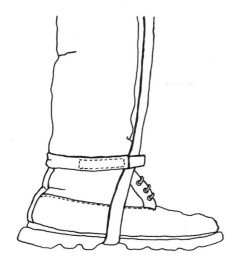

FIGURE 10-7
Chicken loop.

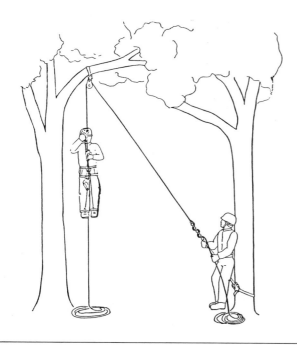

FIGURE 10-8
Ascending practice system.

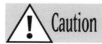

Ascending is a *strenuous activity* to be attempted only by those persons known to be in good physical condition. Those persons with preexisting cardiac or pulmonary conditions, obesity, or other medical conditions that might be exacerbated by exertion, should consult with a physician before attempting ascending.

the ceiling of a building (or a *very strong* tree limb outside) and down to a securely anchored lowering device, such as a brake bar rack or a figure **8** descender.

2. In preparation for the practice, only enough rope hangs vertical for the person to get onto the rope.
3. The lowering device (brake bar rack or figure **8** descender) is locked off until the person begins to ascend. The person operating the braking device allows enough rope through to keep the student high enough off the deck to use his or her ascender but low enough so a fall will not cause injury.
4. An assistant, in addition to a person operating the braking system, can hold the rope below the climber to help the student as he or she begins ascent.
5. When the student completes the ascending cycle, the person operating the braking device lowers the student back to the deck so he or she can get off the rope. *The student must always stop ascending while there is still enough rope to lower him or her to the ground.*

A Three-Ascender System

Figure 10-9 shows a basic three-ascender system using personal ascenders. Because the proportions of each person's body differ, no specific dimensions for the sling attachments can be shown. However, you should tailor the slings for your own use by using the following guidelines:

◆ The seat attachment (with an optional chest harness) should be the top ascender on the rope when you are resting your weight on it. *The ascender must never extend out of your reach up the rope while standing upright in your foot loops or sitting in your harness.*
◆ The ascender for your dominant foot (right foot for right-handed people) should come next on the rope. Its sling should be long enough to allow the ascender to be attached about midthigh when standing.
◆ The ascender for the second foot should be the last one on the rope. Its sling should be just enough shorter than the second sling to allow the third ascender to be immediately below the second ascender when both ascenders' slings are tight.

When all the knots have been tied, make certain that they are contoured well, dressed, and pulled down tightly.

Caution

The operator of the braking device must be thoroughly experienced with its use as a lowering device. The floor under the practice rope should be covered with a mat.

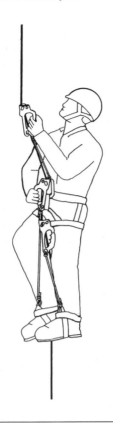

FIGURE 10-9
Basic three-ascender system.

Procedure for Using the Three Ascender System (*Figure* 10-10)

1. For this exercise, use the ascending practice system as described earlier. Before you start, be certain that someone is attending the lowering device and that initially it is locked off tight.
2. With one hand, reach up and pull the main line rope taut. Attach the ascender for the seat harness as high up as you can get it (Figure 10-10, *A*).
3. Attach the next ascender down (the one to your dominant foot) under the seat harness ascender (Figure 10-10, *B*).
4. Attach the third ascender under the second one (Figure 10-10, *C*).
5. To pretest the system, alternately load the seat ascender and each foot ascender to make certain they are holding (Figure 10-10, *D*).
6. If possible, have another person assist you in getting started by having him or her hold the rope down close to the ground. Otherwise, you may have to hold the rope down yourself. This is necessary in getting started because there may not be enough rope weight initially to cause the rope to slide through the ascenders as they are pushed up. Once you have gotten far enough off the ground, the rope weight will cause the rope to automatically slide through the ascenders as they are pushed up.

7. Shift your weight onto the foot stirrups and off the top ascender. Push the top ascender up as far as you can (Figure 10-10, *E*).*
8. Sit down so that you are supported by the top ascender. Take the weight off the next ascender in line by lifting the foot attached to it. Raise this foot ascender up as far as it will easily go (Figure 10-10, *F*).
9. Take the weight off the remaining foot ascender by lifting the foot attached to it and raising the ascender up as far as it will go.†
10. Continue the cycle by repeating steps 7, 8, and 9 until you start running out of rope or you become fatigued. Have the operator of the lowering device lower you back to the ground (Figure 10-10, *G*).
11. Remove all the ascenders from the rope.

Other Ascending Systems

The three-ascender system, detailed here, is one example of an ascending system. There are dozens of different ascending systems in existence that can be used according to such needs as:

◆ Distance to travel up the rope.
◆ Physical strength.
◆ Stamina.
◆ Differences in male and female physique.
◆ Speed.

With a proper amount of research and experimentation, each person can find the type of ascending system just right for him or her. One good place to begin the search for the proper ascending system is in the following book: Padgett A. and Smith B.: *On Rope: North American vertical rope techniques*, ed 2, Huntsville, Ala., 1996, National Speleological Society (see Appendix A).

ASCENDING OVER AN EDGE

Usually the most difficult maneuver in ascending occurs when the person ascending has reached the top of a cliff or a building and has to go over an edge.

As a general rule, as in rappelling, if the strength of the anchors on the main line rope allows it, the higher up the rope is anchored, the easier it is to go over an edge.

The technique for getting over an edge depends on the particular nature of the edge.

---

*Note that when maneuvering your body up so you can raise an ascender, use your leg strength as much as possible. The more you use your legs and feet, and the less you use your arms and hands, the less fatigued you will become.

---

†Note that as you progress up the rope, the person attending the lowering device should slowly let rope out so that you remain a safe distance off the ground. But you should be up high enough so that the rope pulls through the ascender by its own weight as you raise the ascenders.

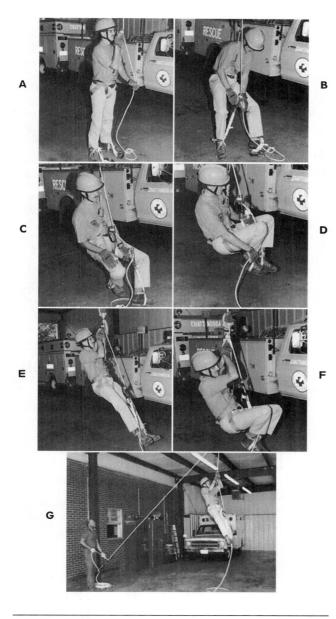

FIGURE 10-10
Using the three-ascender system.

If the Edge Has a Gradual Rollover

1. Ascend until the top ascender is about to make contact with the wall.
2. Push yourself away from the wall with one hand and with your feet.
3. Raise the top ascender above the contact point.
4. Be careful that you do not get fingers caught between the hardware or rope and the wall.
5. As you move upward, and your weight is on the ascender above the contact point, the other ascenders should follow more easily.

If the Edge Is Undercut

1. Ascend until the top ascender is about to make contact with the wall.
2. Bring the lower ascenders up as far as it is comfortable to do so.
3. Try to work the top ascender over the edge by pushing away from the wall with one hand and with the feet.
4. If this is impossible to do, tie off short into the main line rope.
5. Remove the top ascender from the rope and move it up and over the edge and immediately clip it into the rope.
6. Begin ascending again. It is likely that the two remaining ascenders can now be eased over the edge once your weight is on the main line rope above the edge. If this is not the case, then follow the same procedure as you did with the top ascender. *Until you are in a safe and secure position with no danger of falling, never have less than two ascenders securing you to the rope at one time.*

CHANGING OVER

"Changing over" means switching from an ascending mode to a rappelling mode, or from a rappelling mode to an ascending mode, while still on the rope. It is a skill that adds to vertical competency and is particularly useful in emergency situations, such as when you rappel to the end of a rope and find it does not reach the bottom. See Box 10-2 for information regarding equipment.

Procedures for Performing Changeovers
Changing over from Ascending to Rappelling (**Figure** 10-11)

1. For this exercise, use the ascending practice system described earlier in this chapter. Before you start, be certain that a responsible and experienced person is attending the lowering device and it is initially locked down tight.
2. Using a three-ascender system, begin ascending on the rope.
3. When you reach the point where you want to changeover, stop your ascending (Figure 10-11, *A*).
4. Remove your rappel device from your equipment sling and clip it into the second locking carabiner that is attached to your seat harness tie-in point and currently not being used in the ascending system. (If the rappel device is a brake bar rack, lock the carabiner [Figure 10-11, *B*]).
5. Sit down on your seat harness ascender (the top one) so that your weight is on it.
6. Take your weight off the foot ascenders. Move these ascenders back down the rope so that there is slack in the rope between the foot ascenders and the seat ascender. *Do not touch the cam safety levers and do not remove the ascenders from the rope at this time.*

Box 10-2 Equipment Needed
for Changing Over

◆ Two locking carabiners in the seat harness tie-in point; the one that is in use at the time and a spare to be used when changing over.
◆ Harness gear loops or gear sling; the equipment not in use at the time are attached to these (the rappel device while you are ascending, the ascenders while you are rappelling).
◆ Equipment for both ascending and rappelling.

7. Attach the rappel device onto the slack rope between the foot ascenders and the seat ascender. Remove all slack in the main line rope between the rappel device and the top ascender (Figure 10-11, *C*).

8. Lock the rappel device off securely. Make certain there is no slack between the rappel device and the top ascender. (If you have not done so already, lock the seat harness carabiner that attaches the rappel device to the seat harness [Figure 10-11, *D*]).

9. Move a foot ascender back up the main line rope only far enough so that when you put your weight on it, it will remove weight from the seat harness (top) ascender.

10. Shift your weight to the foot ascender and remove weight from the seat ascender.

11. Remove the seat ascender from the rope (Figure 10-11, *E*).

12. Sit down so that the rappel device takes your weight. Remove weight from your foot ascender by lifting your foot (Figure 10-11, *F*).

13. Remove all remaining ascenders from the rope (Figure 10-11, *G*).

14. One by one, remove ascender slings from your body. To secure them, wrap them around the ascender they are attached to and clip them into your equipment sling.

15. Unjam the rappel device and proceed with the rappel (Figure 10-11, *H*).

Changing Over from Rappelling to Ascending (Figure 10-12)

16. Stop the rappel at the point where you want to begin the changeover. Lock off the rappel device securely, following guidelines in Chapter 9, Rappelling (Figure 10-12, *A*).

17. Remove the seat harness ascender (top ascender) from the equipment sling. Clip the sling into the spare carabiner in the seat harness' front tie-in point (the one currently not being used). Lock the carabiner (Figure 10-12, *B*).

18. Place the top ascender on the rope as far up as you can push it. It is important that there be no slack in this ascender sling. One way to achieve

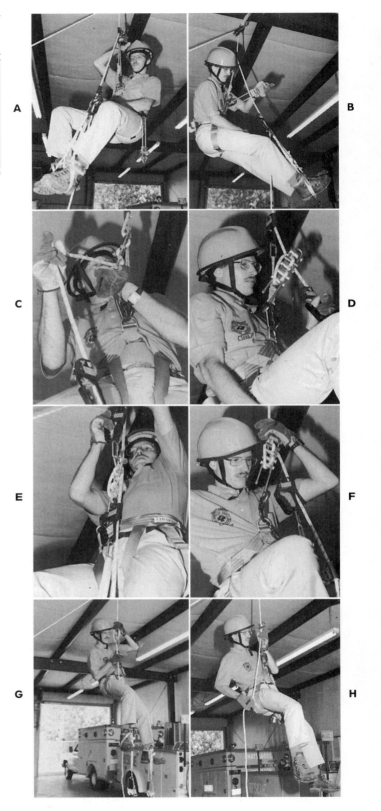

FIGURE 10-11
Changing over (ascend to rappel).

this is to let slack through the descender until the top ascender sling becomes taut.

19. Place the other ascenders on the rope connected to proper slings via the foot. If any of these interfere with the position of the rappel device, then back them off down the rope a couple of feet below the rappel device (Figure 10-12, *C*).

20. When all the ascenders are securely attached, unlock the rappel device and slowly let rope through it. When your weight is off the rappel device, remove the rappel device from the rope and clip it back into the harness gear loop (Figure 10-12, *D, E,* and *F*).

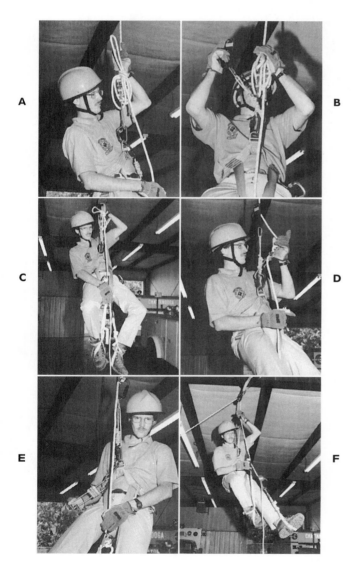

FIGURE 10-12

Changing over (rappel to ascend).

EXTRICATING A JAMMED RAPPEL DEVICE

The ability to extricate a jammed rappel device from hair or clothing without the use of a knife is an essential skill for the high angle technician. The skills and equipment required for this procedure are similar to those used in changing over.

Because of the real possibility of a jammed rappel device, or similar emergency occurring, it is wise to carry the following spare equipment when you are rappelling:

◆ Two ascenders, any type, or two Prusik loops. The length of the Prusik loops will vary according to body proportion.

◆ A spare, large-locking carabiner.

Procedure for Using Ascenders to Extricate a Jammed Rappel Device (Figure 10-13)

1. Using the ascending practice system, begin a rappel.
2. Assume that the rappel device is jammed (Figure 10-13, *A*).
3. Simulate this by locking off the rappel device securely (Figure 10-13, *B*).
4. Remove the seat (top) ascender from your equipment loop and clip the end of the sling into a spare locking carabiner. Clip the carabiner into the seat harness front tie-in. Lock the carabiner (Figure 10-13, *C*).
5. Place the ascender on the rope above the rappel device. Slide it up as far as it will go.
6. Remove a foot ascender from your equipment sling and attach the end of the sling to your foot. Put the ascender on the rope above the rappel device (Figure 10-13, *D*).
7. Put your weight on the ascenders and remove the weight from the rappel device.
8. Remove the obstruction (hair, clothing, and so on) from the rappel device. (Simulate this by unlocking the rappel device and causing it to go slack on the rope [Figure 10-13, *E*].)
9. Replace the rappel device on the rope and lock it off so that there is no slack in the main line rope between the rappel device and the next ascender up.
10. Put your weight on the foot ascender and remove your weight from the seat ascender.
11. Remove the seat ascender from the rope (Figure 10-13, *F*).
12. Shift your weight off the foot ascender and onto your rappel device (Figure 10-13, *G*).
13. Remove the foot ascender from the rope (Figure 10-13, *H*).
14. Remove both ascenders and slings connecting your body, secure them, and clip them into the equipment sling.
15. Unjam the rappel device and continue the rappel (Figure 10-13, *I*).

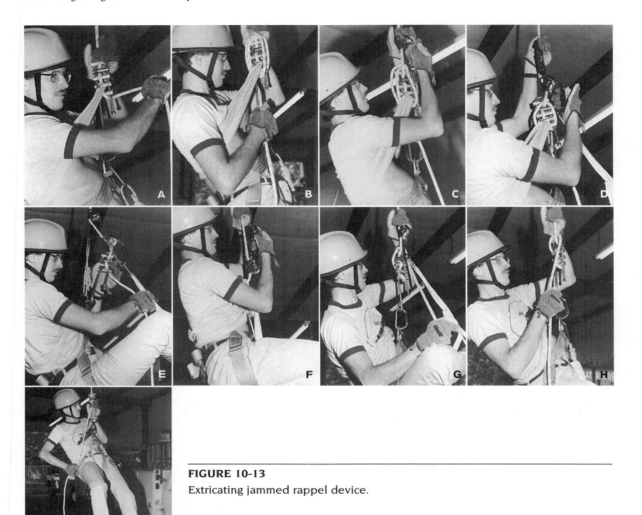

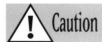

FIGURE 10-13
Extricating jammed rappel device.

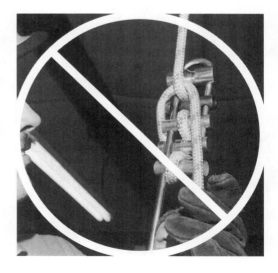

FIGURE 10-14
Avoid trapping rope below top bar.

⚠️ **Caution**

If you are using a brake bar rack, make certain that when you lock it off, the braking hand rope does not get trapped *below* the top bar (Figure 10-14). It must remain *above* the top bar. Otherwise, the device will become jammed when the rope tension comes onto it.

Evaluation Exercises

◆ **COGNITIVE AND AFFECTIVE EXERCISES** ◆

1. What are the two basic types of ascenders?
2. What are the differences between general-use and personal ascenders?
3. Ascenders are attached to the user's body with _____, connectors made either of _____ or of _____.
4. What is the minimum number of ascenders required for ascending?
5. _____ _____ were the first type of rope grab devices used in ascending.
6. The Prusik hitch will operate more efficiently if the rope it is made of is a _____ diameter than the main line rope to which it is attached.
7. Name three possible modes of failure that could occur when using personal ascenders.

8. When you are ascending with a personal ascender, you must never touch the _____ _____ unless you intend the ascender to come off the rope.
9. List at least three characteristics of a good ascending system.
10. In considering the "three points of attachment" rule, what would be two ways in which a person could be attached?
11. _____ _____ _____ is the safety procedure of tying directly into the main line rope.
12. What is the safety feature used to prevent the feet from slipping out of an ascender sling?
13. To conserve strength during ascending, what parts of the body should be used more than other parts?
14. Usually the most difficult maneuver in ascending occurs when a person has to _____.
15. What kind of procedure would be appropriate if you rappelled to the bottom of a rope and found that the rope did not reach the bottom?

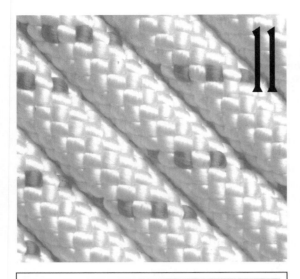

11 The Rope Rescuer

Objectives

At the completion of this chapter, you should be able to:

1. Describe the knowledge and skills needed by a rope rescue technician.
2. Describe what should be the most significant concerns for the rescuer.
3. Describe the low-risk methods to be used in a rescue.
4. Describe the functions of the safety officer.
5. List the important considerations in the care of rescue equipment.
6. Describe the reasons rescuers need to work as a team.
7. List the three levels of rescue operational capability in the NFPA "Standard on Technical Rescue."
8. Describe the role of leadership in a rescue team.
9. Describe the function of span of control in a rescue situation.
10. Describe the role of the incident command system (or incident management system) in rescue.
11. Describe the role of communications in a rescue.
12. Describe the role of preplanning in a rescue.
13. List the steps in planning for the medical aspect of rescue.
14. List the primary medical concerns for the patient in a rescue.

Rope rescue is the providing of aid to those in danger of injury or death in an environment where the use of rope and other related equipment is necessary to perform the rescue safely and successfully. Rope rescue is sometimes called *technical rescue,* and certain aspects of it are sometimes called *high angle rescue* or *vertical rescue.* There are also other related disciplines that may involve some rope rescue skills, but which require additional skills and experience not covered in this book.

Cave rescue, for example, may require rope rescue skills but also involves hazards such as confined space, darkness, chill, and, at times, water hazards. Swift water rescue may involve rope-handling techniques but often requires skills in swimming, boat handling, and knowing the character of running water. Different rope-handling techniques are used in swift water operations to avoid dangers not encountered in high angle work. A seat harness that may be adequate for high angle work could, for example, be dangerous when used in swift water.

ROPE RESCUE SKILLS

A *rope rescue technician* is one who is trained in the necessary skills for rope rescue, has shown that he or she is competent in the skills, and continually trains to maintain these skills. Before the person progresses to qualification in rescue skills, he or she should have evidence of some minimum personal vertical knowledge and skills. He or she should be able to:

◆ Demonstrate the proper use and care of rope.
◆ Demonstrate the proper use and care of other equipment employed in the high angle environment.
◆ Demonstrate the ability to tie correctly and without hesitation the eight knots described in Chapter 6, plus the Munter hitch and the Prusik hitch.
◆ Demonstrate the ability to rig safe and secure anchors.
◆ Demonstrate the ability to safely and confidently belay another person.
◆ Demonstrate the ability to rappel safely, confidently, and under control; the ability to tie off a rappel device to operate safely with hands free of the rope and then return to a safe and controlled rappel; and the ability to operate on the rope with the body in any position, including being inverted.
◆ Demonstrate the ability to ascend safely; the ability to tie correctly, and without hesitation a friction hitch and how to use it, and the uses and limitations of mechanical ascenders; and the ability to safely ascend a fixed rope using both friction hitches and mechanical ascenders.
◆ Demonstrate the ability while on rope to confidently and safely change over from rappelling to ascending and from ascending to rappelling; and the ability to extricate oneself from a jammed rappel device (or similar problem) without the use of a knife.

The rope rescue technician, in addition to personal vertical skills, must train and qualify in other areas before qualifying in the area of rescue. Among these skills are:

◆ Emergency medical skills. Team members should be trained *at least* to a level of DOT first responder (see the section on Medical Considerations for Patients in High Angle Rescue at the end of this chapter).
◆ Team skills. Some examples are litter-handling techniques and lowering and hauling systems.
◆ Communication skills. These include not only the ability to communicate electronically but also the standard voice communications required in specialized team operations such as rescuer lowering and hauling systems.
◆ Other skills depending on the environment, which may include land navigation, snow and ice travel, or survival, for example.

Characteristics of an Effective Rescuer

Although it is difficult to exactly define all the characteristics of an effective rescuer, there tend to be certain traits that do stand out.

One of the most significant traits is the rescuer's concern for the **subject,** the person who is being rescued. The rescuers must realize that the rescue subject is the reason for everyone's being involved in the rescue. This is a human being in distress, a fellow person in physical and, perhaps, emotional pain. A rescuer may contribute to that distress by regarding the rescue subject more as an object than as a person. The rescuers must continually communicate with the rescue subject in their care, even when the subject is unconscious. Hearing is the last sense to go in the unconscious person, and many persons will recall conversations that took place around them when they were unconscious.

Use Low-Risk Methods First

The approach to the subject should be the one that involves the least amount of danger both to the subject and the rescuers.

Some examples of this lower-risk approach include the following:

◆ Always evaluate the situation before approaching it. Hazards to rescuers, depending on the specific environment, could range from hazardous atmospheres, energized wires, falling rocks, to hostile persons.
◆ Don't rush. Rushing into a rescue situation is the sign of an inexperienced rescuer. Rushing causes mistakes that endanger both the rescuers and the subject. Move carefully and meticulously; don't crowd other rescuers.
◆ Choose the least dangerous route to the subject.

◆ In rope rescue, the simplest way of doing the job is usually the most effective way. The more complicated a rescue system is, the greater chance there is of something going wrong.

◆ Instead of setting up operations directly above the subject, where rocks or hardware might fall on him or her (and other rescuers), move slightly off to one side. Keep all nonessential personnel away from the area where they might dislodge rocks and other objects.

◆ Appoint a team *safety officer* to oversee equipment use, anchoring, rigging belays, and personal rappelling, ascending, and seat harness tie-ins. The safety officer should be among the most experienced of the team members and be able to oversee all aspects of the operation.

◆ All rescuers must wear protective gear such as helmets to prevent head injury from falling objects and to lessen injury should the rescuer take a fall. All personnel qualified for high angle operations should be wearing their seat harness so they are ready for any immediate needs.

◆ Before rescue operations begin, set up safety lines. Anyone near the edge must clip into one of them. If there needs to be continued access up and down a steep slope, a securely anchored safety line should be set from top to bottom off to the side from the rescue site.

Prepare for Self-Rescue

Whatever the rescue situation, the rescuer should always keep in mind that anything that can go wrong, *probably will*. Thus, the individual rescuer should always be ready for something to go wrong at any time and be prepared to extricate himself or herself. This preparation should include not only mental preparation but also physical preparation with equipment. Every rope rescuer should carry a small assortment of carabiners, a couple of slings, and either Prusik loops or ascenders for self-extrication from any difficult situation.

Back-Up Other Rescuers

In the same way, each rescuer should be ready at any time to extricate any other rescuer who has gotten into a difficult situation. Whenever any team member is not at work performing a task, all attention should be focused on the activity at hand. Everyone, no matter how intelligent and experienced, has an occasional lapse. All team members should be alert to development of any unsafe condition and be ready to make appropriate corrections.

Commitment to Working as a Team

One of the most important attributes of a qualified high angle person is the commitment to working as part of a team. The difficult and intricate skills of high angle work require teamwork. But it is important that the essential skills be spread throughout the team. If there are only a few people who have the important skills, there is the chance that those few might be absent or disabled when the rescue call comes.

Teams should not think that they are prepared for any rescue if they continually practice on the same rescue tower or same cliff that has convenient places for anchors. The team should make a point of varying their practice sessions in terms of rescue problems and sites. As they become more experienced, they should create practice environments that are deliberately inconvenient and difficult.

CARE OF EQUIPMENT

Just as the sign of good mechanics and carpenters is how they care for their tools, the sign of a competent rope rescuer is evident in the manner in which the technician cares for ropes and equipment. But in the case of vertical gear, it is even more important. For upon these kinds of tools, lives will hang. Among the considerations for avoiding loss and damage to rescue gear include the following:

◆ Do not lay equipment on the edge of a drop. It can easily be kicked or knocked over the edge and be damaged. Or, possibly, cause injury to those working below.

◆ Do not lay equipment on the ground or on the floor. Hardware is easily lost in debris or dirt, and grit damages hardware. Prepare for this when first arriving on the site. Either lay out an equipment tarp or hang a sling on a tree or other beam. All hardware not in use should be placed on the tarp or clipped into the sling.

◆ When working on a vertical face, secure all equipment not in use to your seat harness or gear sling.

◆ Inspect all gear *after* each operation. The time to discover that gear is defective is during inspection time, not during a rescue.

◆ Take all defective gear out of service until it can be repaired.

◆ Belay all lowering and raising of rescue subjects. Any rescuers who request them must be provided with belays.

◆ Ropes need special care (see Chapters 5 and 6).

NFPA STANDARD ON TECHNICAL RESCUE

The *NFPA* standards for rope and related equipment have become an accepted equipment standard. In addition, the fire service has developed performance standards for rope rescuers (see Appendix A, Standards Setting Organizations).

The NFPA "Standard on Operations and Training for Technical Rescue Incidents" (1999 edition) includes the following levels of operational capability in rope rescue: *Awareness.* This level represents a responder with minimum capability. In the course of regular job duties, they may be called upon to respond to, or may be the first on the scene of, a technical rescue incident that can involve search, rescue, and recovery operations.

Operational. This level represents the capability for hazard recognition, equipment use, and techniques necessary to safely and effectively support, and participate in, technical rescue incidents. This can involve search, rescue, and recovery operations but usually under the supervision of technician level personnel.

Technician. This level represents the capability for hazard recognition, equipment use, and techniques necessary to safely and effectively coordinate, perform, and supervise a technical rescue incident. This level can involve search, rescue, and recovery operations.

The NFPA standard on technical rescue allows and encourages departments to develop mutual aid agreements with other organizations where external resources are needed to achieve a desired level of operational capability. Awareness training should prepare responders to know when a situation is beyond their capability and when they need to call for specialized teams with higher levels of capability.

The role of the rope rescue team will vary on department size and the location of the service. Some large urban departments do not see it as reasonable and necessary to train and equip every firefighter to be a rope rescue technician.

What seems to be a common solution in large departments is to treat the rope rescue group as a specialty team, such as is done with many hazardous materials response teams. In this way, the team has its own officers, its own training, and particularly important, its own equipment.

Additional arguments for the creation of a specialized unit include the fact that the members train as a team and respond as a team. With special requirements for membership, there tends to be greater motivation toward skill maintenance and better equipment management.

This specialty team concept may be more difficult to develop in rural areas, where there might be smaller departments and where, often, the team will have to consist of personnel from several different units.

Rope Rescue by Fire Departments

The fire service is increasingly becoming confident and competent with rope rescue skills. This is due in part to the fact that in many areas, prevention and code enforcement has reduced the number of fire calls. In addition, urban areas are being expanded to areas previously considered "backcountry."

Rope Rescue by EMS Units

As with fire departments, the nature of the arrangement for high angle rope rescue skills is often dependent on whether the service is in an urban or rural area. In an urban area, the EMS unit faced with a complicated rope rescue situation might be able to call for a backup from a specialty team, just as they would for a hazardous material or law enforcement problem.

The EMS units may not usually be faced with very specialized rescue situations, such as for high angle, and consequently, will not need the highly specialized training and equipment. However, EMS units in many areas may, in the course of their calls, be routinely faced with special situations such as slope evacuation (see Chapter 14, Slope Evacuation). If the EMS unit expects to deal with such calls, they should be adequately trained and know how to use the gear for slope evacuation. They should also have the awareness training to help them decide when they need to call for specialized teams.

Industrial Rescue

One of the fastest growing specialties for rope rescue is in the industrial environment. This is largely due to regulations on confined space instituted by the U.S. Occupational Health and Safety Administration (OSHA). The OSHA regulations result in part from the large number of casualties in confined space, many of whom were potential rescuers.

Industrial rescue presents special problems for rope rescuers. Many structures present entanglement problems because of interior trays and other obstructions. Rescuers in confined spaces often have to wear breathing apparatus, which present special challenges to movement, endurance, and communications. Confined spaces will often require supplied air hoses for each rescuer, along with retrieval and rescue lines, which result in numerous lines and require an enormous amount of care and coordination to prevent entanglement. The OSHA regulations allow teams to be organized on the industrial site or for employers to use off-site rescue teams. If employers use off-site rescue teams, they must certify that they are properly trained and equipped and capable of a timely response.

Rope Rescue by Law Enforcement

In urban law enforcement, the skills for rope rescue often can be integrated into those experienced tactical teams who already employ high angle tactics for such activities as barricade or hostage operations. The training and equipment are often similar.

In sheriffs' departments, particularly in the western United States, there is often a responsibility for search and rescue. The organizational circumstances will vary. In some cases, paid employees perform the search and rescue tasks. Other departments use a sheriff's auxiliary officer for the team. Some sheriff's offices have a paid member of the department serve as the search and rescue coordinator for the county volunteer teams.

Rope Rescue by Volunteer Search and Rescue Teams

In many areas of the United States, particularly in rural regions, high angle rescue problems have traditionally been handled by volunteer search and rescue (SAR) teams. In the western United States, where this tradition is older and more common, these teams often work under the auspices of the sheriff's department. Often these groups are referred to as *mountain rescue teams* and many are certified by the U.S. Mountain Rescue Association.

In Canada, several provinces, and British Columbia in particular, have a well-entrenched system and tradition of high angle rope rescue teams.

As often happens in EMS and fire, the management of volunteer SAR teams can be different from paid units. The greatest challenge usually comes in two areas: (1) a rapid turnover of personnel and (2) difficulty in motivating members to attend training sessions. The latter problem sometimes can be satisfied with the creation of a certification system. This system requires members to attend a minimum number of training sessions to achieve and maintain their certified status.

Ultimately, motivation may depend on the rate of rescue activity. Those groups answering the greater number of calls are generally the ones that remain viable through the years.

Small Team Management: The Key to Success or Failure

The failure of rope rescue personnel to complete a task in a timely manner can often be laid to the failure of management of the small team situation. The main elements in successful small-team management in rope rescue involve leadership, goals, and strategy.

Leadership

In a rope rescue situation, there should be only one leader. However, there should be several persons on the team who are capable of being a leader when they are needed. The team leader does not have to be a person who can do everything better than everyone else. However, the leader does need the perception of what needs to happen to get the job done and what elements need to be put together to get things to happen in a timely manner.

The rescue leader is not a dictator. A single person is fallible, so the leader must be able to solicit opinions from other experienced members and to use their advice. It is often a good idea in the beginning of an incident for the leader to solicit input from other team members. This helps the leader see any elements he or she may have missed and helps everyone understand what the problem is.

The leader must also be flexible. The rescue situation may change, it may not be what the first call reported it to be, or the first plan may not work. So the leader must be able to develop alternative plans.

The leader must also make certain that team members understand their assignments. One good practice is to have the captain of each group repeat the assignment back to the leader. In some complex assignments, it is useful to write the assignment down on paper for the group captain. This helps make certain that nothing is forgotten.

Goals and Direction

Often, a rope rescue is the solving of a puzzle: how does the team rescue the subject using its rope, hardware, skills, and ingenuity? But for the team to arrive at the answer, it must know the question.

The question, "what are we about to do,?" is presented in the briefing. This briefing should always be given to the personnel who are primarily involved in the operation. They should know what the problem is (subject trapped on ledge), what the overall solution will be (raise the subject with a hauling system), what their unit's task will be (provide an anchor system for the hauling system), and what each person's role will be (have the necessary equipment ready for the riggers).

To best move towards the goal, each task should be assigned to a unit (one or more persons) that has a person in charge who is responsible for seeing the task done and for communicating with the other leaders. Everyone involved in the rescue must have a clear idea of what his or her task is.

Strategy and Allocation of Resources and Time

The focus of the rescue activity, as will be constantly emphasized in this book, must be the subject of the rescue. Thus, the priority must be to have someone take medical charge of the subject and evaluate his or her medical condition as soon as possible.

But while this is happening, all other members of the team should be involved in preparing for the rescue. It will be only in a very large team in which there is someone who has nothing to do.

An effective way to accomplish this task of preparation is to divide the job into specific tasks. Each task is assigned to a subgroup headed by persons responsible to the group leader. Among subgroup tasks would be things such as rigging, anchoring, preparation of the litter, evacuation, crowd control, communications, safety equipment control, and rope management.

The leader, or on-scene coordinator, makes certain that all the actions of the various subgroups are meshing to attain the ultimate goal: the rescue.

Unit Size. One problem encountered in management is that leaders are placed in charge of too many people for them to handle, and they become overwhelmed by making certain that each person completes his or her assigned task. In other words, they do not have a manageable *span of control*. A manageable span of control is generally thought to be from three to five persons. If a task grows in size or complexity so that the span of control is no longer manageable, then the group should be divided into subgroups, each with its own leader.

Putting It Together: A Command System

To make certain that a management system is indeed *manageable* and that it fits with other organizations involved in the activity, there must be some sort of management system. One that is commonly used in North America for the management of emergencies is the ***incident command system (ICS).*** Among many urban fire service personnel, it is known as the *incident management system (IMS).* There are only minor differences between ICS and IMS.

ICS is used for such diverse operations as fires, law enforcement incidents, special events, natural disasters, and hazardous materials spills. It has particular application to incidents involving responses from different agencies or jurisdictions but operates well on incidents as small as auto wrecks.

Figure 11-1 is an example of a rescue operation organized under the incident command system. Most rescue activities occur under the "operations" function of ICS. However, rescuers operating in support capacities would work under the "logistics" function.

One of the most important advantages of the incident command function is its flexibility. The ICS framework can be expanded or contracted depending on the size and nature of the incident. This is particularly important when the response to an incident grows involving many more people. Thus, the organization adapts so that no person gets overextended in his or her span of control.

Safety Officer

In a potentially hazardous activity, a safety officer is a necessity. Because by its nature rope rescue is hazardous, every rope rescue operation should have a safety officer. A safety officer is particularly important in rope rescue because most persons, including leaders, become focused on the complexities of the operation and may not see threats to safety.

In the incident command system, the safety officer is at the level of the incident commander. This means that the safety officer does not get engrossed in other activities such as operations, so he or she can stand back and be objective about any threats to safety. The safety officer must have the right to stop any operation he or she sees as a threat to safety. There should be a safety officer at every geographical location, or sector, where a potentially hazardous operation is taking place.

Some teams rotate the position of safety officer through their members on scene. However, it is essential that the safety officer be an experienced individual who thoroughly understands equipment, rigging, and

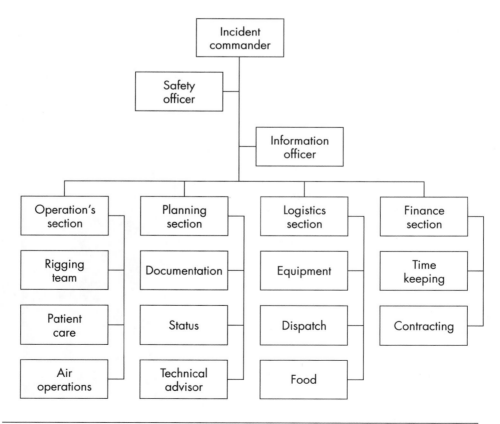

FIGURE 11-1

Incident command system for example incident.

rescue techniques. They must be able to instantly look at a situation and know if something is incorrect. They must always be able to stand back with an objective viewpoint. They must never be pulled into the operation itself.

Safety officers are responsible for monitoring:

♦ Hazards, including hazardous atmospheres and falling debris.
♦ Personal safety equipment, including helmets, gloves, and breathing apparatus.
♦ Rescue rigging, including belays, anchors, rope padding, and unlocked carabiners.
♦ Personal rigging, including seat harnesses, locked carabiners, and knots tied correctly.

Communications

In the high angle rope rescue environment, communications are extremely important for the coordination of the operation and for the safety of all involved. But the conditions in the high angle environment often make normal communications very difficult.

Other sections of this manual describe some standard voice communications used in rope work. But in many high angle situations, the ability to hear voices is severely restricted by distances, by the wind, and by other noise factors, such as falling water.

The solution to this problem may seem to be to use electronic communications, but conventional radio systems are subject to disruption by physical conditions at the rescue site. Typical problems involve the interruption of radio transmission by confined spaces, rock overhangs, structures, and intervening ridgelines. Sometimes the situation can be improved by having all team members switch from "repeater" channels to "simplex" (direct radio-to-radio communications). The simplex communications can avoid the problem of barriers between the communicators and the repeater site. But for simplex to work, the communicators need to be in the same area or working line of sight of one another.

If the team is going to be working with more than one frequency, then there must be a systematic way to keep track of radio channels. If there is no system for channels, the result will be confusion as individuals try to find which channel is usable. At the least, the result is embarrassment; at worst, it will be life-threatening chaos.

If every radio has the same frequency setup, then channel numbers can be used to indicate a frequency ("all units switch to channel 11"). If the frequency setup varies among the radios, then the frequency name must be used ("all units switch to state law mutual aid"). In any case, either the channels must be labeled on the radio, or a frequency sheet must be kept with the radios at all times.

One common problem encountered by rescue team members relates to the management of a radio on a vertical face where both hands tend to be occupied with other activities.

One approach that has been successfully employed by some teams for short-range communications is the voice-actuated headset. Among possible drawbacks are that the units may not fit well with some helmet designs, and they can be put out of commission in close quarters where elements of the system can get snagged or torn off.

One solution that is being increasingly used is a special radio harness that fits across the chest (Figure 11-2). It takes only a simple, short hand motion to key the mike. Although the radio is close at hand, it is also protected and out of the way of much of the activity involved during rope work. By being next to the body, the chest harness keeps radio batteries warm and extends their performance in cold weather.

A nonelectronic alternative is the use of whistle blasts for communications. Obviously these are limited in the degree of information that can be communicated but they are often audible where nothing else works. The exact form of these whistle communications has to be worked out and used in practice beforehand.

One more alternative type of communications exists. This is an even more primitive one but one that might be necessary in certain critical situations. It is what might be called *digital* communication, or the use of a yes-or-no signal.

This kind of system might be called for when a subject is high on a cliff or far across a valley. These are

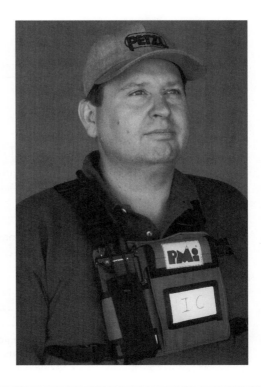

FIGURE 11-2
Radio chest harness.

situations where normal two-way communication is impossible and where the subject does not have a radio.

This digital system works with the rescuers employing a loud hailer to ask questions that allow a "yes" or "no" answer. The subject replies with a flashlight blink or a raised arm.

The Human Side of Communications. Often the greatest detriment to good communication is not an electronic or mechanical failure, but the communicators themselves. In high angle situations, it is particularly essential to communicate in a clear, concise, and specific manner. Does "right" and "left," for example, mean as you face the cliff or building or as you face away from it? In river and stream operations, "river right" is on your right going down stream, while "river left" is on the left going down stream.

It is important to reduce the command vocabulary to as few words as possible and use only those words that are clear, concise, and have few syllables. One should also use the same words for specific actions. As noted in the sections on lowering and hauling systems, the only word for cessation of action is "stop!" Another word should never be substituted, such as "whoa," which could easily be mistaken for *"slow," or even worse,* for *"go."*

Preplanning

Preplanning is the invisible part of rescue. But it is the essential element that can determine whether the rescue operation succeeds in a fairly smooth manner or whether it is cursed with confusion and delay.

A preplan should include the following:

◆ Local rescue needs.
◆ Who has jurisdictional and operational responsibility for rescue in a local area.
◆ How a rescue group fits in and who they report to.
◆ What and who initiates call-out and how it proceeds.
◆ The command structure on scene.
◆ Communications, including frequencies.
◆ How the group relates to other organizations.
◆ Medical control and protocols.
◆ Standardized procedures in approach to the rescue.
◆ How the rescue group conforms to regulations and standards.

The preplan can also provide essential legal documentation to show compliance with regulations and in case of liability challenges. However, it is important that if your group has written operating guidelines, it must adhere to those guidelines.

If you have written guidelines, but do not adhere to them, and then something goes wrong, you could be in as much legal trouble as if you did not have the guidelines. For this reason, it is essential that guidelines be realistic and appropriate to your rescue demands and team personnel.

For example, it may seem idealistic to have the most stringent qualifications for members allowed on rescue operations. But if only a few team members can pass these qualifications, then the high-minded criteria are counterproductive. Or, if the operating guidelines are too specific on techniques to be used, then rescuers may be restricted in dealing with unexpected and changing situations.

Guidelines should be written with the intent of providing to rescuers realistic information on goals, procedures, and safety, while at the same time leaving as much flexibility on techniques they use for achieving those goals.

Most of all, guidelines must be written in an understandable manner and as brief as possible. Otherwise, they will not be read or understood.

MEDICAL CONSIDERATIONS FOR PATIENTS IN HIGH ANGLE RESCUE

The ultimate purpose of performing a high angle rescue is the patient, the rescue subject. Most persons who need rescue will have either injuries or medical problems. Proper medical care and packaging of the patient by rescuers will play a major role in deciding patient survival and recovery. Whether the patient is harmed further by the rescue and if he or she survives the injuries are completely in the hands of the rescue team and medical personnel at the incident site.

This section is a general outline to help the rescue team with developing its approach to the patient in the high angle rescue situation. For more detailed information on the medical care for the rescue patient, consult programs that include rescue medicine and prolonged and delayed patient transportation in their medical programs.

Preparation

The preparation for care of the severely injured patient in the high angle situation is as vital to successful rescue as time spent learning the mechanics of rope rescue systems. There are some essential considerations the rescue and medical personnel should plan for prior to the incident.

Training

Not every person involved in rescue can be qualified at the highest possible medical level. So the rescue team should try to develop resource persons for medical care in the rope rescue environment. The personnel used in this role should have advanced training, under medical control, and practice in advanced skills.

Medical Equipment and Supplies

The process of creating a medical kit for the high angle environment requires careful thought and advance planning. The kit should be appropriate to the provider's level of certification or license. The kit must be usable while hanging in vertical situations and for difficult terrain and weather. The kit must be complete, yet pared down to minimums for weight and packaging considerations.

Experience

Personnel entering the high angle environment for medical care must be extremely familiar with high angle rescue. But they also must be familiar with performing their medical skills in that environment.

Assessment and Interventions

The following section reviews areas that are the most frequent patient concerns in the high angle environment. It also suggests possible interventions by categories of certification by the National Registry of Emergency Medical Technicians (each level being able to perform all of the interventions of the levels below them). A complete discussion of medical care in the high angle environment cannot be fully covered in this book. The following discussion is aimed at the first responder level, with intervention suggestions targeted at each level.

Airway and Breathing Considerations

Airway and breathing are the most crucial concerns in any emergency medical situation. But many patients in high angle rescues have airway and breathing problems. If a patient has an airway blocked by the back of the tongue, by blood, tissue, or vomit, or if his or her breathing stops, he or she will die in a few minutes.

If the patient is unconscious, there must be provisions to maintain the airway. Current medical practice in the United States requires that a medical attendant be with any patient at risk for airway or breathing difficulties. In addition, any patient secured into spinal precautions must have an attendant to intervene in case of airway or breathing compromise. Some questions that must be asked about the patient's airway and breathing status, prior to packaging and moving the patient, include:

- Does the patient have a clear airway?
- Do you need to maintain the airway during the rescue?
- Does the patient have objects in the mouth (gum, tobacco, dentures) that need to be removed?
- Is the patient vomiting or does he or she have the potential for vomiting?
- How will you clear the vomitus during the course of the rescue so that the patient does not aspirate it?
- Is the subject breathing spontaneously?
- Will you be able to monitor breathing throughout the rescue?
- Will you need to assist the patient's breathing before and during rescue?

Airway and Breathing Interventions

Interventions at the First Responder Level

- Open airway with jaw thrust.
- Provide mouth-to-mask ventilations or ventilations via flow restricted oxygen powered (FROP) ventilatory device.
- Administer oxygen via nasal cannula or nonrebreather mask.
- Suction patient's airway with manual suction device.

Interventions at the EMT-Basic Level

- Maintain airway with an airway adjunct (oral or nasal pharyngeal airway).
- Provide ventilations via bag-valve mask (BVM).
- Provide oxygen via assisted ventilations with a BVM.
- Provide suction via manual or powered suction device.

Interventions at the EMT-I Level

- Maintain an open airway with a pharyngeal/esophageal airway device (PEAD), such as the Combi-Tube or PTL devices.
- Provide ventilations via bag-valve PEAD.
- Provide suction through PEAD device.

Interventions at the EMT-Paramedic Level

- Maintain an open airway with endotracheal (ET) intubation, cricothyrotomy device, or surgical cricothyrotomy.
- Facilitate endotracheal intubation with paralytic agents.
- Provide ventilation via bag-valve ET (or cricothyrotomy).
- Provide endotracheal suctioning.
- Administer airway and breathing medication to promote better airway status or improve ventilation status. Additionally, administer Inapsine for the prevention of vomiting during the evacuation.

Circulation

Circulation refers to the continual movement (perfusion) of the blood to the tissues of the body and preventing its loss. A major concern is control of bleeding and blood replacement. The patient must be assessed carefully for signs of shock.

Signs of shock include: increased pulse rate, poor pulses in the extremities, poor skin color and temperature in the extremities, altered mental status, and reduced blood pressure (a late sign of shock).

Some questions that must be asked about circulatory status prior to packaging and moving the patient include:

- Does the subject have a pulse?
- Will you be able to monitor the pulse during the rescue operation?
- Is CPR necessary?

- Will CPR be possible during the rescue operation?
- Does the patient show signs of shock?
- What must be immediately done to treat for shock?
- What rescue procedures will increase or reduce the possibility of shock?
- Is there bleeding and how can you stop it?

Circulatory Interventions
Interventions at the First Responder Level
- Administration of high-flow oxygen.
- Elevate patient's feet at a 15-degree incline.
- Apply direct pressure, pressure points, and tourniquets for external bleeding control.
- Perform cardiopulmonary resuscitation (CPR).

Interventions at the EMT-Basic Level
- Assess oxygenation with pulse oximeter.
- Apply pneumatic antishock garment.
- Apply traction splints to control blood loss from femur fracture.

Interventions at the EMT-I Level. Administer balanced salt solution through large bore peripheral intravenous catheter.

Interventions at the EMT-Paramedic Level
- Administer crystalloid, colloid, or blood products through peripheral or central venous lines.
- Administer circulatory medication to promote better perfusion status.

Head and Spine Considerations

Permanent disabilities to the patient (paraplegia and quadriplegia) could be the result of mishandling by rescuers. Signs of spinal injury include mechanism of injury, numbness and tingling, inability to move an extremity, flaccid muscle tone, shock, absent or difficulty in breathing, and back or neck pain. If the patient has sustained a mechanism of injury that makes spinal injury a possibility, the complete line of the spine from the head to the hips must be immobilized in line. A cervical collar by itself is not effective.

Ambulance personnel traditionally employ rigid backboards, but these are very uncomfortable for long periods and may cause the patient to squirm and counteract the purpose of the immobilization. For long transport periods, a "conforming backboard" such as the KED or the Oregon spine splint may provide better patient comfort and, in the long run, better immobilization. However, the conforming backboard must be properly secured with the patient in the litter so there is no movement either lengthwise or side to side. Any patient who has trauma above the clavicles, trauma with periods of unconsciousness, serious orthopedic injury (that is, femur fracture, pelvis fracture, humerus fracture, and so on), or has fallen 15 feet or greater must be placed into full spinal immobilization. Head trauma is also a source of long-term disability and is quite common in the high angle patient.

Head-trauma patients are prone to nausea, vomiting, altered mental status, and in critical injuries hypertension and bradycardia. Signs of head trauma include: mechanism of injury, periods of unconsciousness, inadequate respirations, skull fracture, facial injury, head cuts, lacerations or bruises, amnesia, and ataxia. Some questions that must be asked about the patient's head and spine status, prior to packaging and moving the patient, include:

- Is there a possibility of head or spinal injury?
- Do you need to perform spinal precautions before you move the patient?
- Should you secure the patient to a spinal immobilization device before placing him or her in a litter for transport?
- Are you prepared to assist the patient's breathing and circulation during evacuation?

Head and Spine Interventions
Interventions at the First Responder Level
- Place patient into full spinal precautions.
- Administer oxygen via nasal cannula or nonrebreather mask.

Interventions at the EMT-Basic Level. Apply traction splints and full spinal immobilization.

Interventions at the EMT-I Level. Administer balanced salt solution through large bore peripheral intravenous catheter.

Interventions at the EMT-Paramedic Level
- Administer crystalloid, colloid, or blood products through peripheral or central venous lines.
- Administer Mannitol to reduce head trauma complications, Solu-medrol to reduce spinal cord disability, and Inapsine to prevent vomiting prior to packaging. Also administer medications for circulatory and respiratory support.

Evaluation Exercises

◆ COGNITIVE AND AFFECTIVE EXERCISES ◆

1. Name seven personal skills that a rope rescue technician should have.
2. Name the reason for everyone being involved in rescue.
3. Name six examples of lower risk approach to use when approaching a rescue subject.
4. List the three levels of operational capability in the NFPA "standard on technical rescue."

5. A manageable span of control is generally thought to be from _____ to _____ persons.

6. What is the standardized management system commonly used for all types of emergencies?

7. In the incident command system, the safety officer operates at what level?

8. Name three things in rope rescue that the safety officer is responsible for monitoring.

9. List seven things that should be included in a preplan.

10. Name three essential considerations rescue and medical personnel should plan for prior to the incident.

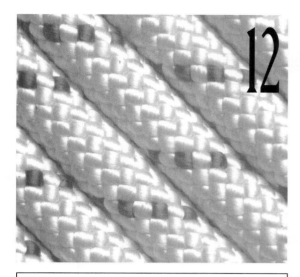

12 Rescue Belaying

◆ *Prerequisites*

Before attempting the activities described in this chapter, you must have demonstrated that you can properly:

1. Use and care for rope.
2. Use and care for other equipment employed in the high angle environment.
3. Tie correctly, and without hesitation, the eight knots described in Chapter 6.
4. Apply the principles of anchoring and rig a safe and secure anchor.
5. Apply the principles of belaying and safely and confidently belay another person using either a Munter hitch or personal belay device.
6. Apply the principles of rappelling: rappel safely, confidently, and under control; tie off the rappel device to operate hands free of the rope and then return to a safe and controlled rappel.
7. Ascend safely; tie correctly, and without hesitation, a friction hitch and demonstrate how to use it; describe what the uses and limitations of mechanical ascenders are; and have the ability to safely ascend a fixed rope using either friction hitches or mechanical ascenders.
8. While on rope, safely change over from rappelling to ascending and from ascending to rappelling; have the ability to extricate oneself from a jammed rappel device (or similar problem) without the use of a knife.

Key Terms

Load-Releasing Hitch (LR Hitch) Any hitch that can sustain major forces without tightening and, with the tension still on it, can be untied and released under control. Among these are the Mariner's hitch, which uses webbing, and the LR hitch, which uses accessory cord.

Prusik Minding Pulley A pulley with specially shaped side plates that help manage Prusiks.

Tandem Prusik Belay Two triple-wrap Prusik hitches of differing lengths set a few inches apart in a series on a belay rope in order to grab the rope in case of main line failure or to hold the load while adjusting the lowering and raising system.

Objectives ▼

At the completion of this chapter, you should be able to:

1. Tie a load-releasing hitch.
2. Rig a tandem Prusik belay system.
3. Operate a tandem Prusik belay system.
4. Rig a Prusik minding pulley.
5. Operate a Prusik minding pulley.

RESCUE BELAYS

Any time you are belaying more than a one-person load, you will need greater control than is available with one-person belay devices.

Some one-person belay systems may work for more than one person if conditions are just right. For example, when a rope runs over an edge, the added friction can help in controlling the load. But there are many varying conditions, such as the belayer's grip strength, that make it difficult to predict how reliable the belay will be. Consequently, some of these devices and techniques are not going to reliably catch the load if there is more than one person's weight on it. In addition, most one-person belay devices are not designed by the manufacturer to catch more than one person's body weight.

Brake Belays

There are a variety of belay systems that can be used for rescue loads, but there are disadvantages to each. Some rope rescue systems use two ropes running through a braking device, such as a brake tube. Other systems employ two brakes, each controlling a rope that is attached to the rescue load such as a litter (see Chapter 15, High Angle Lowering). Two commonly used braking devices in these two rope systems are the brake bar rack and the brake tube. These two brake systems are designed so that each lowering device backs up the other. In essence, each braking device belays for the other one.

There are distinct disadvantages in any rope rescue system. For example, in a two-brake system, the persons operating the brakes must be well coordinated and they must be alert for a failure of the other system.

Another drawback relating to such braking systems relates to "reversibility." When using most brake systems, it is difficult to instantly change direction from a lowering to a haul. For example, it is near impossible to pull rope back through a brake bar rack with most bars engaged. With a brake tube, it is possible to reverse direction, although it may be somewhat difficult in some conditions. If the operation is only going to be a straight lowering, then "reversibility" may not be a concern.

The dilemma with rescue belaying is that there is no system guaranteed to work every time and under all conditions.

The Tandem Prusik Belay

One system that has been shown to work under many rescue belay conditions is the *tandem Prusik belay* system.

The tandem Prusik belay system consists of two triple-wrapped Prusiks anchored securely and placed in line on the belay rope (Figure 12-1). This system is designed so that in case of failure, the Prusiks grab the

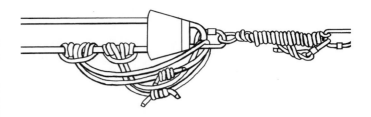

FIGURE 12-1
Tandem Prusik belay system with load-releasing hitch.

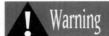

Tandem Prusik belays will not work in all rescue conditions. Prusiks can slip on ropes that are muddy or icy. A Prusik-type belay may not be appropriate in a hazardous environment where a hang up could cause severe injury or death.

The success of a tandem Prusik belay very much depends on the interaction of the material in the Prusik hitch with the rope material. Before relying on a tandem Prusik belay, test the materials you are using for their holding power.

rope. When rigged correctly, they should have a clutching action. This means that instead of an abrupt shock load, as might occur with metal camming devices, there is a more gradual stopping of the load.

Under certain conditions, the Prusiks may not catch. For example, under icy or muddy conditions, the belay rope may slip though the Prusiks without them catching.

The tandem Prusiks can fail under other conditions. For example, in high impact situations, tandem Prusiks can cause the belay line to fail by pinching it until the rope separates. Also, the Prusik material itself can fail, particularly if the wrong size or type of Prusik cord is used to build the tandem three-wrap Prusik belay system.

The success of a tandem Prusik belay very much depends on the interaction of the Prusik cord material with the rope material. To make certain that it will work when needed, you should test your Prusik cord with the rope you will be using in a rescue situation.

The second part of the Prusik belay system is some means of releasing the Prusiks should they jam. There are several means of load releasing, but the one commonly used is the *load releasing hitch (LR hitch)*.

The load-releasing hitch serves two primary purposes:
1. If the belay line becomes accidentally loaded, the LR hitch can be used to shift the load back to the main line.

2. The load-releasing hitch has some shock absorbing capacity.

In addition, the LR hitch can be used for some non-belay situations such as changing over from a raising system to a lowering system or from a lowering system to a raising system.

Constructing the Tandem Prusik Belay System

To assure that the tandem Prusik belay system works as designed, you will need to adhere closely to specifications.

The Tandem Prusiks. The following procedure assumes that you are using ½-inch (12.7-mm) rope for your belay line:

1. Using 3 m (118 inches) of 8 or 9 mm nylon climber's accessory cord, cut 2 lengths:
   - 65 inches (1.65 m).
   - 53 inches (1.35 m).
2. Tie the ends of each of the lengths together into a loop using a grapevine ("double fisherman's" knot), forming two independent loops.
3. Tension both loops. There should be 1¼ inch of tails after tensioning.
4. Place each Prusik with three wraps on the rope.
5. Position the longer of the two Prusiks going toward the load.
6. Position the shorter of the two Prusiks between the first Prusik and the anchor.
7. Wrap both Prusiks in the same configuration on the rope. Position them so the double fisherman's knots are between the Prusiks and the carabiner.
8. Dress the Prusik hitches (see Chapter 6, Knots, on dressing knots). There should be about 4 inches (10 cm) of space between them when both are fully extended from their anchor. The Prusiks should not bump one another except when raising and using a *Prusik minding pulley.*
9. At the anchor, clip the Prusiks into a large locking carabiner. Clip the long Prusik in first, then the shorter one.

The Load-Releasing Hitch (Figure 12-2)

1. Cut about 25 to 30 feet (about 7.5 to 10 m) of 9 mm kernmantle accessory cord.
2. Double the cord.
3. Secure the two loose ends together by tying them into a simple figure 8 knot (Figure 12-2, *A*).
4. Using the middle of the cord, rig a doubled Munter hitch onto the anchor carabiner leaving a short bight. Lock the carabiner (Figure 12-2, *B*).
5. Pull out about 6 inches (15 cm) of the bight from the Munter hitch (Figure 12-2, *C*).
6. Clip the tandem Prusik (load) carabiner onto this bight. Lock the carabiner (Figure 12-2, *D*).
7. Wrap both sides of the cord three times around the bight (bundle of rope) between the two carabiners. Do this wrap smoothly and tightly (Figure 12-2, *E*).

8. To complete the LR hitch, pull the loose ends with the figure 8 knot through the bight left between the bundle of wrapped cords and the load end carabiner clipped into the bight (Figure 12-2, *F*). This load end carabiner is where the tandem Prusiks or other load is attached to the LR hitch.
9. As final security, tie off (or block) the doubled cord with an overhand knot around the bundle. Chain the excess (Figure 12-2, *G*).

Releasing the Load-Releasing Hitch. If the Prusiks jam or become loaded and you need slack, do the following (Figure 12-3):
1. Untie the overhand knot.
2. Pull out the end of the line with the figure 8 knot (Figure 12-3, *A*).
3. Hold one hand tightly over the three wraps.
4. Carefully pull the cord out of the bight (bundle) between the two carabiners (Figure 12-3, *B*).
5. If there is not enough load to pull slack through the hitch, slowly remove a wrap from around the coils. As you remove a lower wrap, hold the upper wrap with your hand (Figure 12-3, *C*).
6. Take off only as much wrap as necessary for the cord to slide and allow slack (Figure 12-3, *D*).

Operating (tending) the Tandem Prusiks. The tandem Prusiks should be tended by a belayer wearing gloves. Keep the following points in mind (Figure 12-4):
- Before a lowering or raising operation, the belayer must inspect the Prusiks to make certain they have been tied correctly, they are neat and dressed, and are the appropriate distance apart.
- The belayer must make certain that the Prusiks are tight on the rope. If at any time during the operation, the Prusiks should become loose, the belayer must immediately call for the operation to "stop!"
- To check for tightness, the belayer should listen for the sound caused between the inside of the Prusik and the sheath of the belay rope as the rope slides through. If there is no sound, the Prusiks will have to be retightened.

⚠ Warning

1. Never release an LR hitch until you are certain the load can be successfully transferred to some other system or will reach the ground before all the cord in the LR hitch is let out.
2. Be certain you will be able to control the load as you release it. In extreme load situations, it might be a two-or-more person job.
3. Keep your fingers, hair, and clothing from getting caught in the Munter hitch.

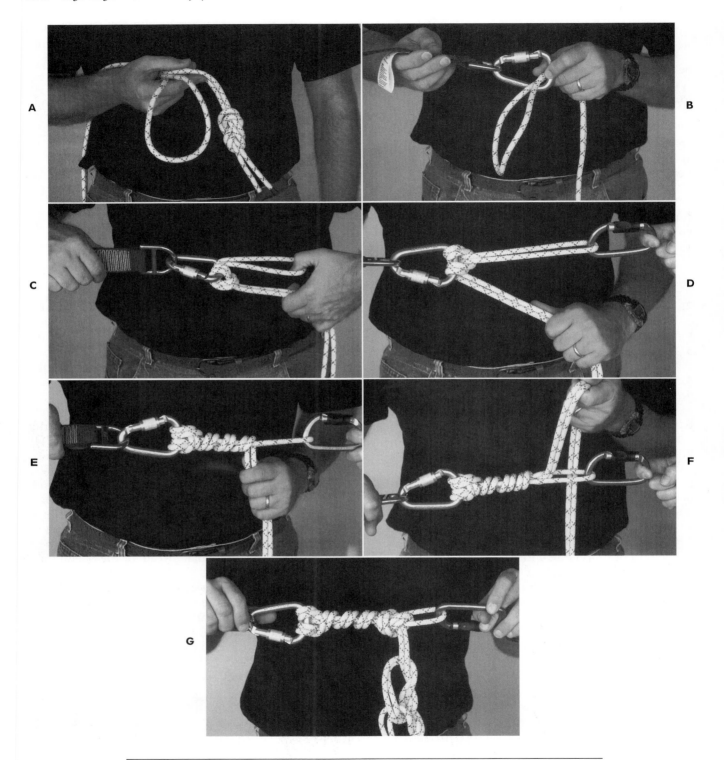

FIGURE 12-2
Constructing the load-releasing hitch.

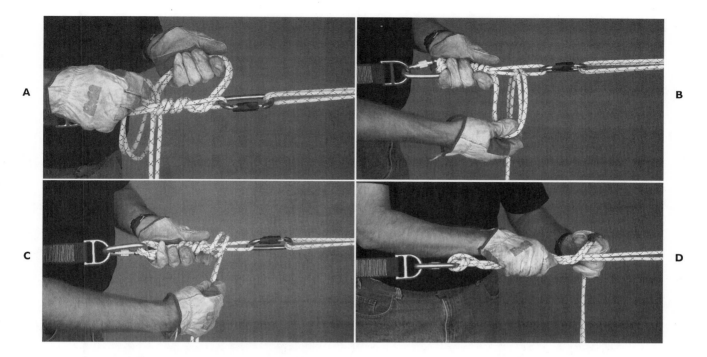

FIGURE 12-3
Releasing the load-releasing hitch.

The basic approach is to keep one hand cupped on the Prusiks as the rope is pulled in or let out. Use the other hand to take up or pull out the belay slack and feel the tension to decide if more or less rope is needed.

Giving Slack or Feeding Out the Belay in a Lower Operation (Figure 12-4)

1. Start with your hands together (Figure 12-4, *A*).
2. Have one hand cupped on the Prusiks to hold them in place and prevent them from coming tight when you don't want them to. This is the *Prusik hand.*
3. With a twist of the wrist of the other hand (the *feeling hand*), pull out about 18 to 24 inches of the rope through the Prusiks (Figure 12-4, *B*).
4. This will form a shallow S curve in your feeling hand between the Prusik hand and the belayed load.
5. As the belay begins to come tight, the S curve will flatten out, thus straightening out your wrist (Figure 12-4, *C*).
6. This is your signal to slide the feeling hand back up against the Prusik hand and again pull out another foot or two of slack forming the S in your feeling hand (Figure 12-4, *D*).
7. Make certain the Prusiks remain snug during the operation. You should be able to hear the Prusiks sliding on the rope (Figure 12-4, *E*).

Taking in Slack or Belaying a Raise Operation

1. Hold the Prusiks in your Prusik hand in a way that keeps them almost but not completely snug against their anchor (Figure 12-4, *F*).

> **⚠ Warning**
>
> Belayers must be alert at all times. Failures often occur with no warning.
> While belaying with tandem Prusiks, do not allow the rope to contact any part of your body other than your hands. You could be injured if the belay activates.

2. Pull any available slack through the Prusiks by applying tension to the belay line with the feeling hand (Figure 12-4, *G*).
3. As slack develops, remove it by sliding the Prusiks forward toward the load with the Prusik hand and keeping tension behind the hitch with the feeling hand (Figure 12-4, *H*).
4. Be careful not to run the Prusiks too tight because it is possible the load can suddenly change direction and the Prusiks would quickly jam. This would require the use of the LR hitch or some other way of unloading them, if the load direction could not be changed back to a raise.

The Prusik Minding Pulley (PMP) The Prusik minding pulley (PMP) is sometimes used in raising operations to help operate the Prusiks (Figure 12-5). The tandem Prusiks, when rigged correctly, catch on the edge of the pulley side plates as the rope enters the pulley. The side plates of the PMP are designed to keep the Prusik knots sliding on the rope and not to

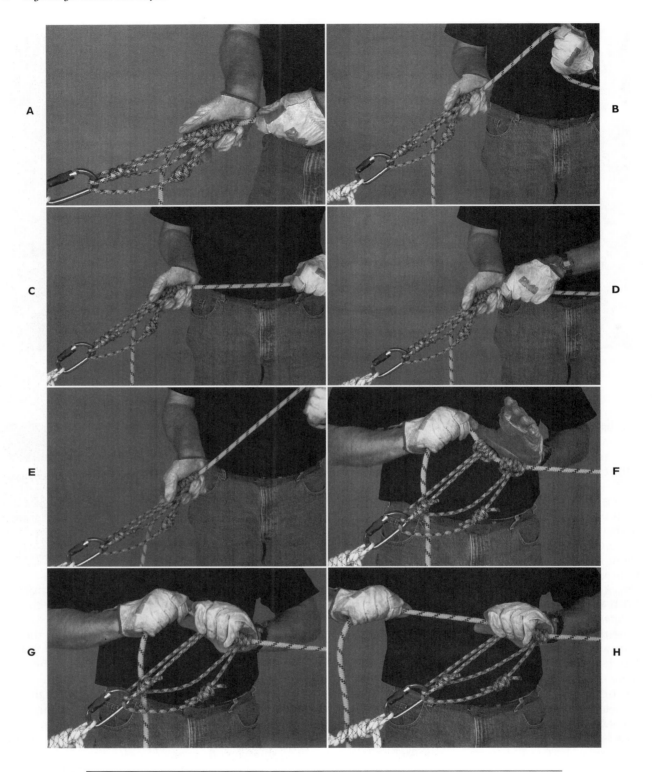

FIGURE 12-4
A-E, Giving slack with the tandem Prusik belay. **F-H,** Taking up slack.

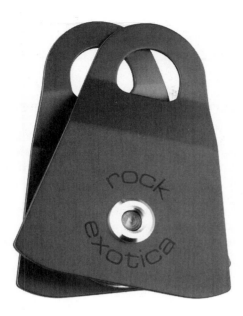

FIGURE 12-5
The Prusik minding pulley.

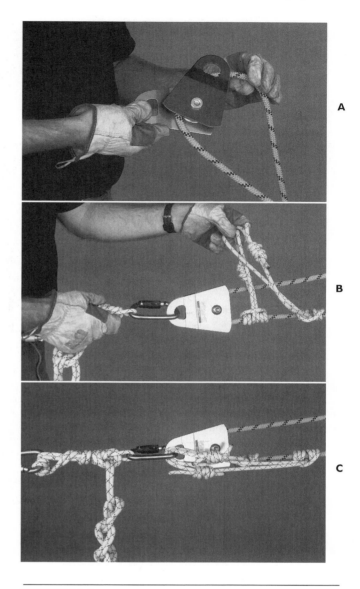

FIGURE 12-6
Rigging the Prusik minding pulley.

bind in the pulley. The PMP is designed so that should there be a failure, the tandem Prusiks will grasp the rope and catch the load.

As with any Prusik safety situation, the Prusiks must be tight enough to grasp if the rope should slip through them. The Prusik minding pulley should have a tender who makes certain that the Prusiks remain tight and properly dressed.

Rigging the Prusik minding pulley (Figure 12-6)
1. Rig the PMP in the same carabiner with the Prusiks.
2. Run one end of the belay rope through the pulley and attach the Prusiks.
3. Rig the Prusiks next to the carabiner spine, with the PMP next to them.
4. To do this, attach the load to the side of the belay rope that has the Prusiks.
5. The near Prusik should only be a finger width or so below the side plate when the Prusik is attached to the pulley's carabiner and slightly snugged up.
6. The far Prusik should be about 4 finger widths below that. More distance makes the system very inefficient.

Operating the Prusik minding pulley (Figure 12-7)
1. As the load is hauled, pull the belay rope through the PMP. Do this by keeping one hand on the rope feeding into the pulley (side with the load) as you pull the rope on the opposite side with your other hand. The Prusiks should "tend" themselves.
2. Your hand grasping the rope on the load side will move toward the Prusik knots.

3. If you have tied the Prusiks so the cord is very loose and the Prusiks have to travel a distance before setting, there may be the danger of shock loading the system. Then, as your hand reaches the Prusik knots, grasp them. Slide them back toward the load to remove slack.
4. Any time you have the opportunity (such as during pauses in hauling), retighten the Prusiks.
5. For best efficiency, keep the angle between the ropes going in and out of the PMP as close to 0 degrees as possible.
6. The belayer must remain within reach of the PMP whenever it is being operated.

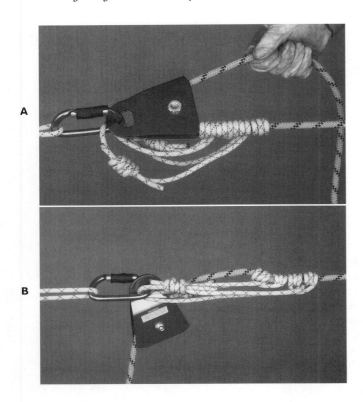

A

B

FIGURE 12-7
Operating the Prusik minding pulley.

Evaluation Exercises

◆ COGNITIVE AND AFFECTIVE EXERCISES ◆

1. What are the two primary problems in using a two-line braking system, such as brake bar racks or brake tubes in a belay situation?
2. What are the primary components of a tandem Prusik belay system?
3. Name three conditions in which a Prusik belay system might fail.
4. What is the main purpose of the load-releasing hitch?
5. What four things should one check for when inspecting a Prusik belay system?

▼ PSYCHOMOTOR EXERCISES ▼

6. Correctly tie a load-releasing hitch.
7. Correctly rig a tandem Prusik belay system.
8. Correctly operate a tandem Prusik belay system.
9. Correctly rig a Prusik minding pulley.
10. Correctly operate a Prusik minding pulley.

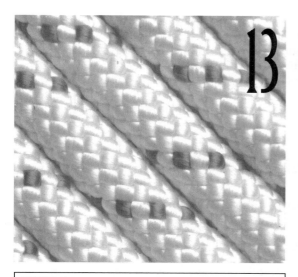

13 Pickoff Rescue Techniques

Key Terms

Pickoff Rescue A rescue in the high angle environment involving an uninjured or slightly injured subject in which a single rescuer usually has direct physical contact with the subject and in which a litter is not initially used in the rescue operation.

◆ *Prerequisites*

Before attempting the activities described in this chapter, you must have demonstrated that you can properly:

1. Use and care for rope.
2. Use and care for other equipment employed in the high angle environment.
3. Tie correctly the eight knots described in Chapter 6.
4. Apply the principles of anchoring and rig a safe and secure anchor.
5. Apply the principles of belaying and safely belay another person using either a Munter hitch or personal belay device.
6. Apply the principles of rappelling: rappel safely and under control; tie off the rappel device to operate hands free of the rope and then return to a safe and controlled rappel.
7. Apply the principles of ascending: tie correctly, and without hesitation, a Prusik hitch and know how to use it; comprehend the uses and limitations of mechanical ascenders; confidently and safely ascend a fixed rope using either friction hitches or mechanical ascenders; confidently and safely change over both from rappelling to ascending and from ascending to rappelling; extricate yourself from a jammed rappel device (or similar problem).

Objectives

At the completion of this chapter, you should be able to:

1. Describe the kinds of conditions in which pickoff rescue techniques might be employed.
2. List the skills and equipment that are required for pickoff rescue techniques.
3. Discuss the rescue considerations and priorities involved in the following pickoff rescue situations: (1) subject wearing seat harness, (2) subject not wearing seat harness, (3) unconscious subject, and (4) hostile and combative subject.
4. Discuss the medical concerns and priorities involved in the pickoff rescue.
5. Safely and efficiently perform a pickoff rescue of a person wearing a seat harness.
6. Securely tie a hasty seat onto a subject harness and either a hasty seat harness with a chest harness or a hasty body harness.
7. Safely and efficiently perform a pickoff rescue of a person not wearing a seat harness.

USING THE PICKOFF RESCUE

Pickoff rescue techniques are procedures in the high angle environment in which a single rescuer has direct physical contact with a rescue subject to remove the person from a hazardous situation. Other persons may be involved in the rescue in support capacities or to perform such vital tasks as belaying. Teamwork and good communications remain essential in pickoff rescue techniques.

Pickoff rescue techniques are usually done without the use of a litter. They often involve the attaching of the rescue subject directly to the rescuer's rappel system. Then the rescuer rappels or is lowered to control the body weights of both rescuer and rescue subject. In certain advanced techniques (not covered in this chapter), rescuers might ascend the rope with the subject attached to his or her ascending system. Also, he or she may lower the subject using a braking device suspended on rope or attached to midface anchors while the rescuer remains in position on the rope.

Pickoff rescue is generally only performed when the rescue subject is uninjured or only slightly injured. It is extremely difficult for only one person without a stretcher to rescue a seriously injured subject without making the injuries worse and incurring potential liability as a result of negligence.

Therefore it is absolutely essential that pickoff rescuers evaluate and stabilize subjects in terms of injury before moving them. The only exception to this is when there is an immediate threat to life such as hazardous atmosphere, explosion, or fire.

A pickoff rescuer, to be able to competently evaluate a subject and treat for injury, should have emergency medical training at least to the level of DOT First Responder and preferably to the level of Emergency Medical Technician or higher.

Pickoff techniques require that the rescuer must begin *above* the subject and then rappel or be lowered to the area of the subject.

Pickoff Rescue Situations

Pickoff rescue techniques might be appropriate where:
- It is appropriate for only one person to perform the rescue.
- There is a shortage of personnel and/or resources.
- The urgency of the situation means there is no time to await additional personnel.
- The benefits of a pickoff rescue outweigh the risks involved.

The need for pickoff rescue might occur in any of the following situations:
- A firefighter's interior exit is blocked during a fireground operation, there is no time to set up a ladder, and there is no opportunity for self-rescue.
- A high-rise window cleaner has had an equipment malfunction and is stranded on the side of a building out of reach of ladders.
- A construction worker has become stranded on scaffolding.
- A potential suicide has climbed to an exposed area to jump but is hesitating.
- A rock climber has fallen and is only slightly injured but needs assistance in getting off the face.
- A sightseer or picnicker has slipped onto a ledge and cannot go up or down.
- A hiker has blundered into dangerously steep terrain and is unable to move because of the danger of falling.

Teamwork and Communications

The term *pickoff* rescue usually involves only one rescuer in direct contact with the person in distress. This, however, does not mean that other rescuers will be kept from the operation. It will be a safer and more efficient operation if other skilled and knowledgeable persons are involved in essential tasks such as belaying, lowering or raising, spotting, and communications.

Also, if the rescue subject is to be rappelled or lowered to the ground, then essential personnel will be needed at the arrival spot to attend to the medical needs of the subject. Several people may also be needed to perform a litter evacuation to an ambulance or other medical care.

Skills and Equipment Required in Pickoff Rescue

In the performance of pickoff rescue techniques, there are often several sets of rope-work skills being performed simultaneously. There are also several different kinds of equipment being used at once.

The success or failure of the rescue will depend on choosing the appropriate system for the rescue. An absolute knowledge of the equipment and the ability to perform the skills are necessary. These abilities only come with constant practice of the skills required for efficient use of the equipment. This expertise and experience will determine whether you can pull it off or if you will be pulled off.

Pickoff rescue procedures can mean multiple ropes in use at once, along with more connecting lines, slings, and equipment. This means an increased challenge in rope and equipment management. The rescuer must have the experience and knowledge to be aware of all the rope, equipment, and webbing in use at once to keep it from damage from rope cross, to

> **! Warning**
>
> Pickoff rescues should only be performed by those specialists who have been trained in the technique and who have demonstrated they have the prerequisites required for training for the technique.

keep it from tangling, and to be able to manipulate without hesitation the specific line when needed.

Anchors and other equipment used in pickoff techniques must be able to withstand the combined weight of two persons plus any shock loading that may be involved.

Before dropping your rope to rappel, you must size up the situation. If the subject is barely hanging on, hitting him or her with the rope could knock him or her off the face. Also, if the rope is close to a panicky subject, he or she could grab your rope, stopping your rappel or causing injury or death to you and/or the rescue subject.

One possible solution is to take the bagged rope with you, attached to your person (see the section Protecting the Rappel Rope that is Below You on page 120, Chapter 9, Rappelling, along with the warning about attaching a bagged rope to yourself). Always make certain there is enough rope in the bag for you to reach the ground.

Your choice of rappel device and how you use it are critical to your ability to safely perform a pickoff rescue. The weight of two persons will be very difficult to control with a single wrapped figure 8. If you decide to use a large figure 8, you will need increased friction, such as double wrapping.

Another problem with using a figure 8 is that it tends to twist the rappel rope, complicating your rope control problems. For greater control, consider using the brake bar rack, which will give you the ability to vary control according to the load.

The Belay Question

In some pickoff rescue situations, a belay may be desirable but it may not always be feasible. In fact, there may be some situations where a belay could encumber the operations or even endanger the involved individuals.

For example, if there were a situation where both the rescuer and the rescue subject each had their own rope, what would happen if both persons were also belayed with additional separate ropes? There would now be a situation in which *four* ropes were coming together. There would be the real possibility of rope tangle and possible damage from rope cross. The problem of rope management would increase as rescuers tried to decide which line went to specific harness tie-in points and how each line would affect other lines as angles changed with the positions of the people involved.

Some situations where a belay might be required could include:

◆ Beginner practice.
◆ Prolonged operations where fatigue is a factor.
◆ Exposure to objective hazards such as falling debris.

The question of a belay is one that will have to be answered through intelligent decision making and based on the specific situations and people involved. That kind of intelligent decision making can only come with the experience gained through practice

with the techniques in differing environments and under varying conditions.

Medical Considerations

The focus of patient medical treatment in the pickoff situation is better described as *assessment* rather than *treatment*. The subject of a pickoff is one usually *excluded* from treatment rather than *included*. The most important feature of medical considerations in the pickoff subject is one of assessment. The subject suitable for pickoff technique would be one with minor injuries, without risk of disability or life threat.

The assessment of the subject should be thorough and complete. Until such assessment is concluded, the subject should have manual spinal immobilization in place.

The format for the assessment of the subject is very simple (Box 13-1).

Box 13-1 Assessment Format

First the following vital signs are checked:
◆ Level of consciousness (AVPU)
◆ General appearance
◆ Airway

AIRWAY
◆ Does the subject have a clear airway?
◆ Do you need to maintain the airway during the rescue?
◆ Does the patient have objects in the mouth such as gum, tobacco, and dentures, which need to be removed?
◆ Is the patient vomiting or does he or she have the potential for vomiting?
◆ How will you clear the vomitus during the course of the rescue so that he or she does not aspirate it?

BREATHING
◆ Is the subject breathing spontaneously?
◆ Will you be able to monitor breathing during the course of the rescue?
◆ Will you need to perform rescue breathing before and during rescue?

CIRCULATION
◆ Does the subject have a pulse?
◆ Will you be able to monitor the pulse during the rescue operation?
◆ Is CPR necessary?
◆ Will it be possible during the rescue operation?
◆ Does the subject show signs of shock?
◆ What must be immediately done to treat for shock?
◆ What rescue procedures will increase or reduce the possibility of shock?
◆ Is there life-threatening bleeding? How can you stop it?
◆ Does the subject have potential life-threatening bleeding?

SPINAL INJURY
Many emergencies in the vertical environment relate to spinal injury:
◆ Is there a possibility of spinal injury?
◆ Do you have to maintain spinal precautions while moving the patient?
◆ Should you secure the subject to a spinal immobilization device before moving?

If the answer to any of the questions in Box 13-1 is that the subject does have a problem with this area of patient assessment, would it be wiser to begin treatment of the subject and move the subject with a litter evacuation rather than a pickoff rescue?

If the subject has very minor injuries (small lacerations, minor musculoskeletal injuries, and so on), it may be advisable to move the subject with a pickoff.

If there is no immediate threat to life, then it may be wise to use an organized rescue team with proper spinal precautions in a litter. Erring on the side of patient care is always the best rule of thumb. For many groups, it takes just as long to perform a safe pickoff as it does to perform a litter evacuation (because this is what many of us practice the most).

Unless immediate life-threatening environmental factors prevent you from doing so, the preceding medical considerations must be made as a minimum *before* moving a rescue subject and must *continue* during the course of the rescue.

RESCUE OF A PERSON WEARING A SEAT HARNESS

This situation assumes that the rescue subject is wearing a secure seat harness that will keep him or her relatively upright during the procedure. See Box 13-2 for required equipment for this rescue.

Pickoff Rescue Practice System

In the beginning practice of pickoff rescue techniques, it is essential that the person acting as practice rescue subject be in a stable position and only a short distance off the ground so there is a minimum possibility of injury from falling.

As the practice sessions move farther off the ground, the practice subject should either be initially tethered or belayed until in a secure position.

Procedure for Performing a Pickoff Rescue of a Subject Wearing Seat Harness (Figure 13-1)

1. Station a practice rescue subject wearing a seat harness in a position of minimum exposure so that he or she would not be injured by a fall. For example, put the person on a low cliff ledge, in the first-floor window of a practice building, or on a structural member, such as a low beam of a bridge or tower.
2. At the top, rig anchor(s) for your main line rope. Your rope will have to be off to the side of the rescue subject with this horizontal distance a compromise between the following: (1) being far away enough so that your rope will not knock rocks or other debris onto the subject, and you can be out of reach if the subject attempts to grab you, and (2) being close enough so that you can easily pendulum over to the subject. Make certain that when the two of you load the system, it does not severely shock load your rope and anchors, and when you pendulum back, it does not excessively abrade software (ropes and webbing), or loosen debris or rock. Remember that the anchors may be subjected to shock loading and they will be loading from different directions. If the pendulum causes a loaded rope to rub unprotected across a sharp edge, the rope may be cut.
3. Wear a sewn, manufactured seat harness with leg and thigh supports. Clip a locking carabiner into the seat harness' front tie-in point.
4. Attach a rappel device to the seat harness carabiner that has both variable friction and enough control to handle the weight of two persons.* Lock the carabiner on the rappel device.

---

*The brake bar rack qualifies on both points. If this is not available, double wrap a large figure 8 with ears. Use the figure 8 only if you know from experience that you can control the combined weight of yourself and the rescue subject. (See the section, Gaining Extra Friction from the Figure 8 Descender on page 105, Chapter 9, Rappelling.) Be aware, however, that this will complicate your personal rigging. If you plan to use this technique in pickoff rescue, practice it beforehand.

Box 13-2 Required Equipment for Rescue of Person Wearing a Seat Harness

- One main line rope with adequate safety factor for a two-person load.
- One sewn, manufactured seat harness with thigh and leg supports for rescuer.
- One rappel device with enough friction to handle the weight of two persons and, preferably, with variable friction.
- Two large, locking carabiners (in addition to locking carabiner already in rescuer's seat harness tie-in point).
- One short (approximately 2 feet) sling with loop in both ends, or an adjustable rescue pickoff strap that will support one person's weight with an adequate safety factor.

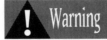 **Warning**

During pickoff rescue procedures, anchors, rope, hardware, and personnel are subjected to sudden increased loads, shock loading, and loads that may come from directions different from those originally anticipated, therefore:

1. Anchors must be rigged for increased and multidirectional loading.
2. Carabiners must be locked, aligned in manner of function, and monitored so that they remain in manner of function.
3. Ropes and slings must have an adequate safety factor.
4. Rescuers must be prepared for sudden increased weight and for providing extra friction on rappel devices.

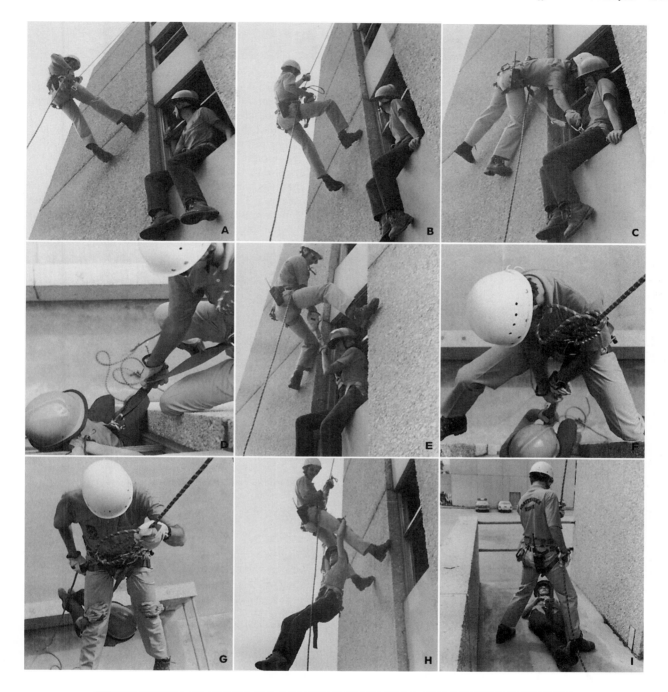

FIGURE 13-1

Procedure for performing pickoff rescue of subject.

5. Clip a large locking carabiner onto one end of the rescue sling. For the moment, leave this first carabiner unlocked. Clip the second large locking carabiner into the other end of the sling. With the sling and first carabiner attached, clip this second carabiner *directly into the rappel device tie-in point* so that the weight of the rescue subject will be taken *directly on the rappel device. Do not clip this rescue sling directly into your seat harness* (Figure 13-2).

6. Lock the carabiner that connects the rescue sling to the rappel device tie-in point. Do not yet lock the carabiner that is in the opposite end of the sling.

7. Begin your rappel and the approach to the rescue subject. As you get close to the individual, rappel slowly or stop just out of the subject's reach. You must now do two things simultaneously (Figure 13-1, *A*): (1) size up the situation (Box 13-3) and (2) communicate with the subject (Box 13-4).

Warning

When performing pickoff rescue techniques, *do not* clip any attachments to support the weight of the rescue subject directly into your own seat harness, primarily for the following reasons:

◆ It can result in painful and, perhaps, damaging pressure on the body of the rescuer, particularly in the groin area.
◆ It will stress a seat harness in an unnatural manner, perhaps resulting in damage and potential failure.

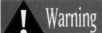 **Warning**

Anytime you go over the edge in a rappel, but *particularly in a rescue*, check for loose personal items or vertical gear. All items and gear must be secured so they will not fall out of pockets, packs, or gear slings.

Other than causing injury to the rescue subject or other rescuers, you may lose an essential piece of equipment just when you need it the most.

Always do a last minute *safety check*. Make certain harness buckles are correctly secured and that all carabiners are locked and aligned in the correct manner of function. Be certain that knots are tied correctly and anchors are secure. Check for any loose clothing or hair that might be drawn into the descender. Be sure that your helmet is secure.

Box 13-3 Sizing up the Situation

WHAT ARE THE PHYSICAL CIRCUMSTANCES?

Is the subject secure or where he or she is in immediate danger of falling?
Is there loose debris above the subject that might be dislodged by your rope?

WHAT ARE THE EMOTIONAL CIRCUMSTANCES?

Is the subject hostile to you?
Is the subject about to leap onto you?
Will the subject follow directions?
Is the subject comfortable in the high angle environment?
Is the subject experienced with high angle work so he or she can assist in the procedure?

WHAT IS THE INITIAL ASSESSMENT OF THE SUBJECT'S MEDICAL NEEDS?

Is the patient conscious and alert?
Is the patient breathing?
Is there uncontrolled bleeding?
Is there a mechanism for spinal injury?
What are the obvious injuries?
What are the patient's physical complaints?

Box 13-4 Communicating with the Subject

◆ Reassure.
◆ Tell the subject who you are.
◆ Tell the subject exactly what you plan to do.
◆ Ask if the subject is injured.
◆ Describe in detail how you will do the rescue.
◆ Describe to the subject how he or she can help:
  1. Do not move until told to.
  2. Do not grab anything unless told to.

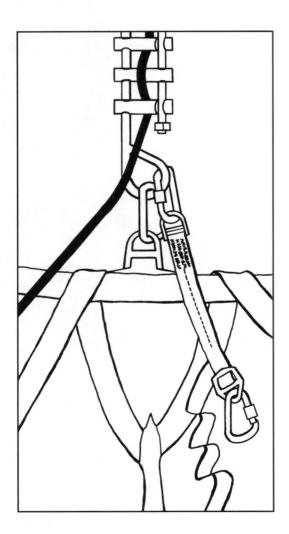

FIGURE 13-2
Arrangement of rescue sling.

8. Stop and tie off your rappel device with yourself about 2 feet above the level of the subject. *Always above.* If you are initially too high to reach the subject, you can always unlock and rappel down a few more inches. But if you are too low, you may not be able to get back up to him or her easily and quickly (Figure 13-1, *B*).

9. Make certain that the subject stays put. If it is feasible, the best position for him or her is to be sitting. While you are talking with him or her, begin your initial medical evaluation.

10. Check the condition of the subject's harness. Make certain that the harness is both undamaged and is correctly fastened. Take the large locking carabiner that is at the bottom of the sling attached to your rappel system. Lean over and clip it directly into the subject's seat harness tie-in point. *Do not clip into any parts of the harness not meant to support the load of the wearer.* If you are too high, rappel down only the distance needed to make the connection. *Avoid slack in the rescue sling* (Figure 13-1, *C*).

11. As soon as you have clipped the rescue sling into the main part of his or her harness, immediately lock the carabiner. You now have the subject secured to your system. If you are using an adjustable pick-off sling, take up all the slack in the sling (Figure 13-1, *D*).

13. Brace with your legs spread wide and your feet against the wall (Figure 13-1, *E*).

14. Tell the subject to do the following:
    ◆ If the subject is not sitting and it is possible to do so, tell him or her to sit.
    ◆ Have the subject place his or her legs together between yours (Figure 13-1, *F*).
    ◆ Have the subject place his or her hands on your legs for support (Figure 13-1, *G*).
    ◆ As the subject holds onto your legs, have him or her very slowly swing down between your legs until his or her weight comes onto the sling. While the subject is doing this, direct him or her, reassure him or her, and brace so that you and the subject do not slip (Figure 13-1, *H*).
    ◆ Tell the subject to hold onto the sling to steady himself or herself. The final position of the subject should be facing you. If the face is not vertical or overhanging, have the subject face the wall to protect head, back, and buttocks from being bumped and bruised. His or her head should be below your buttocks; his or her full weight onto the sling and the rappel device. The sling should remain between your legs during the remainder of the procedure.

15. When the subject's full weight is on the sling and he or she has stabilized, unlock your rappel device and begin to rappel very slowly.

16. Keep the subject below you and between your legs. If you are close enough to the cliff or building face, fend away from it with your feet.

17. As you approach the ground, tell the subject that you want him or her to lie down as his or her body touches the ground. You will straddle the subject.

18. When the subject is lying full on the ground, you are straddling him or her, and you have slack in your rappel device, disconnect the subject from your system by unclipping him or her from the short sling (Figure 13-1, *I*).

19. Remove your rappel device from the rope.

RESCUE OF A SUBJECT NOT WEARING A SEAT HARNESS

Placing a Manufactured Seat Harness on a Subject

There is a good chance that the subject involved in a pickoff rescue will not be wearing a seat harness. In such a case, the rescue procedures are essentially the same, except that the rescuer must either place onto the subject a sewn, manufactured harness or tie a hasty harness onto him or her.

In itself, this placing of the harness for rescue can be a very difficult process. The rescuer will probably be hanging on a rope at a difficult angle (perhaps even upside down), dealing with a frightened and, perhaps, injured subject, under difficult environmental conditions.

Because of these difficulties, the student rescuer should first practice a pickoff rescue on a subject wearing a seat harness and then try a pickoff placing a seat harness on the subject.

A sewn, manufactured harness is preferable to a tied one if one is available, with the following considerations:
    ◆ If the subject is in immediate danger of falling, stabilize him or her as soon as possible by tying the subject off to a secure point.
    ◆ The harness should be designed so that it can be placed onto the subject with as little disruption as possible. In particular, it should be done without the subject's becoming unbalanced by having to step into the harness.
    ◆ It must be quick and easy to put on. It should not have a multitude of buckles, snaps, and adjustments.

Placing a Tied Seat Harness on a Subject

There are a variety of tied harnesses that might be placed on a subject for a pickoff rescue procedure, but the following considerations should be made in deciding which ones to use:
    ◆ The harness should be tied with a minimum of physical disruption to the subject.
    ◆ The harness should be quick and easy to tie under difficult conditions.
    ◆ The harness should be self-adjusting.

The Hasty Seat Harness

The hasty seat harness is one type of seat harness that can be placed on a subject easily with a minimum of disruption. It is created from a length of tubular webbing ranging from 10 to 15 feet long, depending on the size of the subject. The webbing is tied into a continuous loop using a ring bend (water knot) backed up before the rescuer begins the rappel.

Tying the Hasty Seat Harness (Figure 13-3)

1. Approach the subject from behind. Place the loop across the subject's shoulder so that the sides of the loop hang down along his or her side and the top of the loop runs across the back of the subject's neck.
2. With both hands, reach around the sides and under the arms of the subject and the vertically hanging sides of the loop. *From this point until you have the subject clipped into your system you must keep your arms in this position around the subject in case he or she should slip or fall.*
3. Now reach down with either or both hands. Go between the subject's legs *from the front* and grasp the bottom of the loop. Take the loop firmly in both hands.
4. Pull the loop back through the subject's legs and up toward the front of his or her waist.
5. As you pull the loop up through his or her legs, let the top section of the loop running across the subject's shoulders fall down the back. If necessary, you can help this along with your chin or head.
6. Continue pulling on the lower end of the loop. As you pull the slack out of the loop from behind, the webbing will slide down your arms and past your hands to form the harness.
7. To cinch down the webbing, take a loop in each hand and pull each one to an opposite side so that the webbing is contoured around the subject's body. Make certain that the webbing remains taut.
8. Bring the two loops back to the center together and clip a locking carabiner across them together.

A Rescue Chest Harness

Figure 13-4 illustrates a rescue chest harness. This chest harness *must not be used alone.* It must be used in combination with a rescue seat harness, such as the hasty harness. It may also be used with a sewn, manufactured seat harness to help hold a subject upright.

Tying the Rescue Chest Harness.

Figure 13-5 illustrates the tying of a quick chest harness. This can be used in combination with a seat harness for a pickoff rescue procedure.

1. Take a continuous loop of webbing tied with a ring bend (water knot) backed up with an overhand knot.
2. Twist the loop into a figure 8.

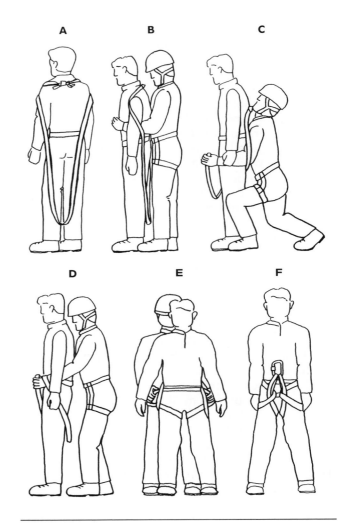

FIGURE 13-3
Tying of hasty seat harness.

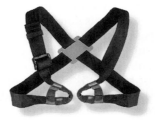

FIGURE 13-4
Manufactured chest harness.

3. Lay the loop across the subject's back with the loop crossing on the back at armpit height.
4. One at a time, put the subject's arms through each loop.
5. Bring each loop to the center of the chest.

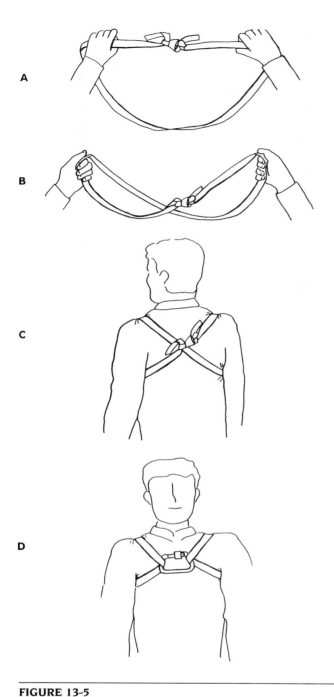

FIGURE 13-5

Tying rescue chest harness.

6. Clip the loops together with a carabiner. Or, if the harness is too loose, pull one loop through the other and clench it down. Clip a carabiner through the long loop.

7. Make certain that the seat and chest system is equalized. Neither the seat nor chest harness should take the full load. They should be stable so that the subject does not "accordion" when the load is applied at acute angles.

Combining the Rescue Chest Harness into the System

8. Clip the carabiner from the chest harness into the end of the rescue loop (where you have previously clipped the carabiner for the seat harness). *Do not clip the two carabiners together* so you will be able to make adjustments in either the seat harness or the chest harness.

RESCUE OF AN UNCONSCIOUS SUBJECT
Medical Considerations

An unconscious subject should be rescued using a litter unless there are overriding considerations such as an immediate threat to life.

In addition to the primary survey for the ABCs *(airway, breathing, circulation)*, there are particular medical considerations associated with an unconscious subject:

- ◆ If there is a particular threat of airway blockage, there must be continued attention to keeping it clear.
- ◆ If unconsciousness is due to trauma (such as a fall) or the cause is unknown, it must be assumed that the subject has a spinal cord injury, and there must be spine immobilization.

Because the subject may not be able to describe his or her injuries, there may be potential hidden injuries, such as fractures.

When a person becomes unconscious, hearing is the last sense to go. So, always talk positively with an unconscious subject, even though you suspect he or she might not be able to hear. This communication may eventually elicit a response and may prevent him or her from becoming combative.

If a litter cannot be used for an unconscious subject, then special pickoff rescue techniques may be employed.

An unconscious subject will not be able to hold himself or herself upright or fend off from the face of a building or cliff. So there must be special considerations for a rescue harness used for an unconscious person:

- ◆ The use of a full-body harness that is sewn and manufactured.
- ◆ The addition of a chest harness to the hasty seat harness.
- ◆ A tied full-body harness.

Requirements for a full-body, combination seat-chest harness include the following:

- ◆ It must hold the subject upright.
- ◆ It must prevent the subject from sliding out.
- ◆ It must be simple to put on, without large numbers of buckles or knots.
- ◆ It must be usable in adverse conditions (cold, dark, wind, and so on).

Evaluation Exercises

◆ COGNITIVE AND AFFECTIVE EXERCISES ◆

1. Describe the general medical condition of the subject when most pickoff rescues are performed.
2. Unless there is an immediate threat to life such as hazardous atmosphere, explosion, or fire, what should a pickoff rescuer do before moving the rescue subject?
3. Name three general circumstances in which a pickoff rescue technique might be appropriate.
4. Give two reasons why before dropping your rope to rappel for a pickoff rescue, you must size up the situation.
5. What is one possible way to keep your rappel rope secure in a pickoff situation?
6. The most important feature of medical considerations in the pickoff subject is one of _____.

7. List the minimum equipment required for the rescue of a subject wearing a seat harness.
8. In a pickoff rescue, where should the end of the pickoff strap that is closest to the rescuer be attached?
9. After you have assembled the gear and rigged for a pickoff rescue, what is the one thing you should always do before going over the edge?
10. What should be your position in relationship to the subject when you stop and tie off your rappel device to perform a pickoff rescue?
11. In addition to the primary survey for the ABCs (airway, breathing, circulation), what are the two major medical considerations associated with an unconscious subject in a pickoff rescue?
12. Name three requirements for a full-body, combination seat and chest harness used for the subject in a pickoff rescue.

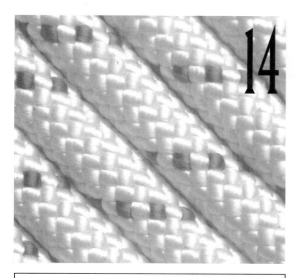

14 Slope Evacuation

Key Terms

Brakeman Person who operates the braking device that controls the rate of descent of a litter in slope evacuation.

Counter Balance Haul System A procedure for hauling that uses a 1:1 ratio and a haul team that moves in a direction opposite to the load.

Haul Team The group of persons who provide the power to raise the load.

Litter Captain The person in slope evacuation who manages the litter team and coordinates the litter movement with other members of the rescue team.

Litter Attendant An individual who helps control the litter or attends to a patient's medical needs during a slope evacuation rescue. Also known as *litter tender.*

Packaging The placing of a rescue subject in a litter to consider primary medical problems and physically stabilize the subject in the litter.

Progress Capture Device (PCD) A rope grab device, general-use ascender or hitch, placed on the rope in a hauling system to prevent the rope (and load) from unintentionally slipping back down as the haul system is reset. The PCD is also commonly referred to as the *ratchet.*

Rope Handler The person in a lowering operation who assists the brakeman with rope management.

◆ Prerequisites

Before attempting the activities described in this chapter, you must have demonstrated that you can properly:

1. Use and care for rope.
2. Use and care for other equipment employed in the high angle environment.
3. Tie correctly, and without hesitation, the eight knots described in Chapter 6.
4. Apply the principles of anchoring and rig a safe and secure anchor.
5. Apply the principles of belaying and safely belay a person using either a Munter hitch or belay plate.
6. Apply the principles of rappelling: rappel safely and under control; tie off the rappel device to operate hands free of the rope, and the return to a safe and controlled rappel.
7. Apply the principles of ascending: tie correctly, and without hesitation, a Prusik hitch and know how to use it; comprehend the uses and limitations of mechanical ascenders; confidently and safely change over both from rappelling to ascending and from ascending to rappelling; and extricate yourself from a jammed rappel device (or similar problem).

Objectives

At the completion of this chapter, you should be able to:

1. Describe what steps are involved in a slope evacuation.
2. List some examples of slope evacuation application areas.
3. Given a selection of equipment, choose what would be used in a slope evacuation system.
4. Describe what considerations are involved in the medical care of a subject during a slope evacuation.
5. Describe what steps are involved in the packaging of a subject for slope evacuation, in both summer and winter conditions.
6. Discuss the functions of the following: litter tenders, litter captain, brakeman, and haul team; then provide examples of their interaction.
7. Discuss the functions of rope, braking systems, safety cam, haul cam, and pulleys in a slope evacuation.
8. List several examples of communications concerns during an evacuation.
9. Identify the elements of a hauling system in slope evacuation.
10. Explain the principles and application of a 1:1 hauling system, a counterbalance haul system, and a 2:1 haul system.
11. Act as a litter tender in a slope evacuation.

Key Terms—cont'd

Slope Evacuation The movement of a rescue subject over terrain so rugged or angled that it requires the litter to be attached to a rope for safety and control. In slope evacuation, most of the weight is taken by the litter tenders. Slope evacuation is also known as *low angle evacuation*.

Tree Wrap A technique of running a rope around a tree trunk to create friction for a braking effect in a litter lowering.

Hauling System A procedure for hauling where the force input into the system is roughly the same as the load being hauled.

Objectives—cont'd

At the completion of this chapter, you should be able to:

12. Package a rescue subject for slope evacuation, following local protocol or the guidelines set forth in this text.
13. Construct the rigging for a litter in a slope evacuation.
14. Rig the braking and belay systems and the safety cam for slope evacuation.
15. Repeat from memory voice communications used in slope evacuation.
16. Act as a member of a haul team in slope evacuation.
17. Act as a rope handler in slope evacuation.
18. Act as a brakeman in slope evacuation.
19. Construct a 1:1 or a counterbalance hauling system for slope evacuation.

THE NEED FOR SLOPE EVACUATION

The term *slope evacuation* may not provoke the image of excitement or challenge that comes with *vertical or high angle rescue*. But it is in many areas the most common type of rope rescue performed by emergency service personnel.

It is often the type of rescue with which emergency service personnel experience the most problems. Many people are inexperienced with slope evacuation and are unaware of the potential problems involved. Consequently, many rescuers are often poorly equipped and trained for the problems and hazards encountered in slope rescue.

The division of where *slope evacuation* ends and *high angle evacuation* begins is not always easily defined. But the essential differences are in the way that the litter and the rescue personnel are used (Box 14-1).

Examples of Slope (Low Angle) Evacuation

Slope evacuation includes any inclined or rugged area over which a litter must be carried and where it is difficult or dangerous to do so without the assistance of a rope (Box 14-2). Under some conditions slope evacuation is also called *broken ground evacuation*.

Elements of Slope Evacuation

A slope evacuation will usually consist of the following elements (Figure 14-1).

The Litter

Requirements

Strength. The litter must be sufficient to withstand stresses of supporting weight of the rescue subject and rescuers while being supported by rope. The litter must also be able to withstand blows from contact

Box 14-1 Differences between Slope Evacuation and High Angle Evacuation

SLOPE EVACUATION
- Litter tenders have most of their weight on the ground.
- There may be three or more litter tenders.
- Rope is attached to one end of the litter.

HIGH ANGLE EVACUATION
- Litter tenders have their weight supported by litter and rope.
- Weight of litter is supported by rope.
- At most, there are two **litter attendants**.
- Litter hangs from vertical ropes.

Box 14-2 Examples of Slope (Low Angle) Evacuation

- Road cuts and fills.
- Loose rocky slopes ("scree" or talus).
- Hills.
- Snow and icy slopes.
- Rugged, broken terrain.
- Urban stairs.
- Industrial environments.

with rocks, trees, and other hard objects. It must help protect the patient.

Tie-in Points. Tie-in points are used to attach ropes, rescuers, and for patient protection. The tie-in points must be easily accessible and have high strength.

Rigid or Semi-rigid. The litter must be rigid or semi-rigid to protect the patient and aid in handling. The litter must also maintain an envelope of protection for the patient despite stresses and unequal loading (Box 14-3).

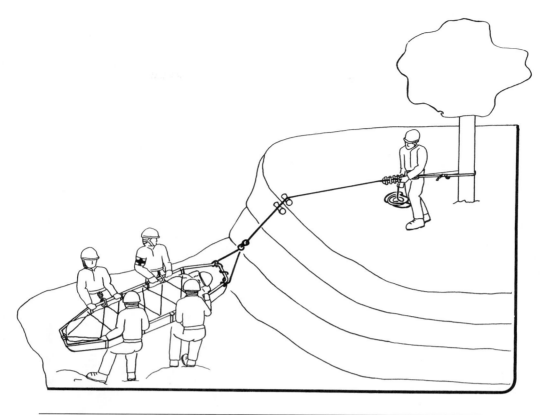

FIGURE 14-1

Elements of slope evacuation.

Anchor System

A safe and secure anchor system is a critical part of any slope evacuation (see Chapter 7, Anchoring, for a review of the criteria for safe and secure anchors).

Rope

To maintain greater control over the operation, most rescuers prefer a rope with a minimum of stretch, such as static (low-stretch) kernmantle. The rope is usually attached to the head end of the litter. Up slope from the litter the rope is attached as in below.

If Litter Is Being Lowered Down-slope

The Rope Runs Through a Braking System. The rope running through a braking system imparts friction to the rope to make the descent of the litter easily controlled by one person known as the **brakeman.**

The Brakeman. The brakeman controls the braking system and the rate of descent of the litter.

If Litter Has to Be Raised Up Slope.
If the litter has to be raised up slope, the rope runs through the hauling system.

The Hauling System. The hauling system enables the litter to be easily raised by the **haul team,** who are rescuers that provide the force to safely and efficiently raise the litter up slope.

 Box 14-3 Examples of Litters for Slope Evacuation

- ◆ Wire basket "stokes-" type litters.
- ◆ Plastic basket litters.
- ◆ Semi-rigid (SKED, Reeves).

Progress Capture Device (PCD). The progress capture device prevents the rope (and litter) from inadvertently sliding back down slope.

Whether Litter Is Being Raised or Lowered

Litter Tenders. The litter tender, depending on slope angle, patient weight, severity of terrain system capacity, and overall risk-benefit, may range from three to six people. Because more people tend to get in each other's way and add weight, there should only be as many attendants as it takes to comfortably and safely do the job. Litter attendants connect themselves to the litter with the litter tie-ins.

Litter tie-ins. The litter tenders are better able to maintain footing and stability by being tied into the litter. They lean back onto the tie-ins, putting their weight onto the litter. In turn, their weight is taken by the rope, braking device, and anchors. Depending on the medical condition of the rescue subject, there may also be a medical attendant.

Medical Attendant. Usually the member of the team with the highest level of medical training and experience is the medical attendant. Depending on the condition of the patient, the medical attendant may be a litter tender or may have to devote full attention to the patient.

Litter Rigging for Slope Evacuation

There are two commonly used techniques for attaching the rope to the head of the litter.

Tying the Main Line Rope Directly to the Head of the Litter

If the length of the slope evacuation is only one rope length and the rope will not have to be detached from the litter during the operation, then the main line rope may be tied directly onto the head of the litter.

Figure 14-2 illustrates a typical system for attaching a main line rope to the head of a litter for slope evacuation. This attachment consists of a very large loop created at the end of the rope by a figure 8 follow through knot. This loop around the end rail of the litter can be created with the following procedure:

1. At the end of the rope that is to be attached to the litter, measure off twice the distance between outspread arms (a total of approximately 10 feet).
2. At this point into the rope, tie a simple figure 8 knot.
3. Run the rope around the head rail of the litter several times so that it evenly spreads the forces along the rail.
4. Bring the end of the rope back to the simple figure 8 knot.
5. Tie a figure 8 follow through knot using the simple figure 8 knot. *Be certain to leave several inches of tail past the knot.*
6. Use this tail to tie a double overhand backup knot (barrel knot).
7. Center the knots so that both legs of the loops pull evenly onto the litter rail.

> ### ⚠ Warning
>
> When connecting a main line lowering or hauling rope to the end rail of a litter, the force must be spread out evenly along the rail by weaving the attachment around the rail multiple times. *Never attach a main line lowering or hauling rope to a single point on the rail of a litter.* Many litters are susceptible to failure if sudden forces pull at a single point of the rail. This is particularly true of litter rails that are butt welded. A sudden force at such points can cause the weld to break and the litter rail to fail.

8. Make certain that the figure 8 follow through knot is dressed and pulled down tightly. After doing this, make certain the backup knot is snugged against the main knot. This technique cannot be used on some types of plastic litters where the

> ### Suggestion
>
> For a more stable tie-in, start the wrap of the litter rail with a clove hitch and end the wraps with a second clove hitch on the opposite side. This will keep the bridle from slipping around as the direction of load shifts and adds some backup if one portion of the litter rail should fail.

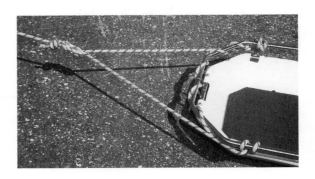

FIGURE 14-2
Direct main line attachment litter.

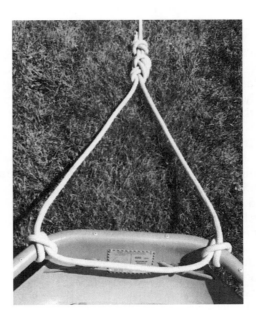

FIGURE 14-3
Tying main line to litter.

plastic material covers the rail at both ends. Figure 14-3 illustrates one technique for attaching a main line to such a type of litter. This technique uses clove hitches at each corner where the litter side rails meet the head end of the litter. Be certain to tie the clove hitches so there is no slack between them in the portion of rope inside the litter.

9. Once the loop for the tie-in is complete, make certain that it is large enough to create a safe angle on the knot (see page 78, Chapter 7, on how wider angles can create greater stress). But the loop should be small enough so it does not easily snag or get in the way.

Tying a Closed Loop Directly to the Head of the Litter

During some slope evacuations involving more than one rope length, the lowering rope will have to be removed and reattached to the litter. In such cases, it is more practical to leave a closed loop of rope tied at the end of the litter. To attach the lowering and haul-ing line to the loop, tie a figure 8 on a bight knot in the end of the main line rope and clip it to the loop with a large, locking carabiner (Figure 14-4).

To create a closed loop in the end of the litter:
1. Take a length of rope about 6 feet long.
2. Run it around the head rail of the litter to spread the force around the rail.
3. Tie the two ends of the rope together with a grapevine ("double fisherman's") knot or figure 8 bend knot.
4. Adjust the grapevine knot so that it is off to the side and not in the center where the main line rope will attach (Box 14-5).

Packaging the Subject for Slope Evacuation

Review the section, Medical Considerations for Patients in High Angle Rescue, beginning on page 145, in Chapter 11, The Rope Rescuer.

The litter attendants should be constantly concerned with the state of the patient's airway and breathing. If there is a threat to the patient's airway, such as vomiting, the attendants must be ready to tip the litter and clear the airway.

Packaging the Subject in the Litter

The major considerations for *packaging* a subject for slope evacuation include:
♦ The medical condition of the subject.
♦ The subject not being further harmed by being carried in the litter.
♦ The subject being protected from environmental factors (cold, wetness, falling debris).

Box 14-4 Alternative Approach: Bowline Knot

If local policy dictates that a bowline knot be used to create a loop in the end of a rope, then the bowline knot may be used in place of the figure 8 follow through knot, but with the following considerations:
♦ Make certain that the bowline knot is tied correctly (see Figure 6-7, page 63).
♦ Back up the bowline knot with a safety such as the double overhand backup knot (barrel knot).
♦ Monitor the bowline knot so that it does not "capsize" when being pulled over an obstruction such as a rock, a tree, a building edge, and so on.

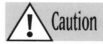

⚠ Caution

The angle made in this loop when it is attached to the main line rope must not be more than 90 degrees. (See Chapter 7, Anchoring.) If the angle is more than 90 degrees, make a larger loop.

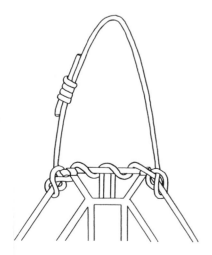

FIGURE 14-4
Tying loop onto litter.

Box 14-5 Alternative Approach: Ring Bend

In the place of rope, tubular webbing may also be used to create the loop. However, you must take care in tying such a loop with webbing because knots tied in it have a tendency to work their way out. Tie the two ends of the webbing together using a ring bend (water knot). *Once the ring bend is tied and dressed, be certain that there is enough webbing protruding past the knot to tie a back up knot.* Because of the tendency of webbing to work out of a knot, the ring bend should be backed up and monitored.

◆ The patient being physically stabilized to not shift whatever the angle or nature of litter movement.
◆ The patient remaining as comfortable as possible because it may be a very long evacuation.

Protecting the Subject in the Litter

Litter Underside. Litter underside is a particular concern in a wire basket litter. This litter is uncomfortable to be in and offers little protection on the bottom from protruding objects, such as twigs, branches, stones, and so on. To protect the bottom and make it more comfortable, line it with material such as a closed-cell foam pad and/or blankets. Be certain to pad hollow spaces along the body, such as behind the knees and the small of the back.

Litter Topside. Topside protection should be for wind, cold, and rain. Additional blankets over the top will help keep the subject warm. But wind and precipitation mean the need for a waterproof and windproof outer layer. One means of providing this waterproof layer is to use a large plastic tarp (15 feet × 15 feet). Lay the tarp out on the litter with a corner pointing toward each end, quickly place the insulation layer inside the tarp and bring the foot end up, then bring the two sides inward (just like a diaper). This "diaper" method is a very good way to protect your patient from weather and provide a vapor barrier effect also. The top portion of the "diaper" can be folded over the patient if he or she can tolerate it, at the top of the litter.

Face and Eyes. Litter patients cannot shield their faces from branches and their eyes from falling debris or rain. Face and eye protection may include a litter shield (but can produce claustrophobia in some patients), a face shield or, at the least, goggles.

Physically Stabilizing the Patient in the Litter

During an evacuation, the litter will be lifted, tilted, and carried at an angle. The patient must be packaged so that he or she does not slip lengthwise in the litter, slide from side to side, or come out of the litter.

Lengthwise Stabilization. Most litters come equipped with some form of foot plates but many of these are unreliable in preventing the patient from sliding down when the litter is inclined. One alternative is the feet tie-in (Figure 14-5), which can be constructed of 1-inch tubular webbing. They should be tied off securely on the side rails to prevent the subject from sliding down in the litter. However, if the subject is suffering from a fracture to a lower extremity, then a foot tie-in cannot be used on that extremity. One approach in this situation is to tie a simple seat harness of the subject using webbing (Figure 14-6). (See page 241 in Chapter 17, Other Tools for Rescue, for instructions on tying a simple seat harness.)

Make certain this does not obstruct blood circulation through the major vessels of the leg to the foot. To make certain that this and other packaging is not obstructing circulation, rescuers must regularly check pulses in the extremities. An alternative is to package the patient into a KED or OSS, thus providing a secure hold on the patient without risk of obstructing blood flow to the feet.

Securing the Subject in the Litter. Litters often come with tie-in straps but they may be inadequate for any of the following reasons:
◆ The buckles may not fasten securely or be strong enough.

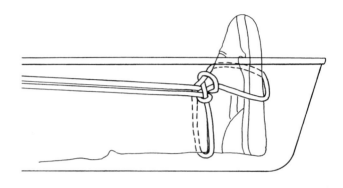

FIGURE 14-5
Foot tie-in to litter.

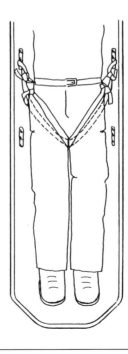

FIGURE 14-6
Thigh tie-in to litter.

- The straps may be old and rotten.
- The straps may be missing.

Figure 14-7, *A* through 14-7, *C* illustrate an alternative technique for securing the subject in the litter:

1. Begin with at least 30 feet of 1-inch tubular webbing. (If webbing is not available, then a rope is an alternative.) Find the center.
2. At the center, attach the webbing with a girth hitch onto the middle of the foot rail of the litter.
3. Lace the webbing back and forth through opposite points along the side rails and toward the head end of the litter.
4. If possible, do not run the line over the main rail. This can expose the line to greater abrasion. With the typical wire basket model, the line may be run around the larger uprights that connect the rail to the body of the litter. On the plastic style stokes litter, a prerigged rope is provided around the inside of the litter for tie-in points.
5. Cinch the line back on itself at the head of the litter as shown in Figure 14-8.
6. Bring the material together and tie it off with a trucker's hitch as shown in Figure 14-8.

Immobilizing the Head

You must immobilize suspected cervical injuries by following accepted medical protocols. If you are *certain* there are no cervical injuries, then you may immobilize the head area of the subject through other means. If the subject is not wearing a helmet, then the head area can be packed with blankets, packs, clothing, or other soft material, then tape the head in place with duct tape across the forehead only. If the subject is wearing a helmet, you must remove it (refer to the helmet removal procedure in *Prehospital Trauma Life Support:* ed 4, National Association of Emergency Medical Technicians, St. Louis, 1999, Mosby.) or it will interfere with both proper spinal immobilization and the patient's airway and breathing status.

! Warning

1. Do *not* lash webbing horizontally across the upper chest or neck. Should the subject slide down in the litter, he or she could be strangled by a line across this area. Instead, return the ends of the webbing back toward the foot area of the litter, as shown in Figure 14-8.
2. Rescuers must constantly monitor the litter lashing. They must check to see if the lashing has loosened and whether it is causing the patient discomfort or loss of circulation.

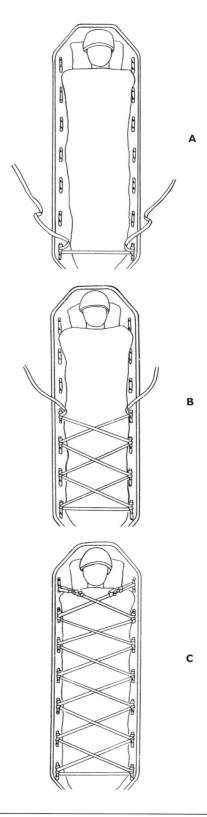

FIGURE 14-7
Lacing subject into litter.

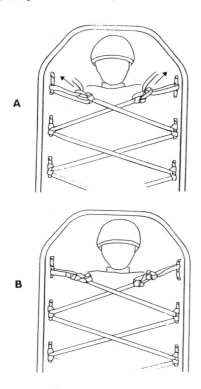

FIGURE 14-8
Avoiding webbing on neck in litter.

Additional Packaging

If the litter has a leg divider, then you must suffi-ciently pad the top of the divider to protect the pa-tient's groin. To prevent side-to-side movement of the trunk, pad the spaces along the sides of the sub-ject with soft material such as sweaters, clothing, blankets, and so on. For the comfort of the subject, pad under the hollows of the body such as behind the knees, the small of the back, and (unless there is cervical immobilization) behind the neck. Also pad bony parts such as the occiput, the back of the skull.

The Litter Team for Slope Evacuation

Before attempting a slope evacuation, a litter team member must realize that slope litter management is very different from managing a litter on level terrain (Box 14-6).

On level, unbroken terrain, the normal number of people carrying a litter is usually six (plus any addi-tional personnel attending to the medical needs of the subject). The full weight of the litter is on them. They are totally supporting their own weight as they maneuver their way across the terrain.

On slopes there may be difficult and treacherous footing, making it difficult to safely handle the litter. Consequently, the approach to litter management on slopes must be different.

Box 14-6 Characteristics of Litter Management on Slopes

- Much of litter and patient weight is taken by the rope.
- Litter movement is controlled by the rope system.
- Attendants have much of their weight taken by the litter and rope system.

Optional Personnel in Slope Evacuation

Medical Attendant. The medical attendant super-vises the medical care of the subject and, where it re-lates to medical considerations, the movement of the subject. He or she is usually positioned at the head of the litter or where best to monitor the patient. Where the slope is at a greater angle, the medical attendant may be safetied into the litter or main line rope with an adjustable sling.

Scouts. The scouts move ahead of the litter to clear a path or warn the team of loose debris, rocks, branches, briars, snakes, and so on.

Litter Tender Positions in Slope Evacuation

Figure 14-1 illustrates the positions for the four litter attendants during slope evacuation. Characteristically they are:
- Bodies turned toward the litter or slightly uphill.
- Depending on the terrain, both hands gripping litter rails, or one hand gripping the litter rail and the other being used for balance.
- Leaning back against tie-ins, their weight taken by the litter and rope system.
- Bodies perpendicular to the slope.
- Allowing rope system to determine litter rate of descent or ascent.
- Equal spacing so they do not bump one another.

Litter Tender Strategy for Slope Evacuation

On the slope above, the brakeman, in communication with the litter team, determines the rate of descent of the litter. The litter team members lean back into their tie-ins and allow the litter and rope system to take their weight. If a litter attendant slips, he or she continues to hold onto the litter rail and pulls his or her body taut on his or her tie-in. The rope system and the other team members can usually keep the litter stable and prevent him or her from falling. The litter team, in concert with the rope, acts as a sort of self-equalizing table and pro-vides stable transportation for the subject.

If more than one litter attendant loses footing or the terrain becomes particularly treacherous, the team captain can call a temporary "stop." This will give the team the chance to regain its stability.

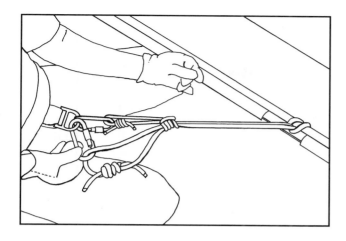

FIGURE 14-9
Litter tender tie-in.

Litter Tender Tie-Ins

The litter attendant tie-ins are critical for maintaining litter attendant stability and position at the litter. The litter attendant clips one end of the tie-in directly into his or her seat harness and the other end directly into the litter rail.

The simplest form of the tie-in can either be:

◆ A daisy chain with multiple clip-in points.
◆ A continuous loop of webbing or small diameter rope.
◆ A section of small diameter rope with a loop in each end.

The daisy chain, or rope or webbing loop, can be clipped into the litter top rail with a large locking carabiner.

Not all locking carabiners have gates that will clear the rails of the stokes-type litter. The larger rails on wire basket models and the rails on plastic litters will accept only certain models of a few carabiner brands. Consult manufacturer and distributor specifications before purchasing carabiners for this purpose.

An alternative to attaching the tie-in to the litter rail with a carabiner is to attach it by girth hitching to the rail. The disadvantage in this technique is that it cannot be removed or attached as quickly as one attached with a carabiner.

Because each person's body proportions, such as trunk size and arm length, are different, the tie-in length will vary. But generally the tie-in will be no more than 2 feet long.

The optimum length for the tie-in should be one that will hold the litter attendant in position to have both hands on the litter rail but maintains freedom of movement.

The Adjustable Tie-in

An option to the fixed length attachment is an adjustable length tie-in (Figure 14-9). The adjustable length tie-in enables the attendant to change the space to adapt to varying circumstances, such as changing terrain and obstructions. It also is an advantage if different team members have to use it.

The adjustable tie-in consists of two elements:

1. A fixed length safety line constructed of 8 to 9 mm accessory cord.
2. An adjustable tie-in of 7 mm accessory cord that uses a triple-wrap Prusik on the fixed line to change the distance between a litter tender and the litter. (To work properly, the Prusik cord must be of smaller diameter than the fixed safety line.)

Constructing the Adjustable Litter Tender Attachment

1. Take an 8 to 9 mm diameter accessory cord 2 m (about 80 inches) long.
2. Tie it in a continuous loop using a grapevine (double fisherman's) knot.
3. Girth hitch one end of the loop onto the litter rail. This end should be on the end opposite the grapevine knot. Where possible, place it where it will not slide on the rail, such as upright attachment points. On some plastic litters there is not as much choice of where to clip in. But one possibility is the spot where the plastic meets the rail. This junction will prevent the carabiner from sliding down toward the foot end when the litter is tilted.*
4. Clip in the end opposite the girth hitch to the litter tenders seat harness with a locking carabiner.
5. Take a 7-mm diameter accessory cord 1 m (about 40 inches) long.
6. Tie it in a continuous loop using a grapevine (double fisherman's) knot.
7. Attach the loop to the safety attachment with a Prusik. The Prusik should be over both strands of the safety attachment.
8. Attach the other end of the adjustable loop to the litter tender's harness using a separate locking carabiner.

Brake and Anchor Systems for Slope Lowering

The braking system is essential for a controlled lowering operation during slope evacuation. It in turn is dependent on secure anchors. (See Chapter 7, Anchoring, for a review of the criteria for safe and secure anchors.)

The location and number of brake and anchor systems depend on whether the length of the lowering is one rope length or more than one rope length.

---

*Note that some recent models of litters with plastic baskets have litter top rails similar to the metal stokes design (one of these is made by Junkin). In these cases, attach the tender tie-ins the same way as with the metal Stokes design.

> ## ⚠ Warning
>
> Older model plastic litters may not withstand the stresses of rope rescue:
> - The plastic material from which their body was constructed is brittle and sometimes fails.
> - The plastic body of the litter is not as well fastened to the rail as later models.
> - Also, sunlight will deteriorate the plastic material in litters stored outside, such as on the roof of vehicles. These litters should not be used in rope rescue.

Slope Lowerings of One Rope Length

A slope evacuation of rope length usually means that only one set of brake and anchors is needed. They are usually placed slightly above where the subject is loaded into the litter.

Lowerings of one rope length are usually easier and less complicated than multilength lowerings because in lowerings of one rope length:
- Only one set of brake and anchors is required.
- There is no changeover to different sets of brake and anchors.
- There are fewer people involved.

Slope Lowerings of More than One Rope Length

Slope lowerings of more than one rope length will usually be more complicated due to:
- Multiple anchor and brake systems.
- Changeovers from one anchor and brake system to another.
- More personnel involved.
- Needing greater coordination in movement of personnel.

In lowerings of more than one rope length, anchor and braking systems will have to be rigged at strategic points down the slope. Among the factors that determine the placement of the anchor and brake systems along the slope are:
- The length of the main line lowering rope, minus the length needed on the lower end of the rope to tie into the litter and approximately 20 feet from the top end of the rope. This must always be kept as spare length before the rope runs out.
- The availability of anchor points.

The rigging of anchors for a braking system can be very time consuming. In a multilength evacuation, the litter team should not be forced to stop the operation each time the rope runs out while waiting for new anchors to be rigged. More preferable is either prerigging or leap frogging.

Prerigging. If there is enough equipment, and enough skilled personnel for anchor rigging, then the anchor and brake systems can be rigged ahead of the litter team.

Leapfrogging. Leapfrogging is the practice of using two sets of rigging teams and brake teams to alternate the rigging of anchors and the operation of the brakes. While the first team is operating the first set of brakes, the second team is rigging the second set of anchors. After the litter rope is detached from the first set of brakes, the first team derigs the first anchors and moves them down to the position for the third anchor and brake system.

Leapfrogging can be a very effective system and can speed the evacuation of a rescue subject. But for it to be efficient, the rigging teams must be skilled at anchoring, knowledgeable of the equipment, and self-reliant. If they do not possess these qualities, then the entire operation may be interrupted as the litter is stopped and rescuers wait for the riggers to finish establishing the next brake and anchor sets.

Braking Systems for Slope Evacuation

Brake Bar Rack. The brake bar rack is useful for slope evacuation in the following circumstances:
- Steeper slopes: The brake bar rack (six bar) usually has adequate friction.
- Terrain that varies between steep and gentle: The brake bar rack can easily vary friction (Box 14-7).

Figure 8 Descender. The large figure 8 with ears can be used in more gentle terrain. Start with the 8 double wrapped to make certain there is adequate friction to control the lowering.

Tree Wrap. The so-called *tree wrap* is a technique rescuers can fall back to for slope evacuation when there is a shortage of equipment for braking systems. It can only be used where there are strong, large diameter trees. The primary disadvantage of the tree wrap is that is tends to increase the difficulty of rope management.

Other disadvantages to the tree wrap technique are that it can cause permanent damage to trees and can contaminate ropes with tree sap. For these reasons, the tree wrap should only be used when no other secure braking systems are available.

Using the Tree Wrap Braking System. Figure 14-10 on p. 178 illustrates a brakeman using the tree wrap braking system.

1. Attach the main line rope to the litter either directly with a large loop at the end of the rope or clipped into a continuous loop that is attached to the litter head rail. The litter should be slightly down slope of the tree wrap location so that the litter does not interfere with the braking operation.
2. If the rope is coiled, stack the rope uphill of the tree with the uphill end of the rope on the bottom

Box 14-7 Alternative Approach: Brake Tube

An alternative to the brake bar rack in slope lowering is the brake tube (see page 212 in Chapter 15, High Angle Lowering).

ADVANTAGE
- Knots can be passed through the device.
- Has good control for lowering.

DISADVANTAGE
- Heavier and bulkier than the rack (group rather than individual equipment).
- More expensive.

 Warning

Before using a tree wrap brake system for slope evacuation, consider the following:
- The tree wrap system must only be used by those who have thoroughly practiced it under realistic conditions.
- It can only be used on *live*, large diameter trees that have strong root systems.

of the stack and the litter end of the rope feeding off the top. If the rope is bagged, deploy the rope bag up slope of the tree with the uphill end of the rope in the bottom of the bag and the litter end of the rope feeding out of the top of the bag.
3. Stand slightly to the side of the tree, with your back to it and the right side of your body pointed down-slope (Figure 14-10, *A*).
4. The rope should be on your side of the tree, running from the stack or bag to the litter, and between you and the tree.
5. With the rope behind you, pick it up and hold it behind you loosely in both hands.
6. Slowly begin to move around the tree backward, still holding the rope as before: loosely in both hands (Figure 14-10, *B*).
7. As you go around the tree, the path of the rope from uphill will be off the stack (or out of the bag), around the downhill side of the tree, through your hands, across your buttocks, back around the lower part of the tree, and then to the litter (Fig. 14-10, *C*).
8. As you need slack, pull it from the rope stack or bag. The ***rope handler*** can assist.
9. Up slope of the tree, you will have to step over the rope coming out of the stack (out of the bag). Keep the rope evenly contoured around the tree and prevent it from crossing itself on the tree (Figure 14-10, *D*).

10. The amount of friction needed depends on the following:
- Steepness of the slope.
- Weight of the litter and the team.
- Circumference of the tree.
A large tree, for example, will rarely require you to wrap it as much as 360 degrees.
11. Once you have enough friction, have the litter team pick up the litter and take slack out of the rope between the litter and the tree. They then lean back into the rope. If there is sufficient friction, they can begin moving down slope with you controlling the speed of their movement (Figure 14-10, *E*).
12. To increase friction, go farther around the tree to wrap the rope more and grip the rope more with your hands.
13. Reduce friction by moving from around the tree, to wrap the rope less, and grip the rope less with your hands.

Rope Management in Slope Evacuation. Good rope management is particularly critical to ensure smooth operation of the brake system in slope evacuation. Without good rope management, kinks in the rope and tangles coming from the stack or bag could jam the brakes and slow the operation or bring it to a complete halt.

To help provide good rope management, a rope handler should assist the brakeman, particularly in a tree wrap lowering. The rope handler assists by feeding the brakeman the rope and removing kinks and tangles before they reach the brakes.

The Belay Question. The question of whether to belay in a slope evacuation must be answered on the scene by trained and experienced personnel. They consider the following questions:
- How steep is the slope?
- Is the footing particularly loose and treacherous?
- Is the slope icy or muddy?
- What would be the consequences of a fall by the litter team?
- Are the main line brake anchors questionable?
- Are there plenty of anchors?
- Is there thick underbrush or large boulders? (The angle made by the main line rope and the belay line in slope evacuation is similar to an advancing wedge. If there is thick underbrush or large boulders, the advancing wedge could tangle.)

Ultimately, rescuers need to answer this question about whether to belay in slope evacuation: would the potential benefit of the increased safety be worth the increased complexity in rope and system management and the increased personnel?

Communications

Good communication in slope evacuation is particularly critical, especially between the litter team and

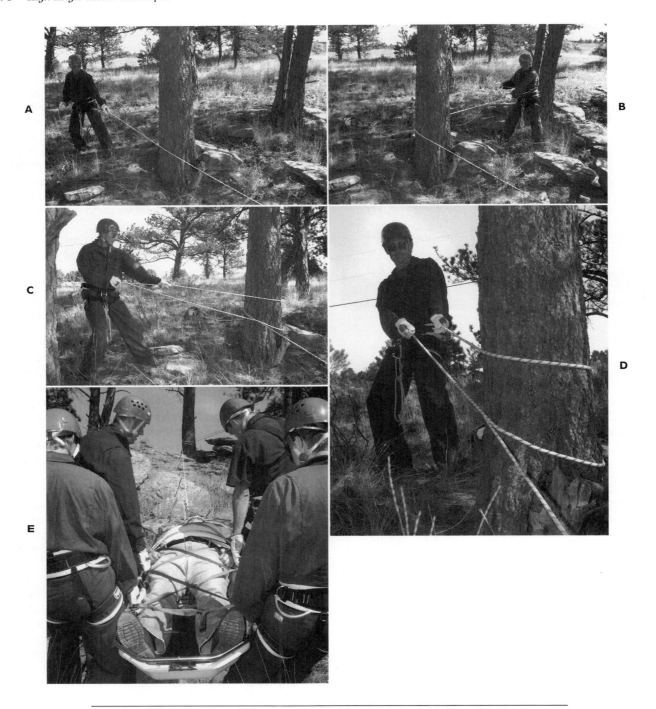

FIGURE 14-10
Using the tree wrap.

the brakeman. It is essential that communication be simple, to the point, and clear (Box 14-8).

For these reasons, voice communications should be limited to a few people. Among these would be the *litter captain* and the brakeman. In those cases where there are problems in communication, such as distance, wind, or waterfall, a relay person may be necessary. Everyone else should keep quiet.

A Typical Slope Lowering

The following sequence outlines the basic elements of a slope lowering operation.

Preparation

Before movement of the litter begins, all major elements of the slope evacuation system should be in place and prepared. You need to check for the following:

Box 14-8 Voice Communications for Slope Lowering

"ON BELAY."

Litter captain to belayer.

"BELAY ON."

Belayer to litter captain.

"DOWN SLOW."

Litter captain to brakeman.
or

"DOWN FAST."*

"STOP!"

Generally the litter captain to the brakeman but may be given by anyone who sees danger or potential problem developing.

"STOP! STOP! WHY STOP?"

This is given by litter captain to brakeman. It is given when, for an unexpected reason and without command from the litter captain, the rope has stopped moving. It could be that the brakeman is still letting out rope, but the rope is jammed somewhere. Obviously the potential for a very serious problem.

"TWO - OH."

Given by the brakeman to the litter captain. It means there is only about 20 feet of rope left. The litter team should set the litter down at a convenient spot so a new brake and anchor set can be established.

"OFF BELAY."

Litter captain to belayer. The litter has been set down in a secure spot. It and the litter team are in no danger of falling.

"BELAY OFF."

Belayer to litter captain.

---

*Note: The "down slow/down fast" command should be repeated by the brakeman back to the litter captain so the captain knows that the brakeman understands. Otherwise the litter may be lowered at a different rate than desired.

♦ The subject has been medically assessed, treated, packaged, and his or her condition is being monitored.

♦ The rope has been properly attached to the litter.

♦ Secure anchors have been set and brakes attached to them.

♦ The rope is wrapped in the brakes and locked off.

♦ The brakeman has the rope in hand and is ready to run brakes.

♦ The rope handler is ready to feed the rope to the brakeman.

♦ Belay line is set in belay device (if applicable).

♦ Belayer is ready to belay (if applicable).

♦ Litter attendants have tie-ins attached to themselves and to the litter and are ready to lift the litter.

1. The litter captain directs the litter team to lift the litter. He or she says, "one, two, three, lift."

2. Once the captain is satisfied all the attendants are ready, he or she says, *"preload."* The team removes slack from the rope by holding the litter downhill against the rope and leaning into their own tie-ins. The brakeman holds the braking system fixed. This is to pretest the system and make certain everything is in order and the litter team has their tie-ins correctly set.

3. If everything is in order, the litter captain gives the voice communication, *"down slow."* The brakeman begins to let the rope through the braking system. The rope handler feeds rope to the brakeman. The litter team leans into the system and moves downhill. (The litter captain may also issue a *"down fast"* if he or she wants to move down slope faster.)

   If anything begins to go wrong, for example, a kink slips past the rope handler and jams the brakes or a litter attendant begins to loose a boot, anyone can call, *"stop!"*

4. The rope handler warns the brakeman that the rope is running out. The brakeman shouts, *"two-oh!"*

5. The litter captain looks for a good place to set the litter down. When the litter is at the place the captain has chosen, he or she communicates, *"stop!"* The captain then directs the team to set the litter down. When the litter is secure and the team in a stable position, the captain communicates, *"off rope."*

If Evacuation Is More than One Rope Length

6. When the litter gets into a spot convenient to the second set of brakes, the team stops there and sets the litter down. The second brakeman and rope handler are already in position.

7. *Alternative A.* The main line rope is now trailing from the litter uphill to the first set of brakes but has been removed from the first set of brakes. If the rope is unlikely to tangle, the brakeman simply attaches the same rope to the second set of brakes. The rope handler will pull the rope down as needed and feed it to the brakeman.

   Alternative B. If the main line rope now trailing uphill is likely to snag, the brakeman detaches it from the litter. The brakeman then attaches a second rope, which is stacked or bagged near the second set of brakes. The team at the first set of brakes will derig the brakes and anchors, recover the first rope as they come downhill, and then rig the third set of brakes and anchors (leapfrogging). If belays are being used, then the second belayer gets ready to belay.

8. The teams repeat the cycle.

9. As soon as the litter team sets the litter down and becomes secure at the end of the first rope length, the first brakeman and rope handler (and first belayer) quickly derig the first brake anchor set. They

then quickly leapfrog down slope past the second brake and anchor set to rig the third brake and anchor (and belay) set. They are ready when the litter team reaches their position and detaches the rope from the second brake and anchor set. This cycle continues until the litter safely reaches an objective such as a road and waiting ambulance, a clearing with a helicopter, or terrain where the carryout may continue.

Hauling

Not all litter evacuations will be going *down* slope. Many of them will have to go *up* slope. Hauling techniques use many of the same principles as lowering. However, hauling systems may involve slightly more complex rope work and may require the use of additional personnel.

Mechanical versus Human Power. There are two general approaches to hauling systems: mechanical power or human power. In the area of mechanical power, there are some powered winches that have been designed for rescue work. With practice at using them and understanding their potential and limitations, these winches can help perform a slope hauling rescue safely and efficiently. As with other types of hauling and lowering systems, there is always the potential for human or mechanical failure, so winches should always be belayed or safetied in some other way.

One danger with powered winches is lack of control and too much power at the wrong time. If there is a jammed litter or a hand caught between a rock and a litter, the powered winch may not slow down until damage is already done. This chapter will concentrate on simple systems that use human power efficiently to haul litters during slope evacuations.

A 1:1 Mechanical Advantage Hauling System. One of the simplest hauling systems to be used in slope evacuation is the *1:1 hauling system.* In essence, the 1:1 simply means that the force needed to haul the

load (litter, subject, and attendants) is about the same as the weight of the load.

Figure 14-11 illustrates the elements of a basic 1:1 hauling system. They include the *litter system*, which is essentially the same as in lowering in that the subject packaged in the litter and the litter team are attached with tie-ins.

The rope system is attached to the head of the litter and in turn runs through a PCD, which is attached to a different anchor from the *pulley*. The pulley is used to change the direction of the rope to a more convenient angle for the haul team, whose members are attached to the main line haul rope by way of figure **8** on a bight knots in the rope or ascenders or Prusik hitches on the rope, which are attached to their seat harnesses.

Pulleys Used in 1:1 *Hauling Systems.* Pulleys used in 1:1 haul systems do not add any mechanical advantage. (In fact, some advantage is lost through the pulley's inherent friction.) Pulleys can, however, make

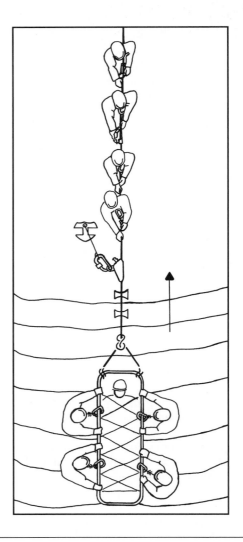

FIGURE 14-11

Elements of 1:1 hauling system.

> ⚠ **Warning**
>
> ◆ Never use a powered winch for hauling human subjects that has not been specifically designed for rescue.
> ◆ Winches not designed for rescue lack the control needed for rescue. There have been severe injuries and deaths in attempts to conduct rescues with conventional powered winches.
> ◆ Always follow manufacturers' instructions when using rescue winches.
> ◆ Practice with rescue winches in realistic conditions before attempting real rescues with them.

things more convenient for a haul team by changing the direction of the rope pull to:

◆ Enable a team to pull along the contour of a hill instead of straight up.

◆ Allow the haul to be in a more convenient place, such as a clearing or along a road (Figure 14-12).

See Chapter 5, Basic High Angle Hardware, for more information on pulleys.

The Haul Team. Haul team members should not be selected on the basis of brute force ability but according to the following:

◆ Intelligence.

◆ Ability to follow commands.

◆ Ability to react quickly.

◆ Sensitivity to feel of haul rope.

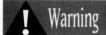

Anchors established for pulley directionals must be stronger than if they were simply supporting a weight equal to the load being hauled. The greater the angle in the rope created at the change in direction, the greater the force on the pulley and the anchor system (Figure 14-13).

Communications for Hauling. The voice communications for hauling movement are initiated by the litter captain (Box 14-9). Except for one special exception, *no one* else initiates communications for hauling. *Everyone else stays quiet.*

The Important Progress Capture Device (A.K.A., "Ratchet")

Whatever the type of hauling system, it is essential that there be a safety system to prevent the litter from falling back down slope in case of mechanical or human failure in the system. One of the commonly accepted safety system devices is the *progress capture device*, which employs a rope grab device such as a Prusik or cam-type ascender.

Using Progress Capture Devices in Steep Slope Evacuation. Progress capture devices should always be connected to a safe and secure anchor system that is, if possible, *separate* from the anchor system supporting the haul system (Box 14-10).

On some models of general-use ascenders there is an arrow with the caption, "up." This is the indicator for direction of use when ascending a rope. *But in hauling systems, this arrow should always point along the rope toward the load* (the litter, the rescue subject). Some older model general-use ascenders do not have this arrow inscribed on the shell. But if you look at

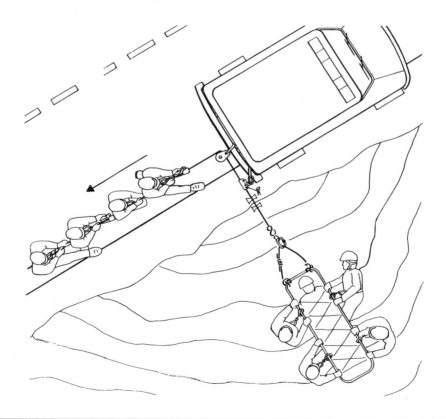

FIGURE 14-12

Making haul more convenient.

Force on a direction pulley's anchor changes with the angle. Maximum load amplification is two times the applied load.

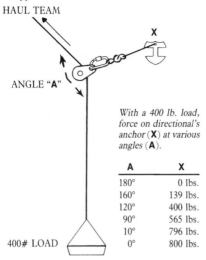

*With a 400 lb. load, force on directional's anchor (**X**) at various angles (**A**).*

A	X
180°	0 lbs.
160°	139 lbs.
120°	400 lbs.
90°	565 lbs.
10°	796 lbs.
0°	800 lbs.

400# LOAD

FIGURE 14-13

Forces on anchors of hauling system.

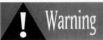 **Warning**

Hauling systems create enormous forces on the rope rescue system. Unnoticed problems can quickly result in catastrophic system failure. Personnel must constantly monitor for potential problems including, but not limited to:

◆ Knots on moving rope that jam in cracks.
◆ Broken gear that causes system failure.
◆ Systems reaching their limit.
◆ Pinned arms and legs.

There must be good communication between team captains and the haul team.

The haul team must be aware that what seems a normal speed for them seems *very fast* for those being hauled (rescue subject, litter attendants). For all these reasons, the haul team must:

◆ Pull slowly unless told otherwise.
◆ At all times, be prepared to stop instantly.

Warning

Never use personal ascenders for hauling systems in which more than one person's body weight may be involved. The use of this type of ascender can result in failure in two potential ways:

1. The frame or other portion of the ascender may fail.
2. The sharp teeth on the cam can tear the rope sheath.

 Box 14-9 The Haul Commands

To avoid potential disastrous confusion, haul commands are limited to a few standardized ones.

"HAUL."

Begin hauling. Needs to be spoken only once. The team will continue to haul until given another command.
or

"HAUL SLOW."

A variation when there is an emphasis on slow movement, such as when the litter is about to reach the top.

"SET."

The haul team immediately stops hauling and gently eases back on the load. This is to set the progress capture device. It may be for reason of safety or, more commonly, to get another bite of the rope.

"SLACK."

The progress capture device is set, so the haul team slacks on the rope. This enables any part of the system to be reset, and the haul team to get another bite on the rope. (If a belay is employed, then the normal belay communications are also used.)
There is one command that anyone may give when they see something going wrong:

"STOP!"

All movement stops immediately. The haul team holds tension until told otherwise.

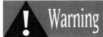 **Warning**

Never substitute voice haul commands unless there is an overriding reason and all team members have previously been informed of the change.

Use only terms that are crisp and distinct and have no chance of being mistaken for other words.

For example, do not replace the word "stop" with "whoa," which can easily be mistaken for "slow," or even worse, "go."

the shell in profile, you will see that the shell vaguely resembles an arrowhead (see Figure 5-19 on page 53). Again, the arrow should point in the direction of the load.

Positioning the Progress Capture Device (PCD). The progress capture device should be on a separate anchor from the hauling system. But it should be close to, and parallel to, the main line rope. This will help prevent shock loading and reduce the slack that interferes with haul system efficiency.

Box 14-10 Note on Terminology

In some previous texts, the progress capture device has been called a "safety cam" or at times a "ratchet cam."

It is inappropriate to call a PCD a "safety cam" because it does not and should not act as a belay. Calling it "safety" can be confusing to some persons.

Although it may act as a "ratchet," "progress capturing" gives a better mental picture of its purpose, particularly for individuals of a nonmechanical state of mind.

A progress capturing device can be either a hard cam (general use ascender) or a Prusik.

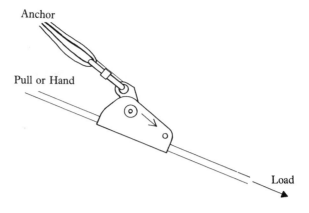

FIGURE 14-14
Setting PCD.

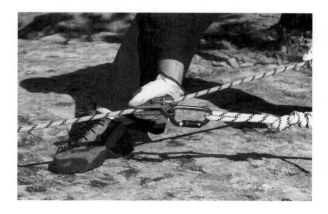

FIGURE 14-15
PCD with tender.

Setting the Progress Capture Device. When rigging the PCD, you have two primary concerns:

1. That the device grabs the rope when needed.
2. That the device not ride up the rope as the rope moves. This could result in dangerous shock loading.

How the PCD is specifically rigged depends in part on the specific type of general-use ascender used and in part on the specific circumstances of the rigging (Figures 14-14 and 14-15).

Free-Running Progress Capture Device. Figure 14-15 shows one method of ensuring that the PCD stays in place and clamps on the rope when needed. *This technique is specific to the use of a general use ascender as a PCD.* The technique uses the services of a person known as the *PCD tender.* As the main line hauling rope moves up, the PCD tender makes certain that the PCD does not travel up the rope. The PCD tender does this by holding the backside of the ascender shell with the palm and with fingers extended out of the way of the cam. He or she holds the shell of the PCD in this manner so that fingers or gloves do not get caught as the PCD suddenly shock loads. A finger caught by the PCD could get injured, and a glove caught in the cam could prevent it from clamping the rope.

Although the use of a PCD attendant can be effective, it does require extra manpower. And there is always the potential for human failure or inattention.

A second technique of using a free-running general use ascender as a PCD is shown in Figure 14-16, *A.* A bungee (elastic) cord is clipped into the empty hole that is usually found toward the "point" of the arrowhead in some general-use ascenders. The other end of the bungee cord is anchored securely to a convenient spot toward the load. A great deal of tension is not required on the bungee cord. But there should be enough to:

◆ Keep the PCD from riding up the rope.
◆ Keep the PCD closed on the rope.

Please note to tie the bungee cord *only to the shell* of the general use ascender and not to the cam itself. Otherwise, the system will not function as needed.

This technique of auto tending of a PCD by bungee will probably not work with Prusik hitches. See Chapter 12, Rescue Belaying, for information on tending Prusik hitches.

A third alternative for setting a general use ascender PCD is shown in Figure 14-16, *B.* This method uses a short piece of cord. It is attached to a weight and the weight is hung so that it will pull the shell of the PCD toward the load.

Spring-Loaded Progress Capture Devices. If a spring-loaded PCD is properly rigged, then the cam will close onto the rope when needed. But the problem remains of how to keep the shell from riding up the rope as the rope moves. Again, the solution would be similar to that of the free-running PCD: a cam attendant, a bungee cord, or a weighted cord.

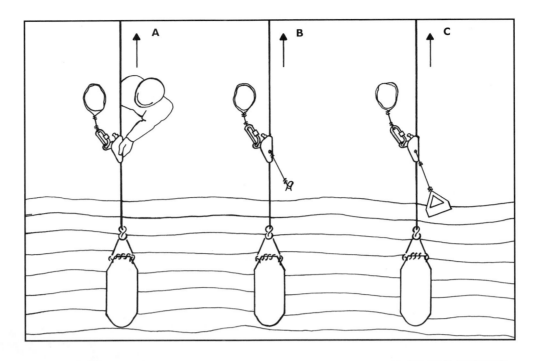

FIGURE 14-16
Setting PCD for automatic.

Prusik-Type Progress Capture Devices. Under certain conditions, a properly used Prusik system may be used as a progress capture device.

For further information, see Chapter 12, Rescue Belaying, and Chapter 16, Hauling Systems.

The Counter Balance Haul System

In any hauling system, the major force that rescuers are fighting is gravity. The counter balance haul system is a method of using gravity to fight *gravity*.

Strictly speaking, a counterbalance hauling system is also a 1:1 haul system. Without considering loss due to friction and other inefficiencies, the force used to haul is the same as the weight of the load it is hauling. But the difference is this: instead of the haul team going off the side (as in the example on page 181) the haul team takes advantage of gravity by going downhill. The load (the litter system) still goes uphill. Figure 14-17 illustrates the elements of a counterbalance haul system. It includes the following:

Litter System. In the litter system, the subject is medically assessed, treated, and packaged in the litter, and his or her condition is monitored. The litter team is attached with their tie-ins.

Rope System. The bottom end of the rope is attached to the head of the litter. As it gets to the top, the rope first runs through the PCD, which is on its own anchor system. Just above the progress capture device, the rope goes through the pulley and anchor system.

Pulley and Anchor System. Note that in this example there are two pulleys:

The first one initially changes the rope direction 90 degrees and then the second pulley changes the rope direction another 90 degrees, so that the rope goes back down the slope.

It might be possible to have only one pulley. But in this situation, two pulleys mean a greater margin of safety and less chance of failure. Remember there are now two loads pulling down slope on the anchors:

1. The weight of the load (litter system).
2. The force of the haul team pulling slightly.

Consequently, there are two pulleys and two anchor systems to share the load. But having these two anchor systems and two pulleys set a distance apart also means two additional advantages:

1. Less chance of the two rope strands tangling.
2. Less chance for the haul team and the litter team to interfere with one another's movements.

A 2:1 Hauling System for Slope Evacuation

Figure 14-18 illustrates a 2:1 hauling system for slope evacuation.

In theory, the force needed by the haul team to move the litter system is only half the force needed in the 1:1 hauling system previously examined. But with the 2:1 hauling system, the haul team will have to travel twice as far.

The 2:1 hauling system is created by anchoring a rope at the top, running it back down to the litter through a pulley that is attached to the litter yoke,

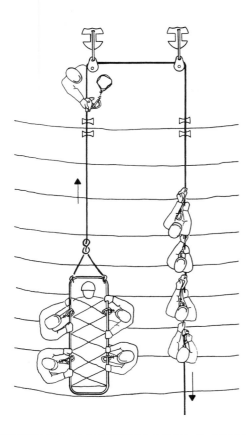

FIGURE 14-17
Elements of counter balance haul.

![Warning]

Although a 2:1 haul system can make hauling easier, it does increase rope management problems:

♦ There are now two strands of rope moving along the same path.
♦ There is a pulley moving, which could easily become jammed on underbrush, trees, rock, and so on. Rescue personnel must be able to reach this pulley, wherever it jams, to free it.
(See Chapter 15, Hauling Systems, for a possible solution to this problem.)

and then running the rope back to the top through a PCD on a separate anchor and near the first anchor. The haul team might be able to pull uphill on the rope, but Figure 14-19 shows them going off to the side, to make it a little easier on themselves. This sideways pull is made possible by running the rope over a *directional* pulley anchored near the anchor point of the top end of the rope.

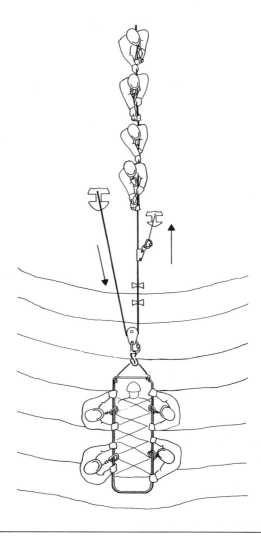

FIGURE 14-18
Elements of 2:1 hauling system.

Other Hauling Systems

Other types of multiple force haul systems may be used in slope evacuations as:

♦ The slope becomes steeper.
♦ Less personnel are available for the haul team.

Drawbacks to Multiforce Haul Systems

Remember that although multiforce haul systems can make it easier for haul teams to move a litter, all of them have some drawbacks, including:

♦ More complicated to rig.
♦ Taking longer to rig.
♦ Creating greater forces on anchors and other parts of the system.
♦ Easier to foul and, perhaps, to fail.
♦ The haul team has to travel a longer distance than with a 1:1 system. Chapter 16, Hauling Systems, examines multiforce haul systems in greater detail.

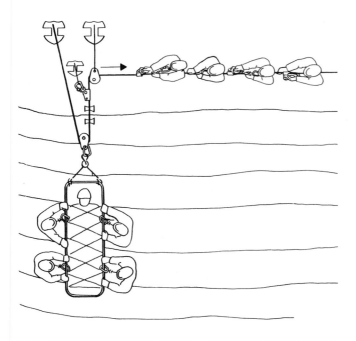

FIGURE 14-19
Side pull on 2:1 haul system.

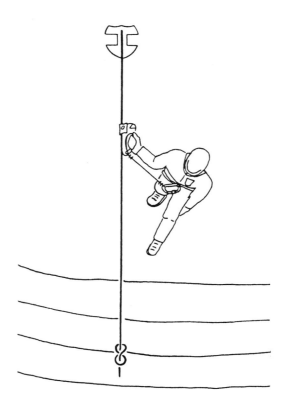

FIGURE 14-20
Personnel safety lines.

Safe Movement of Personnel in Slope Evacuation

One of the problems in slope evacuation is the safe movement of personnel up and down the slope for rigging, medical evaluation, litter rigging, and so on. These people may have problems with footing, thus endangering themselves. But they may also knock rocks or other debris down onto the rescue subject and other rescuers.

To avoid this, one of the first actions on the scene should be the immediate establishment of personnel safety lines (Figure 14-20). These lines should be well anchored and established off to the side. In this way, personnel can travel up and down them without endangering those below.

Once the safety lines are established, personnel can move up and down, either by hand or with descenders and ascender.

Evaluation Exercises

◆ COGNITIVE AND AFFECTIVE EXERCISES ◆

1. List four ways in which slope evacuation differs from high angle evacuation.
2. What could be the consequences of using a single point of attachment to a Stokes litter?
3. Which of the following are *not* considerations in the packaging of the patient?
   A. Spinal immobilization.
   B. Secure strapping.
   C. Protection from environment.
   D. Availability of anchor points.
4. What kind of knot could be used to make a litter attendant tie-in adjustable?
   A. Tautline hitch.
   B. Prusik.
   C. Figure 8.
   D. Bowline.
5. If the lowering requires more than one rope length to accomplish, it is a _____ lowering?
   A. Single pitch.
   B. Multipitch.
   C. Tandem pitch.
   D. Dual pitch.
6. If the lowering requires only one rope length to accomplish, it is a _____ lowering?
   A. Multipitch.
   B. Dual pitch.
   C. Tandem pitch.
   D. Single pitch.
7. Name two factors that will determine the location of brake and anchor systems in a lowering of more than one rope length.

8. What are the duties of a rope handler in a slope evacuation?

9. What are three considerations in deciding whether or not to have a belay in a slope evacuation?

10. Repeat from memory and in sequence the voice communications between the litter captain and the brakeman and the litter captain and a belayer during a slope evacuation.

11. Why should personal ascenders not be used for hauling systems in which more than one person's body weight is involved?

12. When general-use ascenders are used in hauling systems for slope evacuation, which way should the arrow point?
    A. Toward the anchor.
    B. Toward the lateral moraine.
    C. Toward the belay.
    D. Toward the load.

13. Name three potential problems that could develop in a slope hauling system and which members of the team should be on the lookout for them.

14. What is the voice communication that should be given by any member of the rescue team who sees something going wrong during a slope evacuation?
    A. "Halt."
    B. "Belay that."
    C. "Haul slow."
    D. "Stop."

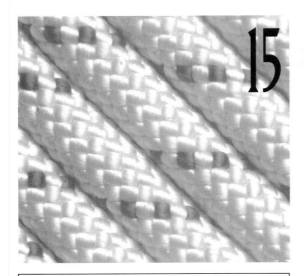

15 High Angle Lowering

Key Terms

Auxiliary Tender The person who rappels or ascends alongside the litter as it is being lowered in order to assist in the rescue. Duties may include medical assessment and/or primary treatment of the rescue subject, assistance in getting the litter over the edge, assistance in handling the litter on the vertical face, and in loading the patient into the litter.

Bridle See *Spider*.

Double Line Lowering The use of two ropes attached to the litter in a lowering rigged so that they may be operated independently to change the angle of the litter. Also called *scaffold lowering*.

Edge Tender The person connected to a safety attachment who works at the edge of a drop in a high angle lowering. His or her duties include assistance in getting the litter over the edge, reducing edge abrasion to ropes and, when necessary, relaying communications between the litter tender and the brakeman.

Load The total combined objects and persons being lowered or raised by a rope in a high angle system. Some examples include a rescue subject, a rescuer, and a subject in a litter with one or two attached litter tenders.

Pig Tail A short piece of rope with which the litter tender attaches to the litter system.

Single Line Lowering The use of one main lowering rope with a belay in litter lowering.

Spider The system of attaching a lowering rope to a litter. A spider usually has four or more legs that connect to various points of a litter to equalize loading. Sometimes called a *bridle*.

◆ Prerequisites

Before attempting the activities described in this chapter, you must have demonstrated that you can properly:

1. Use and care for rope.
2. Use and care for other equipment employed in the high angle environment.
3. Tie correctly, and without hesitation, the eight knots described in Chapter 6.
4. Apply the principles of anchoring and rig a safe and secure anchor.
5. Apply the principles of belaying and safely and confidently belay another person using either a Munter hitch or personal belay device.
6. Apply the principles of rappelling: rappel safely, and under control; tie off the rappel device to operate hands free of the rope and then return to a safe and controlled rappel.
7. Apply the principles of ascending: tie correctly, and without hesitation, a Prusik hitch and know how to use it; comprehend the uses and limitations of mechanical ascenders; confidently and safely ascend a fixed rope using either friction hitches or mechanical ascenders; confidently and safely change over both from rappelling to ascending and from ascending to rappelling; and extricate yourself from jammed rappel device (or similar problem).
8. Apply the principles of slope evacuation: correctly set the rigging in any of the elements of slope evacuation; and safely assume the role of litter tender, haul team member, brakeman, or belayer.
9. Correctly distinguish between one-person and rescue belays; correctly tie a load releasing hitch and demonstrate how to release it under load; correctly rig a tandem Prusik belay system and operate it; correctly rig a Prusik minding pulley and operate it.

Objectives

At the completion of this chapter you should be able to:

1. Define high angle lowering and cite three examples.
2. List and label the elements of a high angle lowering system.
3. Given a list of equipment, select equipment for a high angle lowering system.
4. Discuss the medical considerations for a subject before and during a high angle lowering.
5. Describe the functions of the following positions: litter tender, brakeman, rope handler, belayer, and edge tender.

Objectives—cont'd ▼

6. Describe the functions of rope, braking systems, belay, edge protection, spiders, and litter tender tie-ins in high angle lowering.
7. Identify the need for reliable communications in high angle lowering.
8. Describe the function of knot passing in a high angle lowering.
9. List the differences between single line and double line lowering systems, along with the advantages and disadvantages of each.
10. Repeat from memory the voice communications employed in high angle lowering.
11. Construct rigging for a litter and act as litter tender in a high angle lowering.
12. Construct the rigging for the braking system and act as brakeman in a high angle lowering.
13. Construct the rigging for the belay system and act as belayer in a high angle lowering.
14. Construct a high angle lowering system.
15. Perform a knot pass in a high angle lowering.

THE HIGH ANGLE LOWERING SYSTEM

High angle lowering is also sometimes called *vertical lowering*. Both terms refer to the same principle: the controlled lowering of a rescue subject using a rope. If the subject's injuries are severe enough, the lowering is done with the subject packaged in a litter. High angle litter lowering is usually done with one or two rescuers (litter tenders) attached to the litter, with the weight of the subject, litter, and rescuers supported by the rope.

As the rescuers lower the litter, it may run down against the side of a high angle wall, such as a cliff or side of building or it may be "free" (not touching the wall). This will depend on the nature of the wall where the lowering is performed. If the top of the drop is overhung, the litter will hang out away from the wall. This might be a more difficult operation for the rescuers because they would not have the advantage of pushing against the wall to maneuver themselves and the litter during the rescue.

In some cases where the subject is uninjured or only slightly injured, it may be possible to lower him or her without the litter, either alone or with a rescuer.

Some of the environments in which a high angle lowering might be employed include:

◆ Cliffs.
◆ Buildings.
◆ Industrial sites, either outside a structure or inside a vessel.
◆ Construction sites such as tower cranes.
◆ Other structures such as stacks, silos, or towers.
◆ Vertical caves.

The vertical lowering may take place either on the outside of the structure or on the inside, such as the interior of a silo or tank.

The Lowering System

Figure 15-1 illustrates the basic elements of a vertical lowering system.

The Load

The *load* often will be the subject packaged in a litter. Because of medical considerations and concern for the subject's comfort, the litter is usually lowered in a horizontal position. Also, there is usually less patient anxiety in a horizontal position because he or she mostly sees sky or a ceiling and not the ground.

However, confined space environments or obstructions on the face may require lowering the litter in a vertical position with the head up. The load could also be only the subject, if he is uninjured or only slightly injured. Or the load could be the subject attached to a rescuer.

The Litter Tender(s)

There may be one or two litter tenders. Each litter tender is attached to the litter by at least two connections: a primary tie-in and a safety.

Attachments of the Load to the Main Line Rope(s)

Litter attachments to the rope are known as *spiders*. They are lines that attach at several points to the litter and come together where they are attached to the rope. Spiders usually have at least four legs that attach to the litter, although in some systems there may be as many as six.

The Main Line or Lowering Rope(s)

The main line or lowering rope(s) lines must have a safety factor adequate for the load they are to lower.

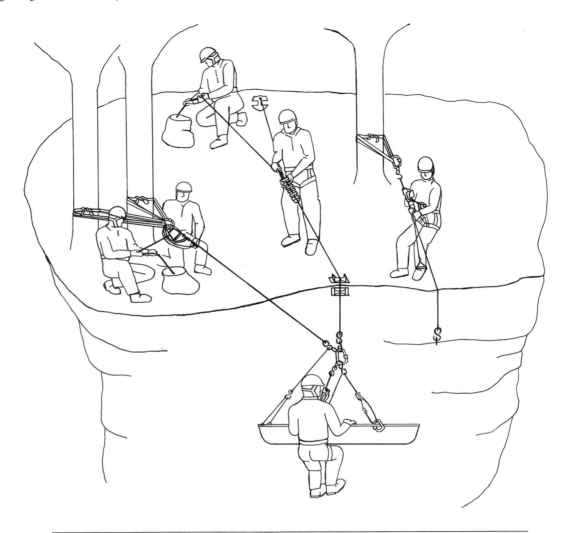

FIGURE 15-1
Basic elements of lowering system.

In some lowering systems, there will be only one main line with a belay. In other systems, there will be two main lines.

Belay System

The belay system is attached to the load and acts as a safety should there be a failure in the main line lowering system.

Brake Device

These are friction devices that are the same as, or similar to, rappel devices. They provide friction on rope running through them to control the descent of the load.

Brakeman

The brakeman controls the speed of the descent of the load by controlling the rope through the brake device.

Rope Handler

The rope handler assists the brakeman by passing the rope to him or her and making certain there are no kinks to jam the brake device.

Belayer

The belayer controls the belay rope through the belay device and catches the load with the belay system should the main lowering system fail.

Edge Tenders

The edge tenders assist the litter tender(s) in getting the litter over the edge of the drop, prevent rope abrasion on the edge, and, if needed, relay voice communications between the litter tender and the brakeman.

Rescue Team Leader

The rescue team leader is the manager of the operation. In the ideal situation, the leader does not get physically involved in actions such as rigging but maintains an objective overall view of the operation.

Safety Officer

The safety officer does not get engrossed in other activities such as operations, so he or she can stand back and be objective about any threats to safety. The safety officer must have the right to stop any operation he or she sees as a threat to safety and must be an experienced individual who thoroughly understands equipment, rigging, and rescue techniques. He or she must also be able to instantly look at a situation and know if something is incorrect, must always be able to stand back with an objective viewpoint, and must never be sucked into the operation itself. Safety officers check for the following:

- Hazards, including hazardous atmospheres and falling debris.
- Personal safety equipment, including helmets, gloves, and breathing apparatus.
- Rescue rigging, including belays, anchors, rope padding, and unlocked carabiners.
- Personal rigging, including seat harnesses, locked carabiners, and knots tied correctly.

Braking Systems for Lowering

The principles of using a braking device for high angle lowering are similar to rappelling. Whether you use the device for rappelling or lowering, the device imparts friction to the rope running through it. And, indeed, some of the devices that are used for lowering are the same as used in rappelling. Some examples are brake bar racks and figure **8** descenders.

But any breaking device used in lowering must provide an adequate margin of control of the load being lowered. A figure **8** descender, for example, may provide adequate control for one person's body weight. But the figure **8** may not provide enough control for loads greater than one person's body weight. For lowering of loads greater than one person's body weight, you will need a device that offers greater friction, such as a brake bar rack (six bars) or a brake tube.

The primary difference between lowering and rappelling is that in most cases of lowering, the friction device remains stationary while the rope moves through it (known as a *fixed brake lower*). In rappelling, the friction device moves, while the rope remains stationary.

Belays for Lowering Systems

In lowering systems, there should be redundancy in the lowering lines so that if one lowering line fails, another will catch the load. This can mean a belay that is apart from, and on a separate anchor from, the main lowering system. Or it can mean two separate lowering lines that back up one another.

In either situation, the systems should be far enough apart so that these two elements do not interfere with one another and become entangled. But they should be close enough together to prevent a dangerous pendulum should the main line fail and the belay be forced to catch the load.

The load caught by a belay in a rescue lowering operation may not fall as great a distance as in climbing. But the lowering must be able to hold the weight of the rescue load plus any force from shock loading. The belayer must use belay devices that enable the belayer to stop the fall of the rescue load.

Communication in Rescue Lowering

As in slope evacuation, the primary exchange of communication signals takes place between the litter tender and the brakeman. If conditions permit, this should be direct communication between the two persons. If there cannot be direct communication because of such factors as distance, noise from machinery or traffic, or waterfall, then a relay person might be required. If *edge tenders* are being used, then one of these persons can be assigned as a communications relay.

Radios

Over longer distances, radios may be a necessity. They also may be required for medical control or for relaying the medical condition of the subject.

The use of the traditional hip-belt radio holsters create some problems in high angle rescue:

- They interfere with seat harnesses and use of equipment.
- They require extensive use of hand and arm motion to use the radio.
- They can result in the radios being dropped.

One solution to these difficulties is the use of a radio chest harness (Figure 15-2). These harnesses, which are commercially available, have the following advantages:

- They are closer, so they do not have to be taken out of the holster for use.
- The chest area is usually free of other harnesses and equipment.
- A simple hand motion can key the mike.

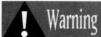

! Warning

In a rescue lowering, a belayer must never use a hip belay or any other belay technique that employs rope friction around the body.

Also, the belayer must never place his or her body as a link in the belay system when rescue lowering (see Chapter 8, Belaying of One-Person Loads).

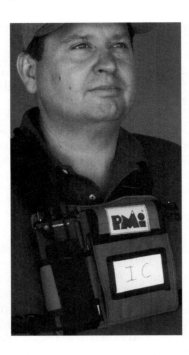

FIGURE 15-2
Chest radio harness.

One other solution to communications challenges is the voice-activated radio. With the mike positioned next to the mouth, transmission occurs whenever someone speaks. One drawback to these radios is that in high winds, the mikes may be keyed by the wind, which prevent communications.

Voice Communication

Direct and reliable communication in vertical lowering is critical for the safety of the patient and rescuers and for the success of the operation. To avoid dangerous confusion, voice communications must be limited only to a few standardized commands necessary for litter movement and for safety.

If the lowering system includes a single line plus belay, then the standard belay commands are included in the lowering commands (Box 15-1).

THE PRINCIPLES OF RESCUE LOWERING

As mentioned earlier in this chapter (see the section Braking Systems for Lowering on page 191), any braking device used in rescue lowering must provide an adequate margin of control of the load being lowered. The first exercise shown for lowering practice uses a figure 8 descender because it is simpler to use in learning the basics of lowering loads. Although the figure 8 may provide adequate control for one person's body weight, it should not be used for loads greater than one person's body weight. For lowering of loads greater than one person's body weight, you

Box 15-1 Lowering Commands

"ON BELAY."
Litter tender to belayer.

"BELAY ON."
Belayer to litter tender.

"DOWN SLOW."
or

"DOWN FAST."
Litter tender to brakeman.

"STOP!"
Generally the litter tender to the brakeman but may be given by anyone who sees danger or potential problems developing.

"STOP! STOP!
or

WHY STOP?"
Litter tender to brakeman. This is given when, for an unexplained reason and without command from the litter tender, the rope has stopped moving. It could be that the brakeman is still letting out rope, but the rope is jammed somewhere. This obviously has the potential for creating a very serious problem and requires an explanation from the brakeman.

"OFF BELAY."
Litter tender to belayer. The litter, rescue subject, and litter tender(s) are on the ground, or in a secure position, and in no danger of falling.

"BELAY OFF."
Belayer to litter tender.

In addition, the following voice communications may also be used when needed:

"SLACK."
Litter tender to brakeman or belayer. The rope is too taut, give us some slack.

"TENSION."
Litter tender to brakeman or belayer. Take up some rope and make it more taut to help us out here.

When a belay is being used, then the tender must specify which line he or she is talking about:

"SLACK ON BELAY LINE."
or

"SLACK ON MAIN LINE."
When the litter has reached the ground, this might also be said:

"OFF ROPE."
Litter tender to brakeman: "I have unclipped the rope from the litter and no longer need the line."

will need a device that offers greater friction, such as a brake bar rack (six bars) or a brake tube.

This practice activity is designed to acquaint the student with the basic principles of lowering but under controlled conditions and using the weight of only one person. This lowering sequence uses a practice rescuer as a load and a figure **8** with ears as a braking device (Figure 15-3).

Lowering One Person Using Figure 8 with Ears (Steep Slope)

1. At the top of a short, approximately 45-degree slope, establish a secure anchor, with an anchor sling attached to it. In the end of the anchor sling, attach a locking carabiner. (If a slope is not available, then use a flight of stairs.)

2. At a separate secure anchor, have a belayer establish a belay station with a sling attached to it. In the end of the sling should be a large locking carabiner with a belay device attached (see Chapter 8, Belaying of One-Person Loads, for additional guidelines on belaying).

3. Have a practice rescuer wear a sewn, manufactured seat harness. Into the seat harness tie-in points, have the practice rescuer clip two locking carabiners. One is for the main lowering line, the other is for a belay. Have the practice rescuer clip the appropriate carabiner into the belay rope and lock the carabiner.

4. With the large figure **8** descender close to where it will be anchored, the brakeman laces the main line rope onto it as shown in Figure 15-4. The small ring should be clipped into the anchor rope with a locking carabiner and the carabiner gate locked. The large ring should be pointed toward the practice rescuer and laced onto the rope going to him or her.

5. The practice rescuer should be facing the brakeman and in a secure position where there is no danger of falling. The practice rescuer takes the main line rope with a figure **8** on a bight knot in it and clips it into a seat harness carabiner. He or she secures it by locking the carabiner.

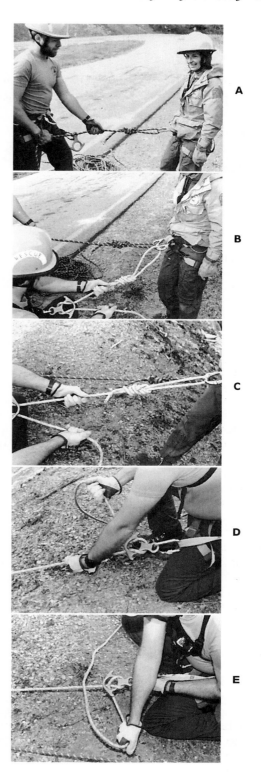

FIGURE 15-3
Figure 8 lowering on slope.

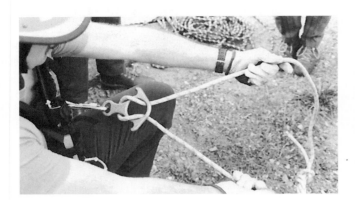

FIGURE 15-4
Figure 8 laced for lowering.

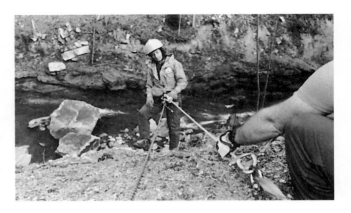

FIGURE 15-5
Brakeman stance for lowering.

6. The practice rescuer takes the figure 8 knot in the end of the belay line, clips into the second seat harness carabiner and secures the carabiner. The practice rescuer initiates the belay sequence (Practice rescuer: "on belay." Belayer: "belay on.")

7. The brakeman pulls the slack out of the section of the main line rope that is between the figure 8 descender and the practice rescuer.

8. For the remainder of this procedure, the brakeman should be wearing gloves. The brakeman's stance should be as shown in Figure 15-5. The following should all be in a straight line: anchor point, anchor sling, anchor carabiner, figure 8 descender, the rope between the figure 8 descender and the practice rescuer, and the practice rescuer's seat harness tie-in.

9. The brakeman's dominant hand (right hand on right-handed people) should be on the slack rope that is feeding into the braking device. This is the *brake hand*. The brake hand must never leave the rope during the lowering operation except when the lowering device is securely locked off. The other hand (the left hand on right-handed people) should be on the rope leading out of the figure 8 descender toward the practice rescuer. This is the *guide hand*.

10. The practice rescuer pretensions the system to make certain that all parts of the system are rigged correctly under load and that no lines will tangle. This also is to remove all slack from the system to avoid shock load when going over the edge. To do this, the practice rescuer calls, "preload." The brakeman holds tension on the brakes, and the practice rescuer pulls slack out of the system.

11. When the practice rescuer is satisfied the rigging is correct, and ready to begin descending, he or she says to the brakeman, "down slow." The brakeman begins slowly allowing the rope

through the figure 8 descender as the practice rescuer walks backward downhill. The brakeman should keep the brake hand approximately 18 inches from the figure 8 descender and slowly allow the rope to slip through his gloved hand.

The guide hand stays lightly in its place on the rope helping to guide the rope out of the figure 8 descender on its way toward the practice rescuer. Where there is temporarily too much friction for the practice rescuer to pull the rope through the descender, the brakeman's guide hand can help pull rope through the device.

12. The belayer must control the belay rope so that there is enough slack in the belay line and it does not interfere with the movement of the practice rescuer. But there must not be too much slack in the belay line, so should the main lowering line fail, the belay line can immediately take the load without severe shock loading.

Locking Off

13. The practice rescuer calls, "stop." The brakeman holds the rope taut, stopping the descent of the practice rescuer. The belayer maintains an "on belay" status.

14. Tying off the figure 8 descender as a braking device is similar to tying it off as a rappel device. *During this procedure, maintain a firm grasp on the brake side of the rope and do not allow the rope to slip through the descender.* With the brake hand, swing the brake side of the rope forward toward the load (practice rescuer) until the brake side of the rope is parallel with the rope that goes out of the descender toward the practice rescuer. Still holding the brake side of the rope taut, swing it farther around in an arc until it is trapped between the large ring of the figure 8 descender and the rope going to the load.

15. To further secure the rope, pull the brake side of the rope firmly down toward the anchor, across

the surface of the figure **8**, and around behind one ear. Pull it firmly between the line going to the load and the large ring and above the line first locked off. Make certain that the rope lies firmly around the device and there is no slack. Bring the brake side of the rope down and around the figure **8** again as before, then behind one ear, but do not place it between the line going to the anchor and the large ring. Instead, form a large bight of rope from the brake side of the rope. Bring the bight up parallel with the rope going to the load. Tie an overhand knot with the bight onto the rope going to the anchor. Be certain that the overhand knot is contoured well, is set firmly against the top of the figure **8**, and there is no slack in the knot (Figure 15-6).

Unlocking

16. Unlocking the brake device is the reverse of tying it off. Untie the overhand knot. Take the bight out of the rope and unwrap it from the figure **8** descender *while making certain that the brake side of the rope remains trapped between the large figure 8 ring and the rope going to the load. Now, while maintaining firm control of the brake side of the rope with the brake hand, untrap the rope and bring it back to its normal position for lowering.*

17. The practice rescuer gives the voice communication, "down slow" (or "down fast"). The brakeman lowers at the appropriate speed, while the belayer maintains control of the belay rope.

Getting Off Rope

18. When the practice rescuer reaches the ground or other intended secure position, he or she calls, "stop." The brakeman stops rope from passing through the descender. (If the lowering rope is too tight for the practice rescuer to disconnect from it, he or she calls, "slack." The brakeman allows some slack to come into the rope.) The belayer maintains the load on belay until the practice rescuer relieves him or her by completing the belay cycle. (Practice rescuer: "off belay." Belayer: "belay off.")

Using a Figure 8 with Ears to Lower a Person down a Vertical Face (Figure 15-7)

1. Choose a short vertical face (approximately 20 feet) where the top breaks over gradually into a steep face. On the first try, do not choose a face with a sharp edge or one that is undercut.

2. Establish a secure anchor point safely back from the edge. *If the brakeman or practice rescuer are too close to the edge they should be attached to a safety line that is connected to a secure anchor point.* If possible, have the anchor point high off the ground. This will assist the practice rescuer in going over the edge. Attach an anchor sling to the anchor point.

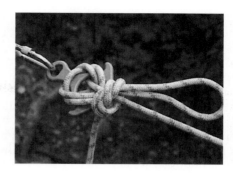

FIGURE 15-6
Locking off figure 8 brakes.

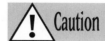 **Caution**

If the practice rescuer is heavy (over 160 lb) the brakeman should make the lowering with the figure 8 descender *double wrapped.*

This anchor sling should be short enough so that the practice rescuer can rig into the main line without being too close to the edge. Have a loop in the end of the anchor sling and clip a locking carabiner to that loop.

3. Establish a separate anchor point for a belay. Securely connect an anchor sling into the anchor point. The anchor point and sling should be established so that when the belayer takes position, he or she has a good field of view of the top and face but is not in danger of falling over the edge. The belayer should be tied into a safety line that is not part of the belay line. (In the ideal situation, he or she should be on a separate anchor from the belay. If this is not possible, then he or she may be on the same anchor point but his or her body must not be linked to the belay system.) (See Chapter 8, Belaying of One-Person Loads, and Figure 15-7, *A*.)

4. On the edge, place an edge roller or a rope pad to protect the main line lowering rope. The edge roller or rope pad should be anchored so that it remains in place and protects the rope as the rope passes over it (Figure 15-7, *B*).

5. Now follow steps 3 through 9 on p. 193 for *attaching the practice rescuer into the belay and lowering system* (Figures 15-7, *C, D,* and *E*).

6. The practice rescuer pretensions the system to make certain that all parts of the system are rigged correctly under load and that no lines will tangle. This will also remove all slack from the system and avoid shock load when going over the edge. To do this, the practice rescuer calls,

"preload." The brakeman holds tension on the brakes, and the practice rescuer pulls slack out of the system.

7. When the practice rescuer is satisfied the rigging is correct, and ready to begin descending, he or she should give the "down slow" voice communication to the brakeman. The brakeman should now slowly allow the rope to pass through the figure **8** descender. The practice rescuer leans back against the rope and begins to move backwards towards the drop (Figure 15-7, *F*).

Getting Over the Edge

8. Getting over the edge will likely be the most difficult part of the operation for the practice rescuer. To make this operation go smoothly, the practice rescuer should remain in close communication with the brakeman. The practice rescuer should not be in a hurry but approach the edge deliberately and slowly. At the edge, the practice rescuer may want to give a "stop" to the brakeman and examine the nature of the situation. The practice rescuer should approach this situation as he or she would a rappel: feet a shoulder's length apart,

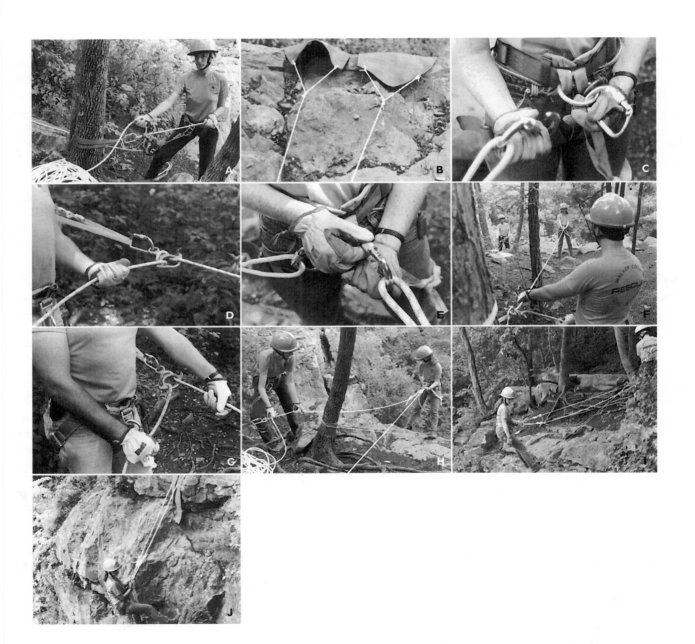

FIGURE 15-7
Figure 8 lowering on verticle.

body perpendicular to the slope, facing the brake-man but looking over his or her shoulder at what is about to come.

9. Follow steps 11 through 17 on p. 194 in lowering one person using figure **8** ears (Figure 15-7, *G, H, I,* and *J*).

Using a Brake Bar Rack to Lower a Practice Rescuer on a Slope

This practice exercise is designed to give the student the feel of lowering a load using a brake bar rack as the braking device. This lowering sequence again uses a practice rescuer as a load (Figure 15-8).

1. Follow steps 1 through 6 on p. 193 (using figure **8** with ears) except do not use a figure **8** descender. Instead, attach the eye of a brake bar rack to the main anchor with a locking carabiner. The rack should be aligned so that the bars are in a horizontal orientation, with the bend of the rack pointing toward the drop. The top bar should be positioned so that its slot that clips onto the frame faces down. Lock the carabiner.

2. Unclip all the bars except for the top bar (the one next to the bend of the rack).

3. Lay the main line rope *on top of* the top bar. *Do not run the rope between the top bar and the rack.* Pull slack out of the rope between the practice rescuer and the top bar. Do this gently so that the practice rescuer is not pulled off balance. With one hand, hold the rack. With the other, pull the rope over the top bar and around the bottom back toward the practice rescuer. At the same time slack is pulled out of the rope between the rack and the practice rescuer, slack should also come out of the anchor sling between the eye of the rack and the anchor point.

4. While continuing to hold the rope taut with one hand, use the other hand to engage the second bar. Slide it up to jam the rope between it and the top bar. As you lace the rope onto the rack, be certain that the rope runs on the side of the bar that is opposite the notch that clips it to the frame of the rack. This keeps the bars pressed against the rack frame.

5. While one hand is holding the second bar in place against the rope, use the other hand to bring the rope around the second bar, as was done around the top bar, so that the rope holds the second bar in place.

6. Continue this procedure until all the bars needed to lower the person down the slope have been laced onto the rack.

7. To lower the brake bar rack, the brakeman's dominant hand (the right hand on a right-handed person) should be on the portion of the rope that is feeding into the brake bar rack. *This is the brack hand. It should never be taken off the rope until the practice rescuer is off rope or the brake bar rack is securely tied off.* The other hand should be on the bars of the rack, cradling them. This is the *guide hand* and it can be used to help change the amount of friction by manipulating the bars.

8. After the rope is laced up in the brake bar rack, take the rope in the brake hand and pull it forward hard in the direction of the load. This should do two things:
   1. Take any slack out of the anchor sling.
   2. Jam the bars together toward the top of the rack.

This is known as the *quick stop position*. It prevents rope from going through the rack. Use this position whenever the lowering has to be stopped quickly.

Now, hold the rack in the quick stop position until the practice rescuer is ready to start being lowered.

Lowering the Practice Rescuer

9. When the practice rescuer is ready, he or she initiates the belay cycle. (Practice rescuer: "on belay." Belayer: "belay on.")

10. The practice rescuer pretensions the system to make certain that all parts of the system are rigged correctly under load and that no lines will tangle. This also is to remove all slack from the system to avoid shock load when going over the edge.

    To do this, the practice rescuer calls, "preload." The brakeman holds tension on the brakes, and the practice rescuer pulls slack out of the system.

11. When the practice rescuer is satisfied the rigging is correct, and ready to begin descending, he or she says to the brakeman, "down slow." The brakeman then begins to allow rope through the brake bar rack. The practice rescuer should lean against the rope to help it move through the brake system. If the rope is not moving through the rack, then the brakeman can encourage it by reducing rack friction.

Changing Friction When Using the Brake Bar Rack for Lowering

12. As in rappelling with the brake bar rack, it is best to begin a lowering with more bars engaged than you expect to need. Once the full weight of the rescuer is on the system, and there is still a need to reduce friction so that the practice rescuer can go faster, first try spreading the bars apart along the length of the rack with the guide hand. The farther apart the bars are from one another, the lower the friction.

    If you still have too much friction, then disengage the bottom bar. Do this in the following way: take the end of the rope in the brake hand and swing in an arc from the quick stop position, first back towards the anchor and then under the rack and toward the load. This releases the bottom bar from under the rope but still has the rope pressing the fifth bar against the other bars.

Now take the guide hand, squeeze the two legs of the rack together, disengage the last bar and move it out of the way. Using the guide hand spread the remaining bars apart to lessen friction.

If there is still too much friction, repeat the procedure with the next bar up, the fifth bar. Swing the rope in an arc in a direction opposite from before so that it uncovers the fifth bar but holds the remaining four bars in quick stop. Unclip the fifth bar and slide it back on the rack toward the eye and out of the way. *Do not lower a load on less than four bars. If the loaded rope is still not moving through the remaining four bars, spread the bars with the guide hand to reduce the friction and/or push the rope through the bars with the brake hand.*

Locking Off

13. The practice rescuer calls, "stop!" The brakeman stops the rope from going through the brake bar rack. The brakeman brings the rack into the *quick stop* position as described on p. 197.
14. If the practice rescuer is to be stopped for an extended length of time, then the brakeman can tie off the brake bar rack. With the brake hand holding the rope in the "quick stop" position, he or she pulls the rope across the top bar and between the curve of the rack and the strand of the rope going to the anchor (Figure 15-9).
15. Next, the brakeman brings the rope back toward the eye of the rack, holding the rope firmly so that it keeps all the bars locked together. The

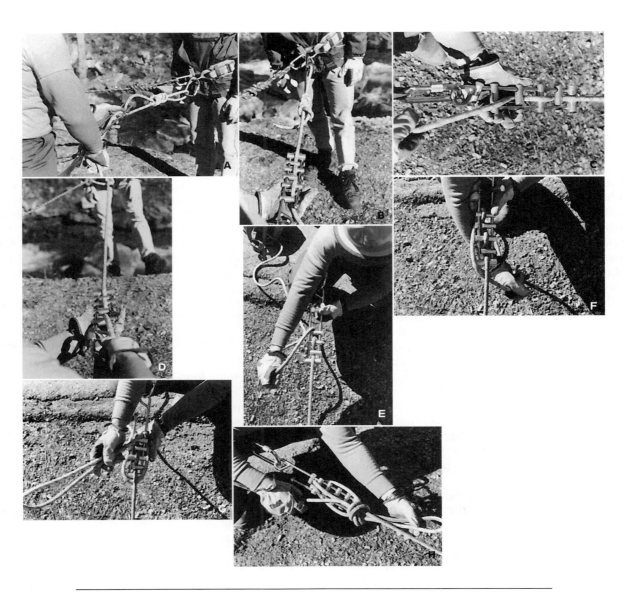

FIGURE 15-8
Brake bar rack lowering on slope.

brakeman then brings the rope through the two legs of the rack and across the bottom bar.

16. Then the brakeman again brings the rope toward the practice rescuer, in the same path as before. The brakeman should pull it firmly so that all the rope strands are taut and the bars are locked together.

17. The brake bar rack should now be locked in the "stop" position. To secure the rope, the brakeman forms a large bight with the strand of rope in his or her brake hand. Use the guide hand to assist in forming this bight.

18. Treating the bight as one strand of rope, tie an overhand knot across the strand of the rope that is going to the practice rescuer. The brakeman should cinch the overhand knot down firmly against the top bar of the rack. *There must be no slack in the strands of rope running over the rack and no space between the bars.* The brake bar rack is now locked off.

Unlocking the Brake Bar Rack

19. The practice rescuer says, "down slow" (or "down fast"). When unlocking the brake bar rack, the brakeman must *always keep a firm grip on the brake side of the rope and allow no slack in the brake side of the rope.* To untie the overhand knot, the brakeman pulls slowly on the braking end of the rope, positioning the guide hand at the center of the bight so that it comes out slowly.

20. With the brake hand firmly on the rope, the brakeman pulls the brake side of the rope in a 180-degree arc until it is pointing in the direction of the anchor.

21. Now, the brakeman, still grasping the rope firmly with the brake hand, pulls the rope from between the two legs of the rack, around the top

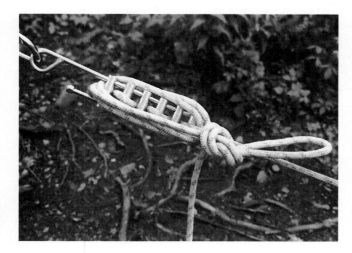

FIGURE 15-9
Locking off rack.

bar and then back to the normal braking position. *The rope must be kept taut by the brake hand during these steps.* With the guide hand, the brakeman spreads the bars apart and continues lowering the practice rescuer.

Getting Off Rope

22. When the practice rescuer reaches the ground or other intended secure position, he or she calls, "stop." The brakeman stops the rope from passing through the brake bar rack. The belayer maintains the load on belay until the practice rescuer relieves him or her by completing the belay cycle: (Practice rescuer: "off belay." Belayer: "belay off.")

If the rope is too taut for the practice rescuer to disconnect the main line from his or her seat harness carabiner, he or she calls, "slack." The brakeman allows some rope through the brake bar rack to allow slack in the main line.

If the practice rescuer has finished with the rope and is ready for it to be used for other purposes, then he or she disconnects from it and signals to the brakeman, "off rope." The brakeman can then pull the end of the rope back to his or her position, remove it from the anchor, or do with it whatever else is needed.

Using a Brake Bar Rack to Lower a Practice Rescuer down a Vertical Drop (Figure 15-10).

1. Choose a short vertical drop (approximately 20 feet) where the top breaks over gradually into a steep face. On the first try, do not choose a face with a sharp edge or one that is undercut.

2. Establish a secure anchor point safely back from the edge. If possible, have the anchor point high up off the ground. This will make it easier for the practice rescuer in going over the edge and for the brakeman to control him or her at that point. The anchor sling should be positioned so that the practice rescuer can rig into the main line without being too close to the edge. However, the brake system should be close enough to the edge for the brakeman to hear voice communications from the practice rescuer. At the end of the anchor sling clip a locking carabiner.

3. Establish a separate anchor point for a belay. Connect a belay sling securely to the anchor point. The anchor point and sling should be rigged so that the belayer has a good field of view of the top and face but is not in danger of falling over the edge. The belayer should be attached to a safety line that is not part of the belay link to the practice rescuer. In the ideal situation, the belayer should be on a separate line from the belay. If this is not possible, then the belayer may be on the same anchor point but his or her body should not be a link in the belay system (see Chapter 8).

4. On the edge of the drop, place an edge roller or rope pad to protect the main line lowering rope. The edge protection should be anchored so that it remains in place and protects the rope as it runs over the edge under load.

5. Now follow steps 1 through 9 on p. 197 for attaching the practice rescuer into the belay and braking systems and for lacing the brake bar rack into the main lowering line.

6. The practice rescuer pretensions the system to make certain that all parts of the system are rigged correctly under load and that no lines will tangle. This also is to remove all slack from the system to avoid shock load when going over the edge. To do this, the practice rescuer calls, "preload." The brakeman holds tension on the brakes, and the practice rescuer pulls slack out of the system.

7. When the practice rescuer is satisfied, the rigging is correct, and ready to begin descending, he or she says to the brakeman, "down slow." As the practice rescuer leans back against the rope and begins to move slowly backwards toward the drop, the brakeman should allow the rope to pass through the brake bar rack. In order for the practice rescuer to move, it may be necessary for the brakeman to spread the bars of the rack apart and, possibly, even remove one or two of the bars. But the brakeman must remember: *as the practice rescuer starts over the edge, and his or her full weight comes onto the rope and the braking system, more friction will be needed in the brake bar rack.*

8. See notes in step 8 p. 196 for guidelines on getting over the edge.

9. On the short vertical drop, continue with steps 11 through 22 on p. 197 (using a brake bar rack to lower a practice rescuer on a slope).

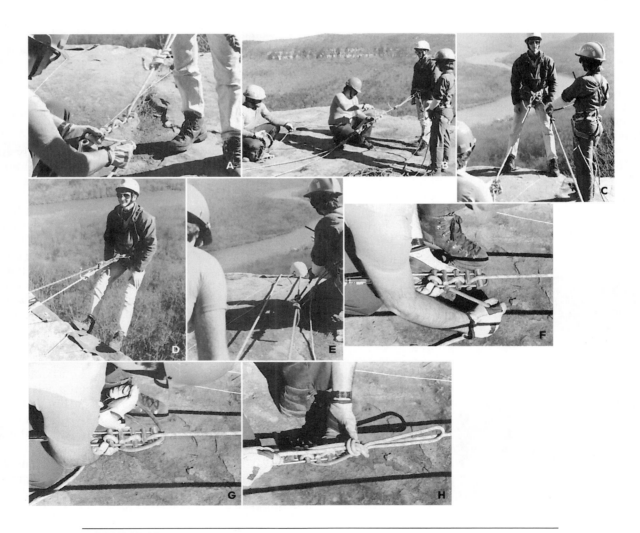

FIGURE 15-10

Lowering on vertical with rack.

LITTER LOWERING SYSTEMS

Litter lowering systems are among the most spectacular of the rope systems. But they are among the most complex. They require superior skills in vertical techniques, in rope management, and in teamwork, as well as a complete knowledge of equipment. For these reasons, litter-lowering systems must be thoroughly planned, worked out, and practiced before they are needed in a real rescue.

Safety Factors in Litter Lowering Systems

Litter lowering systems have higher loads than those systems that involve the load of only one person. The increased loads mean greater stress on the entire vertical system, including ropes, carabiners, knots, anchors, braking systems, and belay system.

These loads include the combined weight of litter, hardware, and other rescue gear; the rescue subject; and one or two litter tenders. (See Chapter 3, "Rope and Related Equipment," on calculating safety factors.)

Position of Litter for Lowering

When possible, a litter is lowered in a horizontal position. This is usually the more comfortable and reassuring position for the rescue subject. It is less likely to complicate most medical conditions and it makes it easier to tend to the medical needs of the subject.

There will be, however, conditions where the litter may have to be lowered in a vertical position. These conditions usually relate to confined space or when obstructions on the face require a small cross section for the litter.

Single Line versus Double Line Lowering

There are many different techniques for lowering litters, but they are generally divided into two types:
1. *Single Line Lowering*
   - One main line for the litter plus a belay line.
   - One litter tender.
2. *Double Line Lowering*
   - Two main lines for the litter. Possibly a belay line.
   - May have two litter attendants.

There are advantages and disadvantages to both systems (Box 15-2).

Litter Rigging for Single Line Lowering

Figure 15-11 illustrates the litter rigging for a single line lowering.

The Spider

The spider joins the main line lowering rope to the litter. It consists of a group of lines that are first attached at separate points to the litter rail and then attached together at the main line lowering rope. The connection where the spiders and main line rope come together is known as the *Master Attachment Point (MAP)*. *For a single line lowering, there should be a minimum of four legs for a spider.*

Spiders can be purchased in the manufactured form or created from webbing or rope. Many litter manufacturers supply spiders but most of these cannot be adjusted for height and litter angle and lack flexibility for different rescue situations.

There are a number of manufactured spiders available that are adjustable for height and angle and have tie-in points for litter tenders. Only purchase pre-made spiders from reputable manufacturers who have specifically designed them for rescue purposes.

Spider Material

Spiders may be constructed either from webbing or rope. Most rescuers who create their own spiders make them from rope because it is easier to handle and allows for a greater variety of knots than webbing.

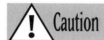

Caution

When using the SKED litter system in a high angle lowering, use the litter's horizontal lift slings as a spider and follow the directions of the manufacturer for their use.

Box 15-2 Advantages and Disadvantages of Single Line vs Double Line Lowering with Belay

SINGLE LINE LOWERING

Advantages:
- Simpler rope work and brake management.

Disadvantages:
- May not have adequate safety factor for weight of two litter tenders.
- More difficult to tilt litter from horizontal to vertical position (requires the loading of the belay line to tilt the litter).

DOUBLE LINE LOWERING

Advantages:
- Can be used where two litter tenders are needed, such as:
  1. Complicated medical management of subject.
  2. Vertical face is too difficult for one tender to manage litter (such as overhangs and gullies).
- Useful where it is necessary to shift orientation of litter.

Disadvantages:
- Greater stress in brake systems and anchors (if both lines run through the same brake).
- More complex rope management.
- May be more difficult to keep litter horizontal if lines come to two different points on the litter.

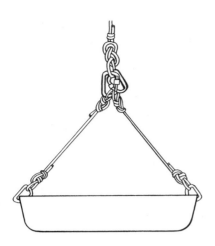

FIGURE 15-11
Litter rigging view from end showing two of four fixed legs.

The lower end of the spider legs attaches to the litter rails with large locking carabiners. The spider should not be tied directly into the litter rail because rope or webbing could abrade through when rubbed over rock. Also, the carabiners give greater flexibility for attaching or detaching the spider to the litter rail.

The carabiner gates should be set inward towards the center of the litter. This helps prevent the lock nut on the locking carabiner from being rubbed open on the face of the cliff or wall. The gates should also be oriented so their locking nuts will close with gravity and not vibrate to an unlocked position.

The spider should be adjusted so that the subject rides in the litter slightly head up (unless there are medical reasons to have the head down). If the subject rides head down, it will add to his or her anxiety and disorientation.

Creating a Spider from Rope

One simple way to create a leg of each spider is from an approximately 7-foot length of rope (Figure 15-11). The rope should be at least ³⁄₈-inch diameter. Tie a figure 8 on a bight knot in each end. Create four of these and make certain that after the knots are tied, the spider legs are all exactly the same lengths.

Alternative Approach: Webbing Sling or Anchor Strip. An even simpler and quicker approach for creating a nonadjustable spider is to use a presewn webbing sling or anchor strap for each spider leg. (See page 74, Chapter 7, Anchoring for information on presewn slings and anchor straps.)

Attaching Spider to Main Line Lowering Rope (Master Attachment Point)

1. At the end of the main line lowering rope, tie a figure 8 on a bight knot.

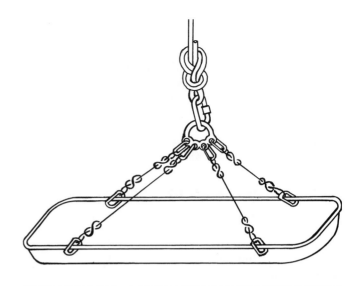

FIGURE 15-12
The rigging plate is an alternative carabiner attachment at the master attachment point.

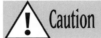

Not all large locking carabiners will fit easily over litter rails. Before purchasing carabiners for this use, measure the diameter of the rail and consult the specifications of the carabiner manufacturer or distributor.

2. Clip a large locking carabiner into this knot. This carabiner must be designed for rescue duty.
3. Now bring all four figure 8 on a bight knots in the ends of the spider legs together. Clip the same carabiner across them and lock the gate.

Alternative Approach: Rigging Plate. An alternative to carabiners at the master attachment point is a rigging plate (Figure 15-12). The rigging plate provides a strong attachment point, while allowing for a variety of rigging points.

1. Attach the rigging plate directly to the main line lowering rope with a figure 8 follow through knot through the large hole.
2. Clip each figure 8 on a bight knot at the top of the spider into its own carabiner.
3. Clip each carabiner into a small hole of the brake plate.

Creating an Adjustable Spider from Rope

Figure 15-13 illustrates an adjustable litter spider made from rope. The adjustable spider can be used in situations where the litter needs to be tilted on its axis. One example of such a situation would be where the cliff is not completely vertical but lies at

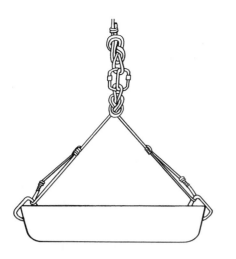

FIGURE 15-13
Two legs of an adjustable litter spider.

a steep angle. To compensate for this angle, but keep the litter and rescue subject on a horizontal, this litter spider can be adjusted.

The materials needed include:

◆ Two lengths of static kernmantle ropes, each 12-feet long. This should be at least ³⁄₈-inch diameter.

◆ Four lengths of Prusik material, each 4-feet long. The Prusik cord must be of appropriate diameter to grip the static kernmantle rope. For example: 7 mm Prusik cord on ⁷⁄₁₆-inch rope, 8 mm on ¹⁄₂-inch (11 mm) rope.

◆ Four locking carabiners with gate openings large enough to fit over litter rail.

1. At the midpoint of each of the static kernmantle ropes, tie a figure **8** on a bight knot. Take the figure **8** on a bight knots and hold them together with the rope strands hanging down. There should be a total of two figure **8** on a bight knots, with four rope strands of equal length hanging down from them.

2. Take the center of each piece of Prusik material and tie a Prusik hitch onto each strand of static kernmantle rope about halfway between the figure **8** on a bight knot and the end.

3. At each of the four ends of the static kernmantle ropes, attach the two ends of a length of Prusik material. Do this with a figure **8** bend (or grapevine) knot.

4. When this is done, there should be four spider legs. Each one should have a loop in its bottom end that is adjustable by sliding the Prusik knot up or down on the static kernmantle material.

5. In each loop at the bottom made by the Prusik material, clip a large locking carabiner.

6. Now hold the completed spider over the litter.

7. Clip each carabiner into a point on the litter rail that gives equalized loading when the litter is loaded.

8. Clip the two figure **8** on a bight knots at the top of the spider into a main line lowering rope with a large locking carabiner for the master attachment point, or attach them to a rigging plate as shown on Figure 15-13.

Rescue Subject Tie-Ins

During a high angle rescue, the patient must be attached to a secure safety and belay system. This system must securely connect the patient, patient packaging, and direct attachments to the spider master attachment point. If the patient is on a spine board, the patient must be securely packaged onto the board, which, as a unit with the patient, is connected to the safety lines. The patient should also be secured in the litter with lacing across the top to prevent shifting in the litter.

The patient should be wearing a harness. A safety sling runs from the subject's harness to the carabiners at the top of the spider MAP. This safety sling is designed to catch the subject if there is a failure in the litter. Always leave slack in the safety sling so the subject will not be pulled upward if the litter tilts.

Litter Tender Tie-Ins

A litter tender tie-in serves the following primary purposes:

◆ To support the weight of the tender so that he or she can have hands free for such tasks as managing the litter and attending to the rescue subject.

◆ To provide safety from falling.

◆ To allow freedom of movement. The tender should be able to move around the litter to clear possible tangles, to clear obstructions under the litter, and to reach all of the subject's anatomy.

Figure 15-14 illustrates a litter tender tie-in system using two ascenders.

The main attachment to the litter system is a "pigtail." It is made of an approximately 12-foot long piece of rope. It is attached with a figure **8** on a bight knot to the carabiners at master attachment point at the end of the main line lowering rope.

The litter tender is attached to the pigtail with two ascenders. One ascender is attached with a sling to the tender's seat harness, while the other ascender is attached with a sling to the tender's foot. To prevent the ascenders from accidentally slipping off the end of the pigtail, the lower end is brought back up and clipped into the tender's seat harness.

This rigging of the pigtail gives the litter tenders the freedom of movement needed in litter lowering. He or she can move with his or her ascenders above the level of the litter to clear possible tangles in the spider rigging. Or he or she can move down below the level of the litter to remove obstructions, such as loose rock.

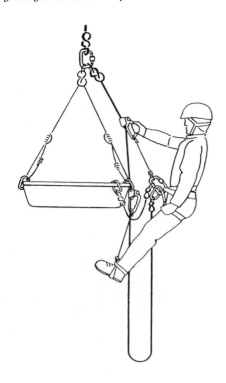

FIGURE 15-14
Litter tender tie-in.

Alternative Approach: Daisy Chain. An alternative litter tender tie-in is a daisy chain. The end of the daisy chain is clipped into the carabiner at the top of the spider, and the litter tender clips into the appropriate "pocket" on the daisy chain to give the proper position on the litter.

The daisy chain tie-in offers these advantages:

♦ It is simple to use.
♦ It can be used by personnel who are not experienced with ascenders.

The daisy chain tie-in offers this disadvantage:

♦ The litter tender lacks the mobility to move below the litter to clear obstructions or perform other tasks.

Procedure for Lowering a Litter (Single Line with Belay)

Use of a Live Practice Subject for Litter Lowering

The use of a live practice subject for litter lowering practice can be very dangerous. There is of course the danger of practice rescuers dropping the practice subject, and in natural areas there is often an extreme danger due to falling rocks. To ensure safety and simplify the operation, first-time litter lowerings should use a dummy or weights in place of a live person.

Many rescue teams, once they have become experienced, do use live practice subjects. They feel that it is important that all persons directly involved in litter lowerings eventually gain experience as the "patient"

strapped into a litter that is being lowered. This will be the only way they can fully comprehend the feelings of the rescue subject.

However, live practice subjects should *only be used after the rescue team has had the amount of quality practice needed to ensure the safety of the person in the litter.*

The Main Line Lowering System

As noted earlier, both the main line anchor and the belay anchor must have a safety factor appropriate to the load that will be on the system.

In addition, the system must be rigged at the top for safety and convenience. On the main line anchor system, the lowering device (such as the brake bar rack) must be attached to the anchor system so that:

1. The brakeman is close enough to the edge to hear voice communication from the litter tender, or there is an edge tender relaying communications between the brakeman and the litter tender.
2. There is enough room at the top between the brakes and the edge so that the litter can be rigged safely and the tender tied in safely.

Belay Systems for Litter Lowering

Figure 15-15 illustrates a belay system for litter lowering. It consists of belay attachments at two points:

1. The belay line is first attached to the master attachment point. This is done by moving back from the end of belay rope approximately 12 feet and tying a figure **8** on a bight knot. Clip a large locking carabiner into this knot and then clip the carabiner into the carabiners that are at the top of the spider in the master attachment point.

   Should anything along the main line system (such as the anchor for the brakes) fail, the belay is rigged to catch at the master attachment point. In this way, it would still maintain the litter in its normal horizontal position.
2. Take the end of the belay line and attach it to the head rail of the litter in the same way as used for the main line attachment in slope evacuation (see page 170).

This is backup for possible failure at the top of the spider. Should this type of failure occur, then the first belay attachment (the figure **8** on a bight knot at the spider) would not catch. The second line of safety would be the belay line attachment at the head of the litter. Should this attachment catch, then the litter would go into a vertical position, with the head up.

Note that all those involved with litter lowerings must keep in mind what would result from the belay's catching the head of the litter and holding the litter in a vertical position.

Never tie the belay line directly onto the subject in the litter. If the belay line caught the patient directly, it would be pulling on his or her harness while the

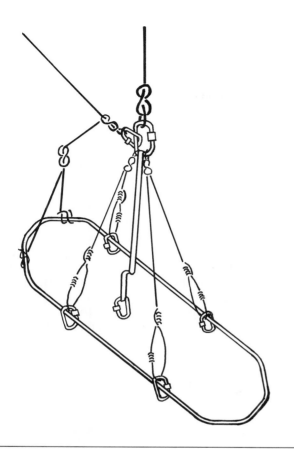

FIGURE 15-15

Belay system for litter lowering.

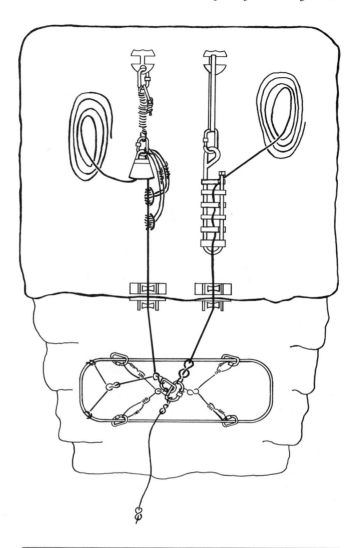

FIGURE 15-16

Litter rigging for lowering.

patient supported the remainder of the load (litter and tender[s]).

The end of the belay rope should go to the head of the litter. This is to ensure that, should the litter go vertical, the rescue subject remains head up.

The litter tender safety sling that is attached to the litter rail should be attached toward the head end of the litter.

Otherwise, if this safety sling is attached at the foot end and the litter goes vertical because of the failure of the spider, the following would occur:

- The tender's pigtail attachment would come loose.
- The litter would go vertical.
- The tender safety would catch at the foot end of the litter.
- The litter tender would be dangling helplessly below the foot of the litter.

Rigging the Litter for Single Line Lowering (Figure 15-16)

1. At the end of the main line anchor sling, attach a locking carabiner. Into this carabiner clip a brake bar rack. The rack should have its eye towards the anchor, with the bend in the rack and the top bar towards the edge of the drop. Lock the carabiner.
2. Rig a belay system.
   - If the lowering is only one person (rescue subject only, no tender attached to the litter system) use a system appropriate for belaying one person (see Chapter 8).
   - If the lowering is more than one person (rescue subject plus tender or tenders), then use a rescue belay system (see Chapter 12).
   - Run a belay rope through the belay system with its end where the litter will be rigged.
3. Lace the main line lowering rope through the brakes (the brake bar rack) with the end of the rope where the litter is to be rigged.
4. Rig the litter for a single line lowering as described above. Attach a four-legged spider to the litter. Have ready a pigtail and a separate safety sling for the litter tender.

5. In the end of the main lowering line, tie a figure 8 on a bight knot. Be certain there are several inches of tail once the knot has been tied and tightened down. Attach all legs of the litter spider to the figure 8 on a bight knot together with a large locking carabiner at the master attachment point. (Or, attach the spider legs with locking carabiners to a rigging plate at the master attachment point.) Attach the litter tender pigtail with a figure 8 on a bight knot to the large locking carabiner (or with a locking carabiner to the rigging plate) in the end of the main line rope. Lock all carabiners. Attach a separate safety sling for the litter tender to the head end of the litter.

6. Connect the belay line to the litter as described earlier, including attachments both to the top of the spider and to the head rail.

7. Load the litter with a dummy or weight equivalent to a large person. Tie the dummy or weights in so that they will not spill out should the litter capsize.

8. Have the litter tender attach to the pigtail with a seat harness ascender and a foot ascender as described earlier. Have the litter tender attached to the end of the pigtail by tying a figure 8 on a bight knot in the end and clipping it into his or her seat harness front tie-in point with a locking carabiner.

9. The litter tender should also attach with a safety sling to a point on the litter rail near the head end.

10. The litter tender initiates the belay cycle. (Litter tender: "on belay." Belayer: "belay on.")

11. Before the litter goes over the edge, the litter tender makes a final check of the rigging.

12. The litter tender pretensions the system to make certain:
    ◆ He or she can visualize that all parts of the system are rigged correctly.
    ◆ No lines will tangle.
    ◆ All slack is removed from the system.

To do this, the litter tender calls, "preload." The brakeman holds tension on the brakes and the litter tender pulls slack out of the system. If all looks good, then the tender prepares for the lower.

13. After checking to make certain that all the other lowering team members are ready and alert, the litter tender says to the brakeman, "down slow." The brakeman begins letting rope through the brake bar rack and the rope handler begins feeding rope to the brakeman. The belayer controls the belay so that there is some visible slack in the rope. The belay rope should not interfere with the litter lowering, but there should be enough tension so that should the main line system fail, the belay will catch the litter system with little shock loading.

Note that at the top, before going over the edge, there may be insufficient weight on the brake system to pull the rope through. So the litter tender may have to lean back, pulling the litter with him or her, while the brakeman lessens the friction. But remember: *once the tender and litter go over the edge, there will be greater weight on the system and greater friction will be needed.*

Getting over the Edge

Getting over the edge is often the most difficult step in litter lowering. The best approach is the slow, deliberate one. Whenever the litter tender begins to feel unbalanced, he or she calls a "stop!" to regain equilibrium. The brakeman and belayer must remain very alert to the needs of the tender.

The general strategy is for the litter tender, attached to the litter, to back slowly over the edge, pulling the litter with him or her. The tender leans back on his connections to the litter system, and in turn, the lowering system.

To make the operation as smooth as possible, the tender should avoid any shock loading of the system. To facilitate this, the brakeman should lower *very slowly* as the litter tender moves back over the edge.

As he or she moves back, the litter tender should try to keep all slack out of the main lowering line, the spider legs, and his or her tie-ins. Leaning back hard against his or her tie-ins will help in part.

If the top of the drop is flat, the tender may have to lift up the litter by the closest rail, with the litter tilted, so that the spider legs are evenly taut.

Should slack begin appearing in the system faster than he or she can cope with it, the tender should call a "stop!" to remove the slack.

It is important to have the slack out of the litter system before you get completely over the edge. Otherwise you will drop and shock load the system, resulting in:
1. Shock loading anchors, equipment, and rigging.
2. Frightening and, perhaps, harming the patient.
3. Possibly injuring yourself.

Alternative Approach: Getting over the Undercut Edges and Parapets

Among the most difficult edges to get over with a litter without shock loading are undercut edges and "parapets" (90 degree) edges.

One possible approach is to set the litter on the edge, belayed and with full tension on the brakes, and then have the litter tender climb around the head or foot end of the litter.
1. Make certain the system is on belay and belayer is alert.
2. Make certain rope is correctly laced in brakes and on tension.
3. Have two edge tenders pick up the litter.
4. As edge tenders move toward the edge, brakeman (or brakemen) slowly allows enough slack for edge tenders to maneuver the litter.
5. The edge tenders set the litter on the edge of the wall.

6. The edge tenders make certain rigging is correct and there is no excess slack.

7. The litter tender checks his or her tie-ins to the litter system.

8. The edge tenders set the litter over the wall with the top rails even with the top of the drop. The brakeman holds the lowering lines tight.

9. The litter tender has upper ascender line as tight as it will go on pigtail. The litter tender, with his or her attachment lines tight, goes over the wall at the head of the litter. The tender leans back into the tight attachment lines and maneuvers around the litter and into position.

10. The litter tender repositions on his or her tie-ins as necessary.

11. The litter tender places his or her feet against the wall, pulls the litter away from the wall, and gets ready for lowering.

Position of Single Litter Tender

The primary duties of the litter tender are:

♦ Attend to the medical needs of the patient in the litter.

♦ Help provide a smooth ride for the patient.

♦ Communicate with and reassure the patient.

♦ Prevent the litter from hanging up.

♦ Shield the patient from environmental factors.

For the litter tender to perform these duties, the best posture is a natural one for sitting in a seat harness, with the litter a few inches above the lap (Figure 15-17). The litter must not rest on the tender's lap or legs. This restricts the tender's movements. Also if the tender's feet are against the wall, then a litter in such a position could settle on the legs and pin them.

Both the tender's hands should be grasping the closest litter rail to help maneuver the litter. If the tender needs to roll the patient (such as to clear the subject's airway), the litter can be rolled toward the tender. The tender reaches across with one hand, grasps the opposite rail, and pulls it over towards him or her to roll the litter and patient.

If the litter is against the wall, then the tender should have both feet against the wall. By keeping feet against the wall, the tender can use the leverage to pull the litter away from the wall by grasping the near rail. This will help keep the litter from bumping against the wall and from snagging.

At midpoint on the wall, the litter tender calls, "stop!" The brakeman brings the brake side of the rope forward toward the load, forcing the bars together and creating a "quick stop" on the brake bar rack. If the stop is going to be a lengthy one, the brakeman has the option of tying off the brake bar rack. But the brakeman should be ready to respond if the litter tender is not initially in position and needs some additional, very short lowerings to reposition the litter.

When litter tender is ready to lower again, he or she calls a "down slow" (or "down fast") and the lowering procedure continues.

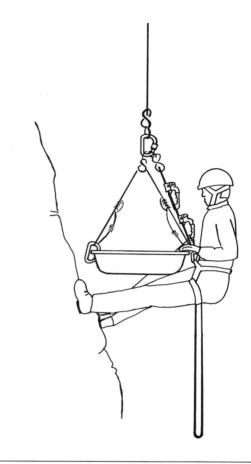

FIGURE 15-17
Posture for litter tender.

Once the litter is on the ground, the litter tender calls a "stop!" If the rope is too taut to disconnect the litter system from the main line, the tender calls, "slack." The brakeman allows slack into the main rope.

When the litter tender is in a secure position with no danger of falling, then he or she concludes the belay cycle. (Litter tender: "off belay." Belayer: "belay off.")

When the litter tender (or others on the ground) have unclipped the litter from the rope and no longer need the line, then the tender gives the voice signal, "off rope." The brakeman (or others at the top) can then pull the rope back up, or, if appropriate, remove it from the anchors.

Positions of Two Litter Tenders

In some situations, such as seriously injured patient or rugged terrain, two litter tenders may be required. In most situations, the medical attendant would be at the head end to monitor patient condition and provide essential care. Some rescue teams also make the medical attendant responsible for the rate of lowering and would be in direct communication with the lowering personnel at the top. At the foot end would be the second tender who would be responsible for manipulating litter around obstructions, pushing brush aside and clearing rockfall.

Note that there are regional variations in how responsibilities are traditionally assigned to litter attendants. But, whichever attendant has responsibility for movement of the litter, that decision must be made before the litter goes over the side.

To help in the medical attendant's duties, he or she would be in position to adjust attachments to best care for the patient. The second tender would be in position to get farther down in order to push litter away from obstructions and to clear away debris.

MEDICAL CONSIDERATIONS FOR PATIENTS IN HIGH ANGLE LOWERING

Review the section, Medical Considerations for Patients in High Angle Rescue, beginning on page 145, in Chapter 11, The Rope Rescuer, and the section, Packaging the Subject in the Litter, beginning on page 171 in Chapter 14, Slope Evacuation.

Loading the Subject into the Litter

The procedures for loading the subject in the litter will depend both on the medical condition and where the subject is to be loaded.

Topside

The actual loading of the subject in the litter will be easier if it takes place on flat ground such as at the top of the drop or on a ledge. Here there may be more manpower to assist and all members of the rescue team are standing on solid footing. However, the litter loaded with a patient may be more difficult to get over an edge for the litter tender. In this situation, the edge tenders can be of great assistance in getting the litter over the edge smoothly and without causing further apprehension and injury to the patient.

Partway Down

If the subject has become injured partway down the face of a wall, then it will be necessary to load him or her in the litter at that point. However, this type of litter loading can be very difficult for the following reasons:

- There is often not much manpower available (there may only be the litter tender).
- With the rescue personnel hanging from his or her harnesses, he or she has difficulty getting leverage. If it is a completely free hanging situation (away from the wall), it will be extremely difficult.

The following are some approaches that can assist in this kind of midface loading:

- Stop the litter lowering before you get too low. It is better to start the loading attempt with the litter

too high because the brakeman can always let a little bit more rope out to lower some. But if you start out much too low, you may not get another chance. And remember that rope, even static kernmantle, will stretch some when the patient is loaded in the litter. Because it is difficult to lift the subject up to clear the litter rails, the optimum level for the litter is equal to the level of the subject.

- Before rigging the litter, have it in line for the subject's position (litter head and foot pointing in same direction as subject's head and feet). If at all possible, have the litter in the correct position before starting over the edge. Otherwise, if the litter has to be turned partway down, the belay and main lowering lines will be tangled.
- A safety line should be clipped into the patient with a seat harness before he or she is moved for loading into the litter.
- Placement of the KED or OSS device on the patient prior to movement will also help a great deal with the movement of the patient.
- Once the subject is in the litter, he or she should have a safety sling run from his or her seat harness to the carabiners at the top of the spider.
- An auxiliary tender will be of great help in loading the litter partway down.

The Use of an Auxiliary Tender

The presence of an auxiliary tender (sometimes referred to also as a *third man*) can be very helpful in litter management and in loading the subject (Figure 15-18). This is particularly true when there is only a single litter tender. The auxiliary tender rappels or ascends on a separate rope system alongside the litter. If local policy or conditions indicate the need, a separate belay may be provided for the auxiliary tender. The auxiliary tender can be of assistance in several critical ways:

- Responding first before the litter lowering to assess the medical condition of the subject and begin primary treatment.
- Assisting the litter tender in getting the litter over the edge.
- Assisting in loading the subject partway down the wall.
- Helping to maneuver the litter around obstructions.

Although the auxiliary tender is on a rappel line separate from the litter lowering system, a tether line running between him or her and the litter may be helpful in keeping close to the litter. This line should be rigged so that the auxiliary tender can easily detach from the litter when necessary.

DOUBLE LINE LOWERING SYSTEMS

In some situations rescuers may choose to use a double line lowering (two lines attached to the litter). The two-line approach can help in the following situations:

- Where it is necessary to change the position of the litter from horizontal to vertical and back

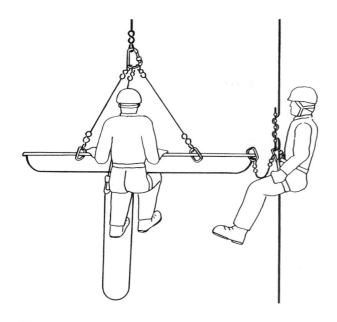

FIGURE 15-18
Auxiliary litter tender.

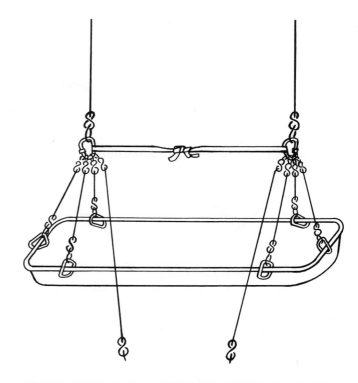

FIGURE 15-19
Spiders for double strand lowering.

again to get it through obstacles on a vertical space or to get through a confined space.

♦ Some two line systems can simplify rigging.
♦ Where two tenders need to be attached to the litter:
1. On an uneven, broken up, vertical face, with obstacles such as overhangs and gullies. These are areas where a single litter tender might have difficulty in managing the litter.
2. Where medical considerations or other concerns relating to the rescue subject are too over-whelming for a single litter tender.

There are two different systems for double line lowering, which include:
1. Both lines are run through one brake.
2. Each line is run through a separate brake, with each acting as a belay on the other.

Spiders for Double Line Lowering

Figure 15-19 illustrates the spider system for a double strand lowering. Note that in this case, there are six legs to the spider. There are three at the head end coming up to meet one lowering rope and three at the foot end coming up to meet the parallel lowering rope.

There are two basic types of spiders that can be used with double line lowering systems:

Single Point:
Both lowering lines come together and are attached at a single master attachment point. In Figure 15-15, the two lines would come into the MAP where one

line now exists. In most cases with a double line low-ering, there would not be the belay line.

Double Point:
Each of the two lowering lines is attached to a separate (usually three-legged) spider component. One is at the head of the litter and one is at the foot (Figure 15-19).

Advantages:
♦ Double point system can give greater flexibility in maneuvering litter in some situations such as get-ting over edge.
♦ Can give maneuverability in changing angle of litter.

Disadvantages:
♦ Potential for high shock loads on dual anchor system if one anchor fails.
♦ May be difficult to maintain the same speed for both ropes if the ropes run through different braking devices and are attached to litter with two-point spider.

Litter Tie-Ins for Double Line Lowering (Two Tenders)

Each litter tender, as seen in Figure 15-19, has his or her own tie-in clipped to a separate lowering rope. As with the single strand lowering, each litter tender is also clipped in with a separate safety line to a point on the litter rail.

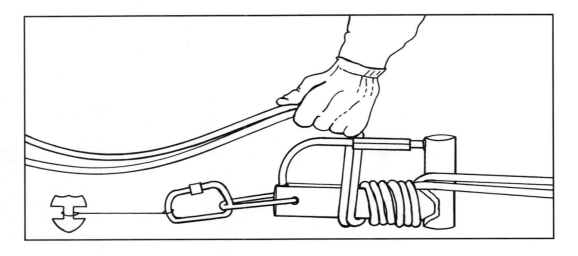

FIGURE 15-20
The brake tube is an alternative to the brake bar rack in double line lowering.

In the case of the double line lowering, only one litter tender gives the voice communications to the brakeman. This is the medical attendant, usually stationed at the head of the litter to best care for the patient.

Brake Systems for Double Line Lowering (One Brake)

Both main lowering ropes should run through the same brake device and be controlled by the same brakeman.

Also, both lowering ropes in a double strand lowering should be of the same diameter, design, and wear. If they are not, they may have different rates of elongation, providing irregular stops when the brakes are applied and different rates of friction that will consequently run through the brakes at different speeds.

An uneven load on the litter may also cause the ropes to run through the brakes at different speeds. This is often the result of the upper torso of the subject being heavier than the lower torso. So the head end of the litter will often be heavier than the foot end.

To even out the loading in a two strand lower, the lighter litter tender can sometimes be placed at the head end and the heavier tender at the foot end.

Alternative Approach: *Brake Tube*

An alternative to the brake bar rack in double line lowering (one brake) is the brake tube (Figure 15-20).
Advantage:
- Knots can be passed through the device (but double lines should be tied so their knots do not pass at the same time).
- Has good control for lowering.

Disadvantage:
- Heavier and bulkier than the rack (group rather than individual equipment).

Changing the Angle of the Litter

The following are steps involved in changing the angle of a litter from horizontal to vertical during a double strand lowering (Figure 15-21):

The litter has already gone over the edge and is being lowered. It is about to reach an area on the wall through which it cannot fit unless it is tilted at a steep angle.

The following sequence assumes that there are different colored ropes going to the head and foot of the litter. In this case, the red line goes to the head, while the blue line goes to the foot.

1. Litter captain to brakeman: "stop!" (The brakeman stops both ropes from going through the brakes.)
2. Litter captain: "down on blue." (The brakeman allows the rope running to the foot end of the litter to run through the brakes but he or she holds the rope that goes to the head end of the litter. As a result, the foot end of the litter goes down, while the head end remains where it is.) Note: If both ropes are the same color, the brakeman will say, "down foot."
3. When the litter reaches the angle desired, the litter captain signals: "stop!" (The brakeman stops the rope going to the foot end of the litter and continues to hold the rope going to the head end. The litter has stopped at a vertical angle with the foot end below the head end. Both litter tenders still hang in the same position but the litter is now parallel to them. They are still able to reach and tend to the needs of the rescue subject.)

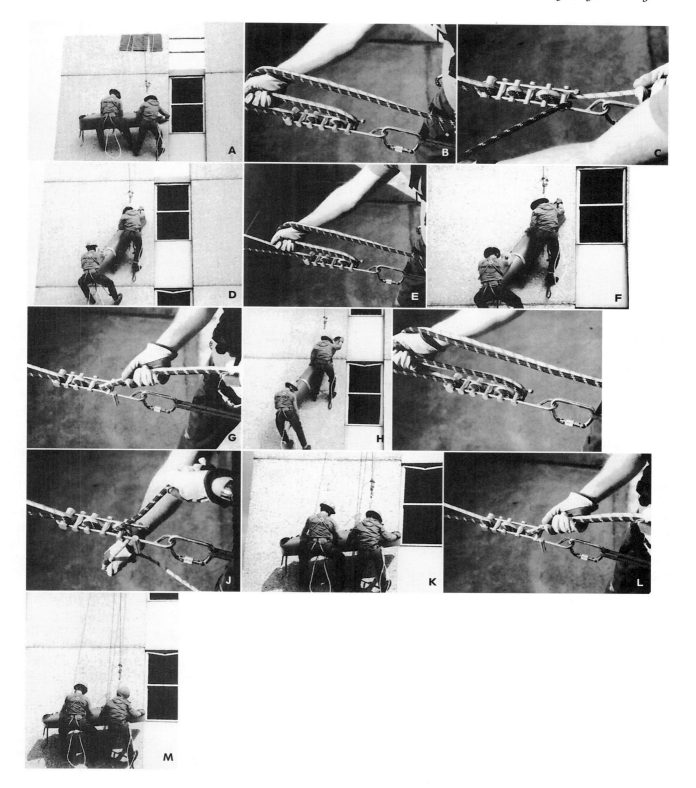

FIGURE 15-21

Changing litter angle during a double line litter lowering.

4. Litter captain to brakeman: "down slow." (The brakeman now allows both ropes to run through the brakes at the same speed. The litter maintains the vertical position it has been set at and continues lowering at that angle.)

To Change the Angle Back to Horizontal

5. Litter captain to brakeman: "stop!" (The brakeman stops all ropes from going through the brakes. The litter stops completely.)

6. Litter captain: "down on red." (The brakeman allows the rope going to the head of the litter to go through the brakes but holds the rope going to the foot. The head of the litter is lowered while the foot end of the litter remains stationary.) Note: If both ropes are the same color, the brakeman will say, "down head."

7. As the head of the litter becomes even with the foot end, the litter captain says, "stop!" (The brakeman stops the rope to the head end from going through the brakes and holds the rope going to the foot end. The litter is now horizontal and not moving.)

8. Litter captain: "down slow" (or "down fast"). The brakeman allows both ropes through the brakes. The litter is lowered in a horizontal position.

Alternative Approach: Continuous Sequence

For the changing of litter angle to work smoothly, it takes practice, teamwork, and good communications. Once a team has become adept at the procedure, then they may be able to skip the "stop/start" steps and keep the litter moving continuously. Such a continuous sequence might run as follows:

1. Litter tender: "down on blue." (Brakeman stops red, continues blue.)
2. Litter tender: "down slow." (Brakeman allows both ropes through brakes.)
3. Litter tender: "down on red." (Brakeman stops blue, continues blue.)
4. Once the litter has become horizontal again, the litter tender calls "down slow" (or "down fast"). The litter continues lowering in a horizontal position.

THE TWO BRAKE LOWERING SYSTEM

Some rescue teams prefer to lower a litter using two brakes instead of a brake and a belay device. In this way, should one anchor fail, the second brake system converts to a belay that can more easily be held by the brakeman, and the device can better be used for a controlled lowering than for a belay device.

The advantage of a double brake lowering is that it shares the load between two anchors instead of one. Also, should one anchor fail, there may be less severe loading because both ropes are under load instead of one having some slack, as would be the case with a belay.

One disadvantage of a double brake lowering is that should one anchor and brake fail, then the second anchor and brake will be subjected to shock loading that will be much greater than twice the original load the surviving anchor and brake had before. The remaining anchor must be able to withstand this loading. The remaining brakeman must be using a braking device that can easily and quickly be adjusted to increase the needed friction. Not all braking devices are capable of quickly giving this needed extra control. The brakeman must be alert and capable of reacting quickly to this possibility.

In constructing a double brake lowering system, the two brake stations should be set close enough together so there is a small angle between the rope. In this way, there would be less of a pendulum should one side fail. Also, both brakemen need to be close together so there is close communication on keeping equal loading on the two braking devices.

Requirements for Dual Brake Double Line Lowering

◆ The size of both spider components must be equal size.
◆ There must be a sling line between the master attachment points. The optimum length of this sling should be long enough to allow the litter to be tilted near vertical if needed but short enough to restrict the two master attachment points from spreading too far apart.
◆ As much as possible, equalize weight on each end of the litter. If using two tenders, use persons of equal size. Or place heavier tender on foot end of the litter. Remember the upper torso of the patient is heavier than the lower torso. Take this into account when balancing weight of litter tenders.

Sizing of Spiders

It is important in a dual line lowering to equalize the size of spiders before starting the lower. The size will depend on physical conditions of the lower. It should be a compromise between the following:

1. Being large enough to, if necessary, load and unload a patient on the midface.

⚠ Warning

When using a tether to connect both three-legged spiders (see Figure 15-19), the litter cannot be allowed to go completely vertical because this could cause the rigging to press against the patient. In such a situation, team members must be alert and ready to call "stop."

2. Being small enough so that the litter tenders can maneuver the litter in difficult terrain, so that the tenders can reach the MAP, and so that the litter does not flop about when trying to maneuver it around obstacles.

Litter Tender Attachments (One Tender)

There are some situations where two litter tenders are preferable. In general these include when there is a critical patient requiring full attention by one tender or where the terrain is extremely rugged.

The use of one litter tender means that there is less weight on the lowering system including the brakes and anchors. There also may be limited numbers of personnel. There are three basic options for a litter tender attachment in a dual line lower with one tender:

1. Have both lowering lines come to a single master attachment point as in Figure 15-13. This will reduce some flexibility in adjusting litter angle.
2. Use two litter attachment points as in Figure 15-19. Attach the litter tender to one master attachment point as with a single line lower.

   The disadvantage to this system is that it will increase the weight on one end of the litter and, therefore, on one set of the brakes. This will make it more difficult to keep the litter horizontal.

   Despite uneven weight distribution, it is usually preferable to place the litter tender on the head end. This gives the tender greater access to the patient. It is also easier for a litter tender to maneuver the litter when at the heavier end.
3. Attach the litter tender to fixed lines equalized between the two master attachment points.

   The disadvantage to this system is that it will make it more difficult for the litter tender to move about.

Passing Knots

If the length of the litter lowering is more than the length of one rope, then it may be necessary to go through a procedure known as *knot pass*. In such a situation, a second length of rope (or more) has to be tied to the first rope in order for the load to reach the bottom. But some brake systems will jam if knots enter them. (See brake tube alternative on p. 210 for an exception.) Therefore a bypass procedure has to be used.

Figure 15-22 illustrates a procedure for passing knots. This system is using a single line lower with a belay (which for clarity, is not shown.)

The following are needed in addition to a regular lowering system:

◆ A separate anchored braking system.
◆ A short length of rope (approximately 25 feet) for interim lowering.
◆ A rope grab for each rope in the main lowering system

1. To avoid delay in the lowering operation, the separate brake system should be rigged and ready before it comes time for the knot pass. The auxiliary braking system is anchored and the short length of rope is rigged into its own brake system. At the end of the short length of rope a figure 8 on a bight knot is tied and a locking carabiner clipped into it. The short piece of rope should be adjusted in its brakes so that the cam will reach the main lowering line just below the main brakes.
2. Before less than 20 feet is left on the first rope, the second main rope is tied to it (with a figure 8 bend knot or a grapevine knot [Figure 15-22, *A*]).
3. Before there is less than 3 feet between the knot and the brakes, the lowering is stopped. *The knot must not get any closer to the brakes. If the system slips and the knot enters the brakes, it will jam and it will take a difficult hauling procedure to get it unjammed.*
4. The rope grab is placed on the main line lowering rope just below the main brakes. If a cam is used, the arrow on the cam should point to the load (down the drop) so the cam grips the main rope. The rope grab is locked on the rope (Figure 15-22, *B*).
5. The auxiliary brakeman holds the auxiliary brakes tight. The main brakeman slowly allows some slack in the main brakes until the load is taken on the auxiliary brake system and the rope through the main brakes becomes slack (Figure 15-22, *C*).
6. Once the load is fully on the auxiliary brakes, the rope is unlaced from the main brake system (Figure 15-22, *D*).
7. The auxiliary brakeman begins to lower on his or her system until the knot on the main lowering is well past the main brakes.
8. The auxiliary brakeman stops the rope from going through the auxiliary brakes. *This must be done before the rope grabs on the main lowering rope get out of reach of the personnel at the top.*
9. Once the knot in the main line is past the main brakes, the main line (now into the second rope) is replaced onto the main brakes (Figure 15-22, *E*).
10. The main brakeman locks off the main brakes. The auxiliary brakeman begins to lower through the auxiliary brakes. The load is taken onto the main line and the auxiliary line goes slack.
11. Once the auxiliary line is slack, the auxiliary brakeman stops rope from going through the auxiliary brakes.
12. The now slack auxiliary line, along with the rope grab, is removed from the main line (Figure 15-22, *F*).
13. The main line lowering continues. If an additional knot needs to be passed, then the auxiliary brake system is reset for it.

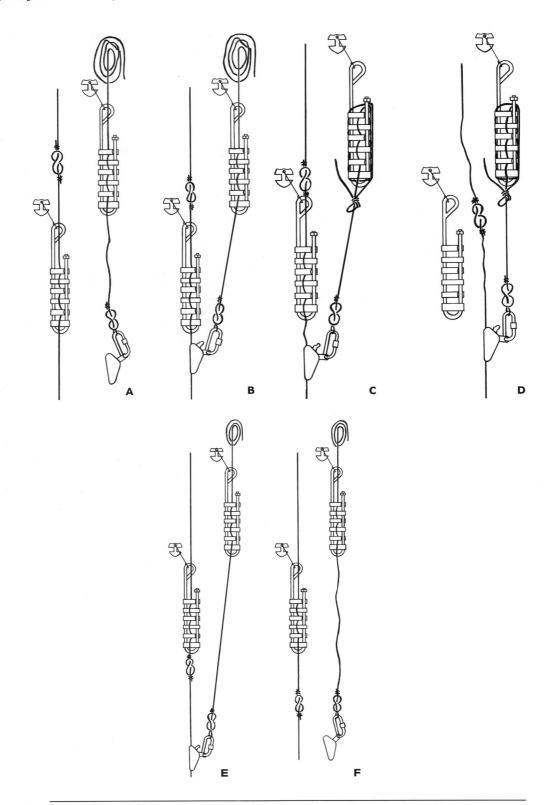

FIGURE 15-22

Passing knot in litter lowering.

Evaluation Exercises

◆ **COGNITIVE AND AFFECTIVE EXERCISES** ◆

1. **List four environments in which a high angle lowering system might be used in a rescue.**
2. **A hip belay may serve as a belay in a rescue lowering system.**
   A. True
   B. False
3. **With a partner, repeat from memory and in sequence the voice signals between litter tender and brakeman and between litter tender and belayer during a high angle lowering.**
4. **In a high angle lowering, the brakeman's dominant hand should be on the slack rope that is feeding into the brakes. This hand is known as the _____.**
   A. Belay limb.
   B. Dominant hand.
   C. Brake hand.
5. **Describe the position of the hands and the rope for a "quick stop" position of a brake bar rack during a high angle lowering.**
6. **When the load goes over the edge during a high angle lowering, what significant change takes place that affects the lowering system and the brakeman's ability to control it?**
7. **List at least one advantage and one disadvantage for the following types of litter lowerings:**
   a) Single line.
   b) Double line.

8. **In a single line lowering, there should be a minimum of _____ legs for a spider.**
   A. Eight
   B. Six
   C. Five
   D. Four
9. **From the list below, select the material that would be needed for a spider used in a single line lowering of a litter.**
   A. Two lengths of static kernmantle ropes, each 12 feet long.
   B. One brake bar rack.
   C. Four lengths of Prusik material, each 4 feet long.
   D. Four locking carabiners with gate openings large enough to fit over litter rail.
   E. Two general-use ascenders.
10. **When a spider is attached to a litter, which direction should the carabiner gate face?**
    A. Outward.
    B. Toward cliff face.
    C. Toward free air.
    D. Toward patient.
11. **Describe the attachment system for litter tender tie-in that includes the use of ascenders to give adjustable height.**
12. **List five duties of the litter tender during a high angle evacuation of a rescue subject.**
13. **List four potential duties for the auxiliary tender during the high angle lowering of a litter containing a rescue subject.**
14. **Name three conditions that might make a double line lowering of a litter with a subject preferable to a single line lowering.**

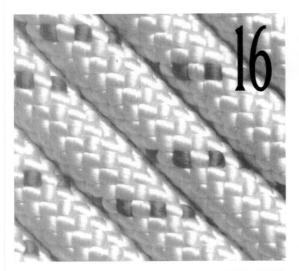

16 Hauling Systems

◆ *Prerequisites*

Before attempting the activities described in this chapter, you must have demonstrated that you can properly:

1. Use and care for rope.
2. Use and care for other equipment employed in the high angle environment.
3. Tie correctly, and without hesitation the eight knots described in Chapter 6.
4. Apply the principles of anchoring and rig a safe and secure anchor.
5. Apply the principles of belaying and safely and confidently belay another person using either a Munter hitch or personal belay device.
6. Apply the principles of slope evacuation: correctly set the rigging in any of the elements of slope evacuation; safely and confidently assume the role of litter tender, haul team member, rope handler, brakeman, or belayer.
7. Correctly distinguish between one-person and rescue belays; correctly tie a load-releasing hitch and demonstrate how to release it under load; correctly rig a tandem Prusik belay system and operate it; correctly rig a Prusik minding pulley and operate it.
8. Apply the principles of high angle lowering systems: correctly rig any of the elements of high angle lowering; safely assume the role of litter tender, brakeman, belayer, rope handler, or edge attendant.

Objectives ▼

At the completion of this chapter, you should be able to:

1. Describe how hauling systems can be used in rescue and describe some typical examples of where they might be used.
2. Describe what constitutes the elements of a haul system.
3. Discuss the functions of the following in a rescue haul system: pulleys, haul cam, progress capture device (PCD), tag line, edge protection, haul team, cam tender, haul captain.
4. Discuss the need for reliable communications in rescue hauling.
5. Describe the principles of a 1:1 haul system, a 2:1 haul system, a 3:1 haul system (Z-Rig), and a 4:1 haul system ("piggyback rig").
6. Discuss how to determine mechanical advantage.
7. Define the difference between theoretical and actual mechanical advantage.
8. Discuss the basic criteria for selecting specific haul systems.
9. Repeat from memory the voice communications used in rescue hauling.

Objectives—cont'd ▼

10. Select equipment to be used in a rescue hauling system.
11. Describe the primary medical considerations in dealing with rescue subjects in hauling operations.
12. Participate as a member of a haul team.
13. Act as a cam tender.
14. Act as haul captain.
15. Act as a belayer for a haul system.
16. Rig a 1:1 hauling system, a 2:1 hauling system, a 3:1 hauling system (Z-Rig), and a 4:1 hauling system ("piggyback rig").

RESCUE HAULING SYSTEMS

Although the knowledge of lowering systems is essential for competent rope rescue personnel, not all accidents take place on high places. In fact, depending on the location, many rescues will involve the raising of rescue subjects out of a lower place. Some examples might include:

◆ Silos.
◆ River gorges, canyons, and escarpments.
◆ Grain elevators.
◆ Sewers.
◆ Tank cars.
◆ Basins.
◆ Utility vaults.
◆ Storage bins.
◆ Fuel tanks.
◆ Air vents.
◆ Mine shafts.
◆ Caves.
◆ Tunnels.
◆ Confined spaces.

Purposes of Hauling Systems

In general, there are two basic reasons for rescuers to employ hauling systems: (1) to make the raising more convenient and safer and (2) to make the raising easier.

Convenience and Safety

The knowledge of hauling systems and the ability to properly use the equipment could mean that rescuers can establish the location of a raising in a place that is more convenient and safer for them.

They could, for example, establish a hauling system that was:

◆ Closer to vehicles and roadway.
◆ Away from rockfall.
◆ Away from potential hostile activity.
◆ Away from bystanders.
◆ Out of view of the media.
◆ At a shorter drop.

Ease

Hauling systems make the job of raising a load easier for the rescue team. They need less force to pull the load, although it will probably take a longer time to raise it.

How Hauling Systems Work

By using hauling systems, you can spread the weight of the load over distance, in this case, over greater rope length.

Note that in Figure 16-1, *A*, on p. 219 a rope goes down a drop of 10 feet and is connected to a load that weighs 100 lb. The rope is directly on the load, and it is a straight haul. So, to bring the 100-lb load to the top requires 100 lb of force (plus some extra force to overcome the friction of the rope on the edge rollers). It will also take 10 feet of rope to do it.

The relationship of how many loads can be moved to the force that it takes to move it is called the ***mechanical advantage,*** or MA.

In reality, rescuers never get the full amount of MA out of any hauling system they rig. This is because some force they exert in the hauling is lost through ways such as friction in the pulleys, rope rubbing against an edge, and rope stretch. The resulting MA that we work with in the field is known as *the actual mechanical advantage.* The MA that we talk about without consideration of the factors such as friction and abrasion is known as the ***theoretical mechanical advantage.*** But to simplify matters, in this book, we will discuss hauling systems in terms of the theoretical mechanical advantage and simply refer to it as the MA.

The actual amount of MA you do get out of a hauling system will depend in great part on how efficiently you can rig the system and on the efficiency of the components such as pulleys you use to build it. There will be several points throughout this chapter on how to avoid the loss of advantage in hauling.

In the simple example in Figure 16-1, *A*, we can calculate the MA as follows:

Weight of load	to:	Force it takes to move load
100 lb	to:	100 lb

So the ratio, or MA, is 1:1

Notice that in this example the length of rope pulled by the rescuers is the same as the distance the load moves.

Now note that in Figure 16-1, *B* there is the same load (100 lb) that needs to be moved up the vertical drop. In this case, the rescuers have attached a pulley on the load (known as a ***traveling pulley*** because it travels with the load). The rope is anchored at the top of the drop. It then runs down through the pulley and back up to the top where the end of the rope is held by the rescuers. So there is now 20 feet of rope and two strands of rope that are moving. As the rescuers pull up the rope, they will pull 20 feet of rope to move the load 10 feet. As a result of having half the load on the anchor and half the load on the side they are hauling, they will pull with a force of 50 lb.

Calculating the MA in this second example looks like this:

Weight of load to: Force it takes to move load

100 lb to: 50 lb

So the ratio, or MA, is 2:1

To see how this haul could be made more convenient, consider Figure 16-1, *C*. Note that the rescuers have now added a second pulley at the top so they can pull the rope horizontally instead of vertically. This second pulley is stationary and is attached to a sling suspended from a tripod, a strong tree, or other similar anchor. This pulley does not add any additional mechanical advantage. As in the second example, there is still 20 feet of rope being pulled, while the load moves 10 feet. In theory it still takes 50 lb of force to move the 100-lb load. So, the calculation is still the same as in the previous example, with a MA of 2:1.

Although the rescuers have not added any MA, they may have made things better for themselves by making things more *convenient* and possibly *safer*. Now they no longer have to stand bunched together on the edge of the drop, awkwardly pulling up on the rope and fighting gravity. With the addition of this stationary pulley (which also acts as a directional), they can now walk back in a line away from the drop as they pull the rope and raise the load.

This illustration is just one example of how convenience and safety must be considered, along with MA, in rigging rescue haul systems.

Ways of Adding to the Mechanical Advantage

The creation of an additional MA can be achieved by increments or by multiplying.

Incremental Addition of MA

Figure 16-1, *D* illustrates a way of moving from a 2:1 MA to a 3:1 MA by changing the system. This particular type of system is commonly called a ***Z-Rig*** because of the general shape made by the rope as it runs through the system.

Note that in the 3:1 system at point "A" there is an anchor to which a pulley is attached. This will be a stationary pulley. Through it runs the main line hauling rope. At point "C" there is also a pulley through which rope runs. But this is a traveling pulley. To this traveling pulley is attached a rope grab with a carabiner. The rope grab in turn is attached to the main strand of the same rope. But the pulley and the rope grab will move as they are pulled by the top end of the rope. The rope grab will grab the rope that goes to the load and pull up the load.

In this system, there are three strands of moving rope. For every foot that the load moves, the haul team must pull 3 feet of rope. The load is supported by three moving ropes, and each rope is supporting approximately $\frac{1}{3}$ of the load. To move the 100-lb load, the haul team must exert a force of approximately 33.3 lb:

Weight of load to: Force it takes to move load

100 lb to: 33.3 lb

So the ratio, or MA, is 3:1

Multiplying the MA

In some cases, the MA of a rescue hauling system can be increased by multiplying it. These are called *compound systems.*

The general rule of thumb is this: when two rescue hauling systems are joined together, the resulting MA is obtained by multiplying the two MAs (Box 16-1). *For Example:* If a 2:1 MA hauling system is joined to a 2:1, the result is 4:1. If a 2:1 MA hauling system is joined to a 3:1, the result is 6:1, and so on.

A 4:1 MA System

To create one type of 4:1 hauling system, take the 2:1 hauling system from Figure 16-1, *B* and add another 2:1 system. Start by adding a second pulley at the end of the rope where before the rescuers were hauling (Figure 16-1, *E*). Now take a second rope and anchor one end of it at point "A2." Run the rope through the second pulley at the end of the first rope and bring the second rope back parallel with itself towards the anchor "A2." The haul team will now pull on the second rope at its free end. As the haul progresses, there will be four strands of rope moving. To move the load up 10 feet, 40 feet of rope

Box 16-1 Exception to the Rule

This is a general rule as applied to the basic rescue hauling systems examined in this chapter. There are some exceptions to the multiplying rule. In certain compound block and tackle systems, for example, the rule may not apply. The most reliable way to determine an MA is to measure the length of rope pulled against the distance the load moves.

must be pulled by the rescuers. To move the 100-lb load, it will take a pulling force of 25 lb:

Weight of load to: Force it takes to move load
100 lb to: 25 lb
So the ratio, or MA, is 4:1

If this were a real situation, then the rescuers could not rig and operate the system as shown in Figure 16-1, *E*. The haul team could not pull up while standing in space, just as the rope could not be anchored in space. But a 4:1 system could still be achieved in this situation if the rescuers were to first add a directional at the edge of the drop as they did in Figure 16-1, *F*. After they rigged the directional

pulley, they could rig a second 2:1 MA system as shown in Figure 16-1, *F*.

First, they would set anchor "A2" a way back from the drop. Next they would pull the top end of the first rope through the directional (and stationary) pulley. Then they would attach the second traveling pulley to the end of the first rope (point "TP3"). After that they would pull the second traveling pulley. They would then pull the end of the second rope back from the edge of the drop and haul on it.

Again, the stationary pulley at the top of the drop would serve only as a *directional* and add no mechanical advantage. But it would provide for greater convenience and safety in the hauling system. The

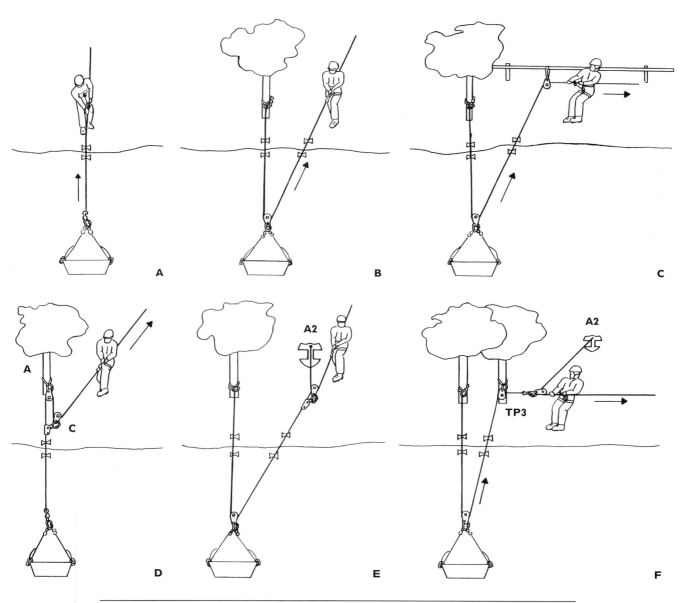

FIGURE 16-1
Calculating MA.

rescuers would now be able to haul by walking back away from the drop. The situation for MA in Figure 16-1, *F* would still be the same as in Figure 16-1, *E:*

Weight of load to:	Force it takes to move load
100 lb to:	25 lb
So the ratio, or MA, is 4:1	

Elements of Hauling Systems

The Role of Rope Grabs in Hauling Systems

In hauling systems, devices called *rope grabs* are used to grip the rope. These devices are usually either one of two types: general-use ascenders (sometimes called *hard cams*) and friction hitches (usually a Prusik hitch).

The Nature of the Rope Grab

The following is a comparison of the major advantages and disadvantages of general-use ascenders versus the Prusik hitch.

General-Use Ascenders. General-use ascenders are also known as *hard cams.* They work by a metal

---

⚠ Warning

Personal ascenders must not be used in rescue hauling systems. Personal ascenders are designed only for one person's body weight. They are not designed for the high stresses resulting from the multiplication of forces that take place in hauling systems. The use of personal ascenders in hauling systems can result in tearing of the rope or in the structural failure of the ascender. Either one of these can result in the failure of the entire system.

A rope grab, depending on its position in the hauling system, will serve the following purposes:

1. To grasp the rope so it can be pulled by the hauling system. This is known as the **haul cam.** An example of a haul cam is at point "C" in the 3:1 hauling system in Figure 16-1, D.
2. To hold the rope while the haul team resets itself to get another bite on the rope. This is known as the *progress capture device* (PCD) or *ratchet cam.*

⚠ Warning

Never use a hard cam or a single friction hitch for a belay in rescue hauling. Under shock loading, a hard cam could cause the rope to fail, while a single friction hitch could fail. See Chapter 12, Rescue Belaying.

---

cam pressing the rope against the metal shell of the ascender. The two most well-known brands are the Petzl Rescucender (Thompson Manufacturing, Inc.) and Gibbs (Gibbs).

Advantages:
◆ Easy to use.
◆ Can be rigged to reset "automatically."
◆ Can be manipulated quickly, even when used as a progress capture device.

Disadvantages:
◆ Can cut through rope when under extreme stress.

Friction Hitches. The most commonly used friction hitch is the triple-wrapped Prusik hitch. The accessory cord used to make the friction hitch should be of smaller diameter than the rope it grips (such as 8 mm cord for 11 mm rope) but have an appropriate safety factor for its use.

Advantages:
◆ If correctly used, it will not cut the rope but gradually stop the rope in a "clutching" action.

Disadvantages:
◆ May be more difficult to manipulate.
◆ Slippage under load can cause friction heat. This can result in melting and failure.
◆ May not catch in icy or muddy conditions.
◆ Wide variation in the types of Prusik material used and in the ability of personnel to use it.

No rope grab device or technique is perfect for every rescue situation. Every rope grab device has some drawbacks. Any device, including hard cams or friction hitches, can be made to fail if they are improperly used or if the system is stressed beyond what it is designed for.

Because hard cams can be made to fail under high shock loading, some rescue teams prefer to use the tandem Prusik system as an alternative rope grab device for the main line in hauling systems (Figure 16-2). During some tests, the tandem Prusik system was shown to have greater energy absorption capability than a number of other methods for belaying large loads.

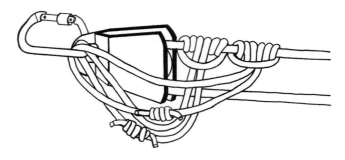

FIGURE 16-2
Tandem Prusik system.

In a low-impact fall, tandem Prusiks are designed to catch the load and spread the force of absorbing the energy of the fall over a greater area of the rope while not harming the rope.

In a more severe fall, the Prusiks may grab the rope, and the surface of the Prusik material melts, creating a "clutch" effect that can absorb the energy of the fall.

In a very severe fall, it is possible for the Prusik cord to melt through completely and fail, to break, or to pinch the main line to failure.

Much of the data indicating the advantages of the tandem Prusik system has been gathered in tests dropping a rigid weight for 1 m (3 feet) in free air. Some rescuers feel that these specific test situations are beyond what most rescuers are going to experience in real rescue situations. In these specific tests, there are no edges, faces, or directionals to help absorb the energy of the fall, nor is there the elasticity that might exist in anchor systems using slings or rope.

Positioning of the Progress Capture Device (PCD)

For the PCD to offer the greatest protection against failure in other elements of the hauling system, it should be positioned as far forward of the hauling system (toward the load) as possible, while still being safely in reach of the rescuers.

For example, if the rescuers are hauling a load up a vertical drop, the PCD should be close to the edge but not over it and out of reach.

It is important to remember that should anything else in the hauling system fail (anchors, hauling team, haul cam, pulleys, and so on) the PCD is the last hope to grab the main line rope and prevent the system and the rescue load from falling. For this reason, *the PCD cam should be on a very good anchor.*

Alternative Approach: Placing the PCD to the Rear Using a Z-Rig. In certain cases, it may not be possible to place the PCD forward of the hauling system. One such situation would be where there are no anchors available for doing so. It is possible when using a Z-Rig (3:1 MA) to place a PCD in *back of* the hauling system (Figure 16-3).

Rigging the PCD in Hauling Systems. Review material on ascenders in Chapter 5, Basic High Angle Equipment, and in Chapter 13, Pickoff Rescue Techniques.

When rigging a progress capture device, it should be set so that its anchor and anchor sling are as much in line as possible with the rope it is grabbing. This should be done without interfering with or jamming the rope (Figure 16-4, *A*). If the PCD is rigged too far off to the side of the rope it is protecting, there will be too much slack in the PCD's anchor sling. This will result in two problems (Figure 16-4, *B*): (1) it can result in dangerous shock loading of the PCD, its sling, and its anchor, and (2) the hauling team will lose some of

the purchase it has gained when it sets the PCD to reposition for another bite.

Setting of a Progress Capture Device Cam. When rigging a PCD, there are two primary concerns:
1. The PCD must clamp on the rope when needed.
2. The PCD must not ride up the rope as the rope moves. This could result in dangerous shock loading.

How the PCD is specifically rigged depends in part on the specific type of rope grab used and in part on the specific circumstances of the rigging (Figures 16-5, *A* through 16-5, *C*).

Free running (not spring-loaded) general-use ascender. Figure 16-5, *A* shows one method of ensuring that the ascender stays in place and clamps on the rope when needed. This technique uses the services of a person known as the *cam tender.* As the main line hauling rope moves up, the cam tender makes certain that the ascender does not travel up the rope. This is done by holding the backside of the shell with the palm and with fingers extended out of the way of the

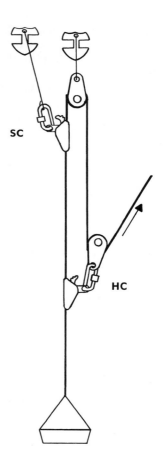

FIGURE 16-3

Alternative position of progress capture device.

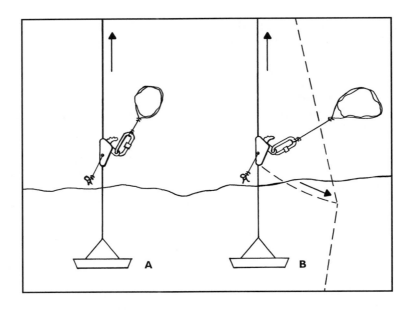

FIGURE 16-4

Alignment of progress capture device.

cam. He or she holds the shell of the ascender in this manner so that fingers or gloves do not get caught if the ascender suddenly shock loads. A finger caught by the cam could get injured, and a glove caught in the cam could prevent it from clamping the rope.

Although the use of a cam tender can be effective, it does require extra personnel. And there is always the potential for human failure or inattention.

A second technique for using a free-running cam as a PCD is shown in Figure 16-5, *B*. A bungee (elastic) cord is clipped into the empty hole usually found in the "point" of the arrowhead. The other end of the bungee cord is anchored securely to a convenient spot toward the load. A great deal of tension is not required on the bungee cord. But there should be enough to keep the ascender from riding up the rope and keep the cam clamped on the rope.

Tie the bungee cord *only to the shell* and not to the cam itself. If the bungee is tied to the cam, the cam might not close when you want it to.

A third alternative is shown in Figure 16-5, *C*. This method uses a short piece of cord. It is attached to a weight and the weight is hung so that it will pull the shell of the cam toward the load.

Avoiding Edge Friction in Hauling Systems

One of the most common problems in the rigging of hauling systems is one that often goes unnoticed until it causes problems. This is rope friction over the edge of the drop and elsewhere in the system. Because ropes in hauling systems are often highly loaded, this can result in two significant problems:

1. The friction can get very high and can result in a tremendous increase in load for the haul

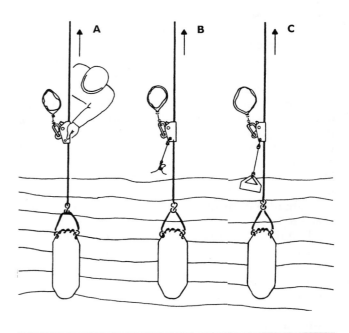

FIGURE 16-5

Setting progress capture device on automatic.

team. Edge friction in hauling is often greater than lowering over the same edge.

2. It can result in severe damage to the rope and other equipment.

Possible solutions to edge friction include edge rollers and directionals, changing the haul rope position, the use of rope padding, or load reduction.

Edge Rollers. Edge rollers may often be the most efficient solution to edge friction. However, they must be centered under the rope and securely anchored at each side. Otherwise, they can easily be turned over as the rope moves slightly from side to side.

Directionals. To protect against edge friction, a directional pulley must hold the rope above the edge. Two ways of doing this are with a tripod (Figure 16-6) or, in a natural area, with a very strong tree.

Changing the Position of the Haul Rope. To change the position of the haul rope, either move the haul system to where the edge is less sharp or move the rope at a higher angle above the edge so there is less friction.

Rope Padding. This may only slightly reduce the friction problem. But it could significantly reduce the damage to the rope (see Chapter 4, Care and Use of Rope and Related Equipment, for tips on padding ropes).

Load Reduction. Keep loads as light as possible. If at all possible, for example, use one tender instead of two on a litter that is being hauled.

The Role of the Haul Team. See page 181, Chapter 14, Slope Evacuation, for information on the haul team.

Tag Lines. A *tag line* can be used for better control of a load. A tag line can prevent the load from hanging up during a hauling operation. Tag lines can be used both from the bottom and then used for getting a load over the edge. A tag line is particularly helpful in hauling litters where the line can be attached to the foot of the litter (Figure 16-7).
    Among the ways that a tag line can be of assistance are:

- ◆ To position a litter when it is hauled through a confined space.
- ◆ To keep a litter from getting snagged on an overhanging edge.
- ◆ To hold a litter away from a wall to ensure a smoother ride for the rescue subject in the litter.
- ◆ To prevent the litter from spinning on free-hanging hauls.

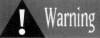 **Warning**

Be certain that overhead directionals are set on a very strong anchor. Some overhead directionals create, in effect, a 2:1 hauling system on the anchor, creating higher forces on the anchor than the weight of the load.

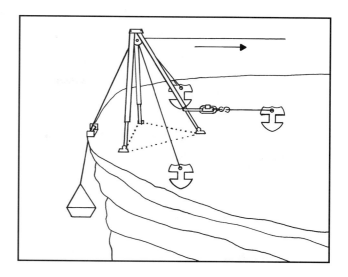

FIGURE 16-6
Tripod used as directional.

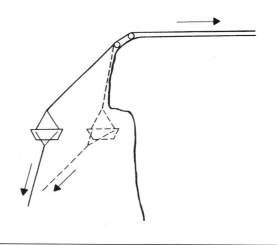

FIGURE 16-7
Tag line on litter.

Getting Over the Edge. Getting a litter over an edge when hauling can be very difficult. It should be done slowly and carefully because a hung-up litter can overstress elements of a hauling system and cause failure.

1. Before starting a haul, tie short tag lines on both the foot and the head of the litter.
2. At the top, station edge attendants *securely tied in.*
3. Make certain the litter attendant is in the best position for getting his or her feet under the litter and against the face (Figure 15-17).
4. Before the litter makes contact under the edge, stop the haul.
5. Have the litter attendant hand a tag line to each of the edge attendants, one at the foot and one at the head of the litter.

6. Restart the haul *very slowly* and be prepared to stop instantly should the litter hang up. If the litter gets hung up and cannot be freed, you may have to slack off on the system to free it.

7. As the litter attendant pushes his or her feet against the face and pulls the litter rail away from the face, the two edge attendants help to pull the litter up and over the edge.

Communications. See page 179, Chapter 14, Slope Evacuation, for information on communications used in hauling systems.

The Rigging and Use of Hauling Systems in Rescue

A 1:1 MA *Hauling System*

Figure 16-8 illustrates a 1:1 hauling system for raising a load up a vertical drop.

Minimum Equipment Requirements
◆ One main line rope.
◆ One anchor sling.
◆ Two locking carabiners.
◆ One rope grab (progress capture device).
◆ Separate belay systems appropriate for the load being hauled.

Rigging the 1:1 System
1. At the top of the drop, establish a secure anchor point well back from the edge. Into this anchor point securely attach an anchor sling. Into the end of the anchor sling, clip a locking carabiner. Into the carabiner clip a pulley. This pulley is the directional through which the rope will run. This directional should be located so that the haul team will be able to move the rope in a convenient direction.

2. Thread the main line hauling rope into the pulley. Tie a "stopper knot" in the end of the rope so that the rope will not slip completely through the pulley and fall over the drop while you are doing other rigging. This could be a simple figure **8** on a bight knot. Or you can secure the rope by temporarily tying off the upper end.

3. Drop the lower end of the rope over the edge. The lower end should be close to where the load is to be hauled.

4. Establish a separate anchor point for the progress capture device. This anchor should be very strong. It also should be located close enough to where the main line rope will run but slightly off to the side of it so that the PCD and its anchor sling do not tangle with the rope. Attach an anchor sling securely onto the anchor point. Into the end of the anchor sling attach a locking carabiner. Into the carabiner clip the progress capture device.

Warning

Hauling systems can create tremendous stress on rope, hardware, and anchors. Hauling team members and other rescuers must keep in mind that forces exerted by the hauling team will be multiplied on portions of the system. If, for example, a haul team exerts a force of 1,000 lb into a 4:1 system, the resulting force on portions of the system could be around 4,000 lb. Higher MA systems could result in even higher forces.

These forces can develop quickly. Should there be a mishap, such as a jammed knot or tangled equipment, system failure could quickly occur.

All rescuers must be aware of the forces they are creating and be constantly on guard against problems that are developing.

If a haul suddenly becomes difficult, do not simply pull harder. The system may have become jammed, and harder pulling may cause a failure. Stop the haul and examine the system for problems.

As with all rescue operations, there should be one person acting as a safety officer overseeing the safety for rescuers and rescue subjects.

5. Attach the progress capture device onto the rope. If it is a general-use ascender, it should have its arrow pointing toward the load. Be certain that after placement on the rope and after the rope is loaded, the PCD creates very little bend in the rope. If there is a great deal of bend in the rope created by the PCD, it means that the PCD is creating a great deal of rope friction that will increase the load for the haul team.

6. Examine the area where the rope will run over the edge. If there is edge friction, place an edge roller under the rope or rig a suspended directional. If neither one of these is available, carefully pad the rope.

7. Establish a belay system on a separate anchor point. The anchor system should be appropriate to the type of load (that is, one person or rescue load).

8. Attach the lower end of the main line rope to the load. Remove slack in the main line rope between the PCD and the load.

9. Attach the lower end of the belay rope to the load. Make certain that there is the proper amount of slack between the load and the belay device.

10. Position the haul captain so that he or she has, if possible, a field of view of both the load and the haul team. If near the edge, the haul captain should be tied into a safety line.

11. Position a cam tender to make certain that the ascender will not travel up the rope and that it will set on the rope when it is supposed to. (Or

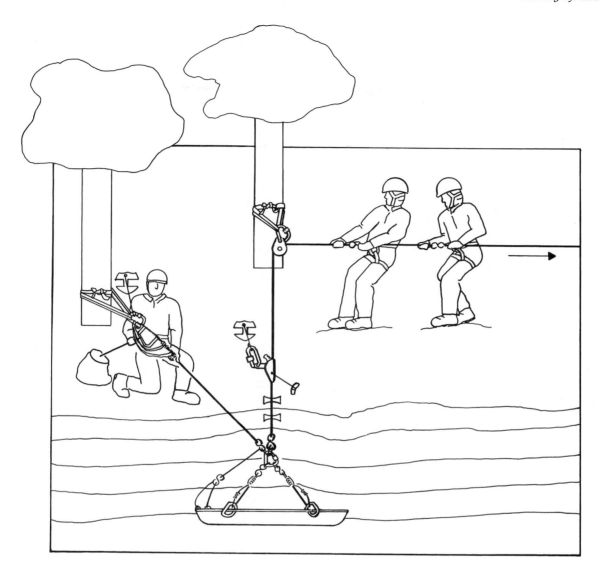

FIGURE 16-8
1:1 hauling system.

set the ascender for "automatic" with a bungee cord or weighted line. If this is done, then some-one, such as the haul captain, must have the ascender in view to make certain that it sets when it is supposed to.)

12. Position a belayer with the belay system ready to establish the load on belay.
13. Position the haul team with the rope in their hands, ready to haul.

Beginning the Haul

14. When ready to be hauled, the person on the load (practice rescuer or litter tender) initiates the belay cycle.
15. When everyone is ready, the person on the load says, "haul slow" (or "haul fast"). The haul captain then relays the communication to the haul team: "haul slow" (or "haul fast").

16. When the haul team goes as far as it can, or the system needs to be reset (and the load has not reached the top), the haul captain says, "set." The haul team immediately stops hauling and slowly eases back so the progress capture device catches. The cam tender makes certain that the PCD is set (if the cam is rigged for "automatic," the haul captain or other assigned person makes certain it will set).
17. The haul captain then says, "slack." The haul team instantly reverses direction and moves back up the rope to take another "bite."
18. The haul captain then says, "haul," and the cycle continues until the load reaches the top.

Getting the Load over the Edge

One of the most critical and difficult parts of a haul sequence is getting the load over the edge. As in rappelling and lowering, getting over the edge can be particularly difficult if it is sharp and/or undercut. But in hauling, the problem can be even more difficult and potentially dangerous. By the time the load is near the top, the main line rope tends to be pulling at a low angle that forces the load against the edge. This also tends to increase the friction of the main line rope on the edge. All these things increase the stresses that are already present in a haul system.

As in rappelling or lowering, the one factor that significantly affects the degree of difficulty of bringing the load over the edge is the angle the rope makes from the load to the anchor point when the load is at the edge. This will range from the most difficult for a horizontal angle (the anchor on the same level as the load when it is at the edge), to the easiest for a vertical angle (the anchor above the load when it is at the edge). There are various ways of increasing this angle including raising the level of the anchor to establishing a high directional. But remember *hauling systems tend to create greater stress on anchors and other elements of the system, so any elevated anchors or directionals must be able to take this stress.*

The use of a tag line can be very helpful in these situations. As the load reaches the top, the tag line can be handed over from persons below to an edge attendant. The edge attendant can then use the tag line to help pull the load over the top.

In addition, the following procedures can be helpful in getting the load over the edge, while avoiding equipment failure and potential serious injury:

- As the load approaches the edge, the haul captain says, "haul very slowly." The haul team moves very slowly and is prepared to stop instantly.
- If a size up of the situation at the edge is needed, the haul captain says, "stop!" The entire hauling process stops while the haul captain evaluates the situation.
- All personnel should be on alert to problems or stresses developing at the edge. Anyone who sees such a situation can call, "stop!"
- The use of edge attendants can be very helpful in getting the load over the edge. This is particularly true with litters, which are very prone to getting snagged. (All edge attendants must be securely attached to safety lines.)

Hauling from a Confined Space

Figure 16-9 illustrates the use of a 1:1 hauling system to perform a rescue from a vertical confined space. This system employs a large tripod. The chains that come with a tripod should also be used at the base of the legs.

Additional features of this 1:1 haul system include the following:

- The tripod must be securely anchored by a "back tie," in the direction *opposite* to the direction of the haul.
- A pulley (directional) is attached via a sling anchored to the apex of the tripod.
- A PCD is also attached to a separate sling that is anchored at the apex of the frame. The PCD should be lower down and closer to the ground. But it should be high enough so that it does not interfere with getting the load out of the hole.
- A tag line should be attached to the load. Initially this is used by the rescuers below to position the load so that it does not snag on the edge. Once the load is out of the hole, however, a rescuer at the top will need to control the tag line. He or she will use the tag line to swing the load from over the hole to where it can be safely detached.
- Once the load is at the top, the haul team will have to give slack, and the cam tender will have to release the cam so the load can be moved from over the hole.

A 2:1 Hauling System Without the "Diminishing V"

The problem with a conventional hauling system with a traveling pulley on the load (see Figure 16-1, *B*) is that it creates a "diminishing V" by having the rope run around the traveling pulley. This "diminishing V" tends to get easily snagged on brush, rock, building

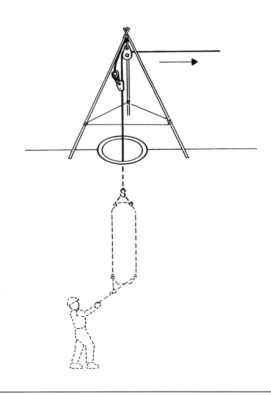

FIGURE 16-9

1:1 haul from confined space.

projections, and other objects as it advances. Another problem is that there are two strands of rope going over an edge to create additional friction.

One solution to the problem of the "diminishing V" that still has a 2:1 MA is shown in Figure 16-10.

Note that there is only a single haul line attachment going to the load, as would be the case in a 1:1 hauling system.

However, after the rope has gotten to the top, a short 2:1 hauling system is attached to it with a haul cam. By keeping the "diminishing V" smaller and at the top, the system is less likely to snag. And if it does, the rescuers are able to reach it to free it.

Setting Up a 2:1 System

1. Follow steps 1 through 9 for setting up a simple 1:1 MA hauling system.
2. At the top, and where rescuers can reach it, attach a haul cam onto the main line rope. This should be placed above the PCD (between the PCD and the anchor). To get the greatest amount of bite possible, the haul cam should be close to the PCD. But it should be far enough away from it so that the two cams will not jam during hauling operations.

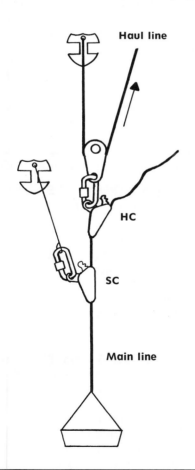

Haul line

HC

SC

Main line

FIGURE 16-10

2:1 hauling system.

Onto the haul cam clip a locking carabiner. Onto the carabiner clip a pulley.
3. Take a shorter second rope (the haul rope) and fold it in half. Attach one free end of the haul rope to an anchor that is in the direction to be pulled.
4. Thread the haul rope through the pulley that is attached to the haul cam.
5. Pull the second strand of the haul rope back parallel with the first strand that goes to the anchor. The haul team will pull on the second strand of the haul rope.

Hauling with the 2:1 System Attached to the Main Line

6. If there is a shortage of personnel for this operation, the haul captain may be stationed at the haul cam to manipulate it. He or she should have a good field of view of the operation. If enough personnel are available, a person should be assigned to be haul cam tender.
7. Follow steps 11 through 16 in setting up a 1:1 hauling system.
8. When the haul captain says, "slack," the haul team instantly reverses direction and moves back up the rope to take another bite. As they do this, the person attending the haul cam resets the system. If this is a hard cam, this is done by grasping the carabiner attached to the haul cam and pulling it back down the rope toward the load. If it is a friction hitch, grasp the knot and pull it down the rope. With the other hand, pull on the main line rope so no slack develops on the main line rope between the haul cam and the load.
9. When the haul team reaches its original position, the team is ready to begin another haul cycle.

Rigging a 3:1 Haul System (Z-Rig). Figure 16-11 illustrates a 3:1 haul system. This particular 3:1 system is also commonly known as a *Z-Rig* because of the approximate shape that the rope makes as it goes through the system.

Minimum Equipment Requirements
◆ One main line rope.
◆ Three locking carabiners.
◆ Two pulleys.
◆ Two rope grabs (one for hauling, one PCD).
◆ Separate belay systems appropriate for load being hauled.

Rigging the 3:1 System
1. Establish an anchor point that is above the load (point A1 in Figure 16-11). Into this anchor point, securely attach a sling. Into the end of the anchor sling, clip a locking carabiner. To this locking carabiner, clip a pulley. This anchor system should be well back from the edge of the drop to allow space for setting up the haul system.

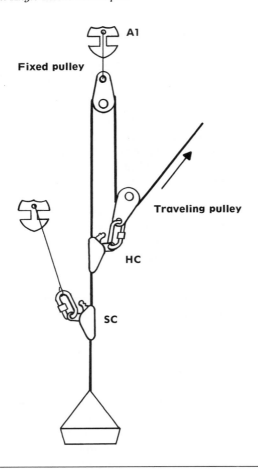

FIGURE 16-11
3:1 hauling system.

7. Bring the upper end of the main rope back in the direction of the load and run it through the pulley that is on the haul cam.
8. Now again reverse direction with the upper end of the rope and bring it back toward the first anchor and parallel with the other two strands. This will be the hauling end of the rope. Remove all rope slack from the hauling system.
9. In this configuration, the haul must be back toward anchor 1 and parallel with the other strands of the rope. Otherwise, if it is off to the side, some advantage will be lost. If, because of limited space or some other reason, the haul team must go off in another direction, then set a directional, using a stationary pulley so they can. In this way, the only advantage lost will be the small amount due to the friction of the directional pulley.
10. Follow steps 11 through 15 for setting up a 1:1 hauling system on pages 224-225.
11. Before the two pulleys at A1 and HC come together, the haul captain says, "set." The haul team immediately stops hauling. The PCD tender makes certain that the PCD has set. (If the PCD is rigged for "automatic," the haul captain or other assigned person makes certain it will set.)
12. The haul captain says, "slack." The haul team instantly reverses direction and moves back toward the load with the rope still in their hands. As they do this, the person attending the haul cam resets the system. He or she does this by grasping the carabiner attached to the haul cam and pulling it back down on the rope until it reaches the PCD (or pulls the Prusik knot back down the rope).
13. When the haul team reaches its original position, the team is ready to begin another cycle.

A 4:1 Hauling System (Piggyback System)
Minimum Equipment Required
◆ One main line rope.
◆ One hauling rope (50- to 100-feet long, depending on space available for the haul).
◆ Three locking carabiners.
◆ Two pulleys.
◆ Two rope grabs (one for PCD, one for hauling).
◆ Separate belay systems appropriate for load being hauled.

Rigging the Piggyback System (Figure 16-12)
1. Attach the main line rope to the load. Secure the upper end so that it does not accidentally slip over the edge.
2. Establish a strong anchor point for the PCD. This should be close enough to where the main rope will run but slightly off to the side of it so that the PCD and its anchor sling do not tangle with the rope. Attach an anchor sling onto the anchor point. Into the end of the anchor sling, attach a locking carabiner. Into the carabiner, attach a

2. Thread the main line rope onto the pulley that has been anchored.
3. Lower an end of the main line rope to the load.
4. Establish a separate anchor point for the PCD. This should be close enough to where the main rope will run but slightly off to the side of it so the PCD and its sling do not tangle with the rope. Attach an anchor sling onto the anchor point. Into the end of the anchor sling, attach a locking carabiner. Into the carabiner, clip a general-use ascender (or attach a Prusik loop onto the rope and attach the sling to the carabiner).
5. Thread the PCD onto the rope. If it is a general-use ascender, it should have its arrow pointing toward the load. Be certain that after placement on the rope and after the rope is loaded, the PCD does not create much of a bend in the main line rope. If there is a great deal of bend created by the PCD on the rope, it means a much higher load for the haul team.
6. At a point just above the PCD, place the haul cam (HC in Figure 16-11). If a general-use ascender, the arrow should point toward the load. Clip a locking carabiner into this haul cam. Into the locking carabiner, clip a pulley.

general-use ascender (or tie a Prusik to the rope and clip the end of the sling into the carabiner).

3. Establish an anchor point for the hauling system (point A2 in Figure 16-12). This anchor point should be in line with the load and well back from the edge to allow room for the haul system. Attach a sling to the anchor point. In the end of the sling, attach a locking carabiner.

4. Take the haul rope (the shorter line). Find the center. At the center of the rope, tie a figure **8** on a bight knot. Clip the figure **8** knot into the locking carabiner on the anchor sling.

5. After tying the figure **8** on a bight knot, you have two strands of the hauling rope. Take one leg of the haul rope back in the direction of the load. At about ⅔ of the way down this leg of the haul rope, create a bight. Put a pulley on the rope at this bight. Into the pulley, clip a locking carabiner. Into the carabiner, attach a rope grab. It must be attached on the main line rope above the PCD (between the PCD and the top end of the main line rope). If the rope grab is a general-use ascender, the arrow on the shell should point toward the load. This is the point where the hauling system "piggybacks" onto the main line rope.

6. On the same leg of the haul rope where you have attached the rope grab, find the free end of the rope. In this end, tie a figure **8** on a bight knot (point P2 in Figure 16-12).

7. Into this figure **8** on a bight knot, clip a locking carabiner. Into the carabiner, clip a pulley.

8. Take the second leg of the haul rope. Bring it down to the pulley you have just clipped into the first leg of the haul rope. Thread the second strand through the pulley.

9. Now pull the end of the second strand back toward the anchor for the hauling system (point A2 in Figure 16-12). This is the end that the haul team will pull on.

10. Follow steps 11 through 15 for setting up a 1:1 on pages 224-225.

11. Before the two pulleys at P2 and A2 in Figure 16-12 come together, the haul captain says, "set." The haul team immediately stops hauling. The PCD tender makes certain that the rope grab will set. (If the rope grab is rigged for "automatic," the haul captain or other assigned person makes certain it will set.)

12. The haul captain says, "slack." The haul team instantly reverses direction and moves back toward the load with the rope still in their hands. As they do this, the person attending the haul cam resets the system. This is done by grasping the carabiner attached to the haul cam and pulling it back down on the rope until it reaches the PCD (or pulling the Prusik knot back down the rope).

13. When the haul team reaches its original position, the team is ready to begin another cycle.

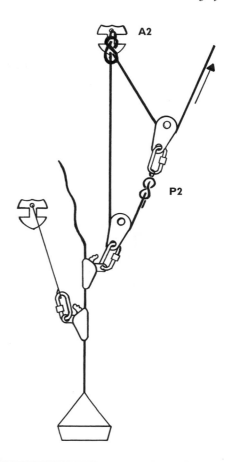

FIGURE 16-12
4:1 hauling system.

General Considerations for Rescue Hauling Systems

As with any rope rescue technique, hauling systems must be adapted to the rescue circumstances and environment and not the other way around. Although thorough knowledge of equipment and techniques is good, you should not necessarily always rig the most complex system that you know. In fact, the simplest system that is workable under the circumstances will often mean an efficient and successful rescue.

The following are some considerations to be made when deciding on a hauling system:

- Necessity of speed: A simple system will often mean:
  1. It can be set up quickly.
  2. The haul itself can be done quickly.
- Few persons available for a haul team may necessitate a higher MA, and therefore a more complex system.
- Large numbers of personnel for haul team use a simpler system. A higher MA system with a large haul team means potential for overloading and system failure.
- Small amount of gear available for rigging usually means a simpler hauling system.

- Cluttered area for hauling means hauling systems are more likely to get snagged. A simpler system may be less likely to get jammed.
- Limited room for haul team. If possible, use simpler system. Limited space will mean constantly resetting the system, and delay in the rescue.
- Higher loads may necessitate a higher MA (more complex system).
- Lighter loads mean possibly using a smaller MA (less complex system).

Evaluation Exercises

◆ COGNITIVE AND AFFECTIVE EXERCISES ◆

1. Name five situations in which rescue haul systems might be used.
2. What are the two basic reasons that rescuers employ hauling systems?
3. Define mechanical advantage.
4. How does theoretical mechanical advantage differ from actual mechanical advantage?
5. Assuming a load of 400 lb, what would be the force needed for a haul team to move it in a 1:1 hauling system? In a 2:1 hauling system? In a 3:1 hauling system? In a 4:1 hauling system?
6. Which of the following can be used to create additional mechanical advantage in some hauling systems:
   A. Stationary pulley.
   B. Traveling pulley.
7. In a basic rescue hauling system, if a 2:1 haul system were added to another 2:1 system what would likely be the resulting mechanical advantage? What would be the MA be if a 2:1 haul system were added to a 3:1 system?

8. What should personal ascenders *not* be used for in hauling systems?
9. What should be the position of the progress capture device in relationship to the other elements of the haul system?
10. What might be the possible consequences of rigging a progress capture device so far to the side of a main line rope that it creates a significant bend in the rope?
11. What are two consequences of edge friction on a rope in hauling systems?
12. Name two ways of reducing such edge friction.
13. What technique can a rescue team use to help control the movement of a litter that is being hauled and to help prevent it from becoming snagged?
14. List the minimum equipment required to rig a 1:1 hauling system. In a 2:1 hauling system. In a 3:1 (Z-Rig) hauling system. In a 4:1 ("piggyback") system.
15. What can be a significant problem with a 2:1 hauling system that uses a traveling pulley attached to the load?

▼ PSYCHOMOTOR EXERCISES ▼

16. Draw a 2:1 hauling system using a traveling pulley on the load. Label the parts and the forces acting on the system.
17. Draw a 3:1 hauling system using a Z-Rig. Label the parts and the forces acting on the system.
18. Draw a 4:1 hauling system using a "piggyback" rig. Label the parts and the forces acting on the system.

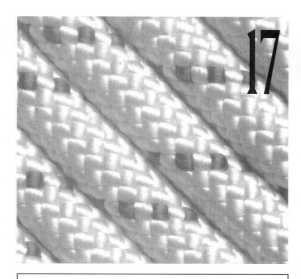

17 Other Tools for Rescue

Objectives ▼

At the completion of this chapter, you should be able to:

1. Describe how each of the following plays a role in the flight characteristics of helicopters: collective, cyclic, antitorque, ground effect, density altitude, and center of gravity.
2. Define "in ground effect" and "out of ground effect" and tell why they are important to a rescue operation.
3. Describe the duties and responsibilities of a helicopter pilot.
4. Describe the danger zones for a helicopter.
5. Describe basic safety rules for working around helicopters.
6. Identify the limitations and hazards of flying a helicopter in the mountains.
7. Describe how to select and set up a helicopter-landing zone.
8. List the procedures for entering and leaving a helicopter during a "hot loading" and in a one-skid landing.
9. List the limitations and dangers associated with a helicopter hover.
10. List the limitations and dangers associated with helicopter hoist systems.
11. Describe considerations for patients before helicopter transport.
12. List the considerations for nets or baskets used in helicopter rescue.
13. Describe the operation of a helicopter short haul.
14. List the medical considerations for a patient who is to be transported in a helicopter short haul.
15. Describe the limitations and dangers of tied emergency seat harnesses.
16. Tie the following emergency seat harnesses: diaper harness, homemade harness, and quick-don harness ("Swiss seat").

Key Terms ▼

Antitorque The use of a helicopter tail rotor to prevent the aircraft from spinning out of control.

Center of Gravity The point where a helicopter is in balance. The center of gravity can be visualized by drawing an imaginary line from the center of the main rotor to the bottom of the aircraft.

Collective The mutual effect of changing pitch on helicopter rotor blades to create more or less lift. The collective is managed from a control on the left of the pilot.

Cyclic The control of helicopter direction of flight by changing the tilt of the main rotor.

Danger Zone The area around a helicopter where there are physical hazards or the pilot's view is restricted.

Density Altitude Pressure (barometric) altitude corrected for temperature and humidity. Density altitude has a profound effect on the helicopter lift and performance.

Ground Effect The condition that occurs when a helicopter hovers close enough to the ground to compress air below itself. The result is increased lift and decreased power requirements for the helicopter and often means the aircraft can hover in a more stable manner. When a helicopter achieves this effect, it is said to be hovering in ground effect (HIGE).

Hot Loading/Unloading A condition where the pilot keeps the rotor turning during loading or unloading of the aircraft.

Key Terms—cont'd

▼

One Skid Landing A condition where a helicopter touches the portion of one skid to the ground to load or unload personnel. It is done where the terrain is unsuitable for a full landing. Also known as a *toe-in*.

Hoisting Vest ("Screamer Suit") A one-person rescue device made of fabric that wraps around a person's torso like a large diaper. It is connected to a line that hauls a person in operations such as helicopter rescue.

Horse Collar A one-person rescue device, usually used in helicopter rescue.

Hover A condition in which an airborne helicopter is maintained in a near motionless position.

Jungle Penetrator A metal device with a tapered end that has arms that swing down on which one or two persons can ride. It is connected to a line that is hauled in operations such as helicopter rescue.

Short Haul A helicopter extrication technique in which a person, or persons, are connected to a rope attached to a helicopter and the aircraft lifts off with a person or persons carried below it.

HELICOPTERS

Helicopters are increasingly being used in rescue, tactical, and aeromedical operations. When helicopters are properly used, they can speed up a rescue operation and reduce the number of persons involved in the operation. However, there are many constraints on helicopter use that rescuers must be aware of. Also, helicopters can be potentially dangerous to both rescuers and patients, so their use requires knowledge and adherence to safety rules and being alert to dangers at all times.

The following section is presented to familiarize you with helicopter operations and safety. Helicopter operations vary locally, depending on specific training, local environment, and the particular aircraft in use. Consequently, specific skills for helicopter operations can be gained by local use.

If your organization does not have helicopters, you should strive to develop an association with helicopter units. In this way, you may work for mutual training and understanding to develop confidence in one another's abilities.

One thing that helps the survival of people in a risky business, such as helicopter piloting, is distrust of the unknown, in particular, the unknown abilities of unknown people.

How Helicopters Fly

Helicopters have some very special aerodynamic characteristics that enable them to perform in the way that they do. But these characteristics also make helicopters vulnerable in other ways.

Collective

Each main rotor blade acts like an airfoil, similar to an airplane wing. As the rotor blades whirl through the air, they create lift. The pilot can vary the pitch of the blades and their rate, or rpms, to create more or less lift. Under the right conditions, this causes the helicopter to rise or drop. The *collective* is managed from a control on the left of the pilot.

Cyclic

The main rotor can be tilted to create a direction of flight. If it is tilted forward, then the helicopter, under the right conditions, will head in that direction. The *cyclic* is controlled from a column on the right of the pilot's seat.

Antitorque

A helicopter with only a single main rotor would spin helplessly in the direction opposite to the turn of the main rotor. To solve this problem, many helicopters use a tail rotor to provide thrust in a direction opposite to the spin of the main rotor in order to stabilize the aircraft. The more power that goes to the main rotor, the more power must go to the tail rotor for counter thrust. The *antitorque* is controlled by pedals at the pilot's feet.

Some newer helicopters use an internal system in the tail ("NOTAR") to create a counterthrust without the need for an external tail rotor.

Some larger helicopters have two main rotors spinning in opposite directions, so they do not need tail rotors.

Ground Effect

When helicopters are close to the ground, their hovering is helped by a cushion of air they compress below themselves. This is called *ground effect* and usually is less than one half the rotor diameter distance from the ground. Ground effect greatly assists in the ability of the helicopter to *hover* in a safe and stable manner (it is called *hovering in ground effect*). Hovering in ground effect increases lift and reduces power requirements

However, ground effect only works well in stable situations, such as a smooth, level, and firm ground surface. If the cushion of air is disturbed, such as uneven terrain, then the ground effect becomes unstable.

Density Altitude

The ability of a helicopter to lift itself is affected by the density of the air. If it is a hot day, or if the altitude is high, the air is less dense and the helicopter has less ability to lift itself. A particularly dangerous combination is a hot day at high altitude. When the margin is close to the line, a small change, such as the additional weight of one person, can make the difference between a helicopter lifting off successfully or crashing.

Center of Gravity

Maintaining weight balance in a helicopter is critical to an efficient and safe operation. The balance of a helicopter is determined around its *center of gravity*. The center of gravity can be visualized by drawing an imaginary line from the center of the main rotor to the bottom of the aircraft. Whenever the weight causes the center of gravity to shift, the aircraft will be difficult to control in flight and in landing. Cargo and passengers must be secured so they do not shift during flight and possibly cause dangerous shifts in the center of gravity. External loads must also be rigged so that they do not significantly disrupt the helicopter's center of gravity.

Roles and Responsibilities
The Pilot

Rescuers must realize that the pilot is in command of the ship. The pilot is the one who makes decisions that affect the safety of the machine and the people in and around it. This includes if and when conditions are right for take off, who approaches and boards the aircraft and when, where people sit on the aircraft, whether gear will be taken aboard and how it will be stowed on the aircraft, and if the mission is to be completed or aborted. If the pilot is uncertain about the people or other conditions in a situation, he or she not only has the right but the *duty* to avoid involvement of the aircraft and crew.

In short, the pilot has the final word. The pilot is the one who knows best the limitations of the aircraft, the flight conditions, and the crew.

No one should approach the helicopter without the permission of the pilot. This is often given through a visual sign such as the "thumbs up." To be certain you are the one being given permission, never approach the aircraft without direct eye contact with the pilot.

Crew Chief

On a larger aircraft, the crew chief performs many of these duties that might otherwise be done by the pilot.

Copilot

On larger helicopters, a copilot may be involved with navigation, communication, and crew coordination. During hovering operations, the pilot may have attention focussed on things outside the aircraft, so the copilot will be responsible for monitoring the aircraft's engine and performance instruments.

Observer

Some helicopter operations using smaller aircraft may include the person commonly called the *observer*. The observer may relieve some burdens on the pilot by assisting with some important responsibilities:

- Directing the pilot into the target and advising of rotor clearances.
- At the landing zone, stationing yourself to keep spectators and other persons from helicopter *danger zones.*

Helicopter Safety

Each year, there continue to be many helicopter mishaps that result in injury and death. Although some of these mishaps relate to mechanical failure, most of them relate to human error. These errors occur both among inexperienced personnel and among personnel who have long experience with the aircraft but who have become so casual about aircraft operations that they have dangerous lapses in attention. Consequently, those persons who work around helicopters must not only educate themselves about the dangers but also continually remind themselves about the dangers.

Danger Zones

Figure 17-1 illustrates the common *danger zones* of a helicopter as you would look directly down onto the aircraft from above. The 12 o'clock position is to the front of the aircraft, the 6 o'clock position is to the rear, the 9 o'clock position is on the left axis, and the 3 o'clock position is on the right axis.

Helicopter danger zones relate both to the physical hazards on the aircraft and to the pilot's restricted field

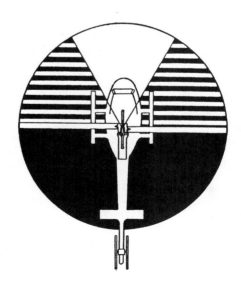

FIGURE 17-1

Danger zones of a helicopter.

of view. Note the shaded area behind the 9 o'clock/ 3 o'clock axis in Figure 17-1. This is the *pilot's blind area*, and no personnel should approach the aircraft from this direction.

With full power on, the threat from the main rotor may not be obvious. As they slow down, however, many main rotors will droop closer to the ground, as low as head high in some models.

The other danger relates to the main rotor on sloping ground (Figure 17-2). When a helicopter sits on sloping ground, anyone on the up hillside will be automatically placed closer to the rotor blades. Consequently, when on sloping ground, always approach a helicopter *from downhill.*

Tail Rotor

Another primary hazard is the tail rotor. It poses a great danger for two reasons:

1. The tail rotor in operation is often whirling at such high speed that in the noise and excitement, the rotor is unnoticed and people walk into it.
2. A sudden wind gust moves the helicopter on the ground, or the pilot makes a quick take off and shifts direction, mowing down a person or persons on the ground.

Consequently, to avoid contact with the tail rotor follow these rules strictly: (1) never approach a helicopter from the rear and (2) never go around the rear of a helicopter to get to the other side.

Unsecured Objects and Debris

Take special care with objects that project above head level. These include radio antenna, litters, weapons, skis, ice axes, and probe poles. These could make contact with the main rotor and could cause serious injury or death to you. They could cause the rotor to fragment, resulting in serious injury or death to other persons. Objects such as these should be carried low and parallel to the ground. In some cases, the helicopter crew will load them in external cargo areas.

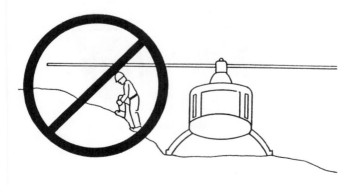

FIGURE 17-2
Rotor danger on sloping ground.

Objects, such as hats and helmets, which could be caught by rotor wash and be sucked into the rotor, must be thoroughly secured.

Rotor Wash. As the helicopter approaches for a landing, the rotor wash will blow all lightweight objects away to either be sucked into the rotor or tail rotor, or cause them to take flight and have to be chased cross country. Such lightweight objects include caps, maps, tents, tarps, loose clothing, empty packs, sleeping bags, clothing, and helmets.

In addition, rotor wash will blow up a massive amount of dust and other debris. Unless you are wearing eye protection, turn away from the landing area to avoid eye injury. Also, keep vehicles away from the landing zone (LZ) because the rotor wash blows debris that can crack windshields and damage paint.

Additional Helicopter Safety Rules

- Everyone working near helicopters should wear a helmet with the chin strap fastened.
- Do not smoke within 100 feet of a helicopter.
- Always buckle up when inside the aircraft.
- Never stand under a helicopter or in its landing/takeoff zone unless you are authorized to attach sling loads or assist in hoist operations.
- When working in a helicopter LZ, wear eye protection against blowing dust and sand.
- After you exit a helicopter always make certain that seat harness buckles are secured inside the aircraft and the door is firmly closed.
- Wear protective clothing. Cover arms and legs to protect from debris blown by rotor wash. Fabrics such as Nomex, cotton, and wool are preferable to fibers such as polyprolene or polyester that melt in flash fires. Boots should be of all leather and cover the ankles. Gloves should be all leather or combination leather and Nomex. All passengers should wear a helmet and eye protection.

Mountain Flying

Among the greatest tolls on rescue helicopters is mountain flying. Some veteran pilots have described mountain rescue flying in North America as being scarier than combat flying in Vietnam.

There are two primary reasons for mountain flying being so treacherous: (1) aircraft performance limitations at high altitude and (2) crosswinds and down drafts.

Aircraft Performance Limitations at Altitude

As you ascend in altitude the air becomes less dense, so the helicopter rotor has less to "bite" into, reducing its capability to lift the aircraft. During warm weather, the air also becomes less dense, meaning even less lift for the aircraft. Thus, a hot summer day at high altitude is a dangerous environment for a helicopter.

The standard for measuring the capability to support an aircraft in flight is called *density altitude*. Density altitude is calculated using the pressure altitude corrected for temperature and humidity. The most important elements in the calculation are altitude and humidity. An increase in altitude and temperature means that density altitude goes up. As density altitude goes up, the rotor blades have less air to increase lift, and performance and capability decreases. Therefore the pilot must increase engine power, and the aircraft must carry less people, cargo, and fuel.

From calculating density altitude, the pilot or crew member can then decide the amount of personnel, cargo, and fuel that the aircraft can safely carry or land with at a given altitude. The higher the density altitude, the more difficult it is for the helicopter to hover both in ground effect and out of ground effect.

Use caution in judging a helicopter ceiling from manufacturer specifications. These are often the ideal, calculated from stripped-down models flying only with a pilot. If the same helicopter has rescuers aboard, and its full complement of gear and equipment, the ceiling may be considerably lower. Other considerations include fuel load, winds, and condition of the aircraft's power plant.

Cross Winds and Down Drafts

Mountains tend to make their own weather, which may be more unpredictable than at lower altitudes. Veteran pilots who have been flying for years in mountains are often able to predict what these conditions may be. But it is often the veteran pilot who gets caught in them.

Landing Zones

One thing that helicopter pilots tend to distrust is LZs with which they have had no previous experience.

The primary reason for this is that unless they know the ground personnel well and trust their judgment, there is no way they can be sure those persons setting up the LZ are fully aware of the hazards and needs of the aircraft. The following are some general considerations for the creation of LZs.

Selection of Landing Zones

Terrain. Helicopters do not do well when landing and, in particular, when taking off at a complete vertical. They operate better and safer when landing and taking off at a slope and, as with fixed-wing aircraft, into the wind. Before pilots land and take off, they need to bring the aircraft to an in-ground effect hover for more control of the aircraft. Unlike fixed wing aircraft that land and stop, helicopters must stop and land.

Figure 17-3 illustrates an ideal terrain for a helicopter LZ. Note that the terrain slopes down both on the approach and takeoff sides, and the landing and takeoff are into the wind. Obviously, there must be adequate space at the top for the landing and maneuvering of the aircraft.

Size. The bigger the LZ is, the better. For smaller helicopters, an LZ the size of a football field would be a good start. Consider both the takeoff and landing needs, as well as potential engine failure.

Debris. Natural debris such as dust, gravel, pine needles, leaves, and light snow can obstruct vision and create hazards including potential mechanical failure.

Obstruction. The landing zone should be free of vertical obstructions. Any such obstruction that cannot be removed must be reported to the pilot, and, if possible, marked or lighted. Particularly dangerous

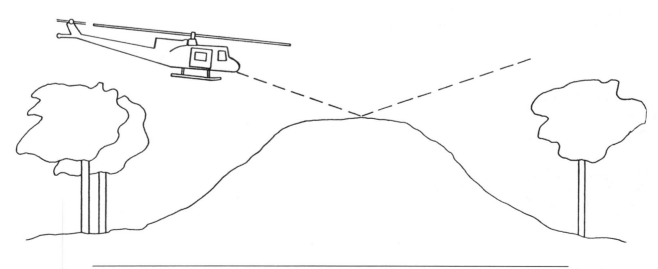

FIGURE 17-3
Ideal terrain for helicopter LZ.

obstructions are utility lines, which are often invisible to the pilot.

Meadows with Tall Grass. Tall grass dissipates a helicopter's in-ground effect, creating dangers in landing, takeoff, and hovering. Tall grass can also obscure hazards such as rocks, stumps, and bogs.

Snow. Loose, dry snow may be kicked up by the rotor wash and blind the pilot. This may cause dangers both in takeoff and landing.

Wet snow may also cause dangers by adhering to the skid or landing gear. This may require more power for takeoff, and when the snow adhesion to the undercarriage breaks unevenly, the aircraft can roll on takeoff.

Water. An additional problem in LZs is that there is often less stable ground effect for a helicopter over water. This can be particularly dangerous at higher altitudes. There have been a number of tragedies in which helicopters at high altitude have taken off or approached for landing over a mountain lake and crashed into the water.

Preparation of Landing Zones
Remove Debris. Remove or secure all debris or loose equipment.

Remove Nonessential Personnel. Remove all persons except those who are completely essential for the landing, loading, and takeoff of the helicopter. Those who are loading must not approach the aircraft until the pilot or crew chief signals them to do so.

Wind Indicators. Pilots will need to know the wind direction both on landing and takeoff. Many services use smoke grenades for wind indicators, but some pilots do not like them because they feel smoke obscures their view of an area. One alternative is tying bright-colored trail tape on posts and other uprights. Other less-effective possibilities for wind indicators include the throwing of dirt, pine needles, leaves, or snow into the air.

When pilots arrive at an unfamiliar LZ, they will commonly make one or more reconnaissance passes to decide the best approach and if a landing can be made safely.

Communications with Pilot

If radio communication is available, then ground personnel should communicate to the pilot basic and essential information such as wind direction and speed, air temperature, and any hazards in the area.

Pilots will usually not depend on visual signals from ground personnel they do not know. However, there are a few basic signals that may be helpful to the pilot.

It is essential to have only one person in charge of the landing zone and communication with the pilot.

The LZ chief should be wearing bright clothing, such as an orange vest so he or she can be identified from the air. The LZ chief should stand at the end of the landing zone with the wind to his or her back and the arms extended toward landing area. This person should maintain position during landing and keep eye contact with the pilot during the landing.

Another important visual signal is the "wave off," used to warn the pilot from landing due to hazards. The person giving the signals repeatedly waves arms from horizontal to crossed over head.

Night Landings
The objective of night-landing lights is to provide adequate orientation without blinding the pilot.

Long-Distance Orientation. Strobes or emergency vehicle lights may stand out among other distracting lights and orient the pilot from a distance. As the pilot begins the approach, these and other bright lights should be extinguished because they can be blinding.

LZ Marker Lights. For marking the LZ perimeter, pilots prefer low-intensity lights, such as chemical light sticks. Avoid flares because they are too bright and are a fire danger.

Box 17-1 asks questions that are essential before a night landing or any flight.

Helicopter Insertion/Evacuation Techniques
Full Landing

Where the terrain allows a suitable LZ, and where the weather allows for it, the full landing is usually

---

 Box 17-1 Twelve Standard Aviation Questions that Could Save Your Life

1. Is this flight necessary?
2. Who is in charge?
3. Are all hazards identified and have you made them known?
4. Should you stop the operation or flight due to:
    ◆ Communications?
    ◆ Weather?
    ◆ Turbulence?
    ◆ A lack of personnel or training?
5. Is there a better way to do it?
6. Are you driven by an overwhelming sense of urgency?
7. Can you justify your actions?
8. Are there other aircraft in the area?
9. Do you have an escape route?
10. Are any rules being broken?
11. Are communications getting tense?
12. Are you deviating from the assigned operation or flight?
When in doubt—don't!

From U.S. National Park Service Aviation.

the most desirable for the insertion or evacuation of personnel.

After the landing, the personnel must await signals from the pilot or crew chief to approach or exit the aircraft. Passengers, whether approaching or exiting the aircraft, must take the same precautions: secure all equipment, do not project any equipment into the rotor, keep heads down, stay in view and eye contact of the pilot, and *move forward in the pilot's view away from the aircraft and avoid the tail section.*

As you enter the aircraft, hold onto the door to keep it from being blown against the helicopter. The door is not weight supporting, so do not use it to pull yourself in. When entering the aircraft, avoid bumping any controls or the pilot.

As soon as you are in your seat, fasten and adjust the seat belt and shoulder harness. Be certain you know how to unfasten the seat belt before take off.

Keep the seat belt/shoulder harness fastened until you have landed and the pilot has signaled for you to exit. As you leave, refasten the seat belts behind you. *Be certain that no seat belts or shoulder harnesses are hanging outside the door.*

Hot loading or unloading is a condition where the pilot keeps the rotor turning during loading or unloading. It may be necessary for a variety of reasons, most commonly the following:

◆ Speed (for example, a critically injured subject, wildland fire, or other threat).

◆ Questionable LZ (for example, the pilot keeps the rotor rpms up to avoid the skid slipping off rock).

◆ Tactical reasons (for example, the LZ may be exposed to weapons fire).

One-Skid Landing

Some helicopter services may employ one skid ("toe-in") landings where the terrain is unsuitable for a full landing. Personnel enter and leave the aircraft by moving carefully and deliberately across the skid in use so they do not upset the equilibrium of the aircraft (Boxes 17-2 and 17-3).

Keep in mind the "commitment rule." Do not commit to the helicopter until you are in it. Commit to the ground once you are definitely on it. One significant problem in hot loads and skid loads is people trying to hang on to the helicopter if it needs to move.

Hovering Tactics

To maintain a hover, the helicopter must use significantly more power, so payload of personnel and cargo has to be reduced. Even worse is when a helicopter has to hover out of ground effect. When a helicopter must hover out of ground effect, or descend and ascend vertically, such as in a narrow canyon, it is flying at "maximum performance" operation. The helicopter is completely dependent on power, it has less stability, and its margins of safety are reduced. These are among the most dangerous situations in which a helicopter can operate and they should be avoided.

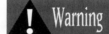 **Warning**

Hovering is one of the least desirable maneuvers for the helicopter pilot because it places the ship in a very vulnerable and unstable situation. Several factors create this situation:

◆ In a hover, the helicopter is being kept in the air only by the collective (angle of the rotor blades) and engine rpm.

◆ In a hover, the aircraft lacks the forward momentum that could add to its lift and carry it away both from its own destruction and the danger to people below it.

◆ In a hover, the helicopter may be endangered by its own rotor wash that may be recirculated to create an unstable air mass.

For these reasons, helicopter hover time must be kept to a minimum.

 Box 17-2 Basic Sequence for Unloading

1. The ship slows and touches the skid on the passenger side of the ship. The pilot maintains the engine rpms to keep the ship level and makes certain that the ship has been stabilized.
2. The pilot signals that the ship is stabilized. The passengers unfasten their seat belts.
3. One at a time, the passengers move carefully onto the skid.
4. Carefully, they step off and beyond (never between the skid and the helicopter).
5. They remain in a crouch on the ground until the helicopter clears the area.

 Box 17-3 Basic Sequence for Boarding

1. Stay crouched until the pilot has steadied the ship.
2. Move close to the skid while watching the pilot. Do not touch the skid until the pilot signals.
3. When the pilot signals, place one foot on the skid and grasp the doorframe. Your movement must be slow and deliberate. Do not switch feet on the skid. Move slowly and deliberately through the door placing your other foot inside the ship.
4. Follow through by moving your first foot from the skid. Take your seat and fasten the safety belt.

Hoist Systems

Hoists are based on either hydraulic or electric winch systems and are usually found in medium to heavy aircraft, such as the Huey and Blackhawk series. Although they add convenience to some helicopter operations, winches require a well-trained and experienced team.

Their failure is usually due to one of the following reasons:

- Cable break. The cable has been overstressed previously, and the defect was undetected. When loaded, the cable fails catastrophically.
- Failure in the winch mechanism. This can occur when the winch mechanism fails catastrophically as the cable is being wound, or the cable has been completely extended but the mechanism is unable to draw it in.

Belayed Hoists. Some helicopter services belay the hoist with a separate line. The separate line is usually a nylon rope that would be the same as is used in a high angle environment.

There are some complications involved in belayed hoists. Some of these include potential tangling, the need for additional personnel for the belay, and communications problems. With newer, more reliable hoist systems, hoist belays are being used less than before.

Hoisting Vest ("Screamer Suit"). The *hoisting vest* is a net-like device constructed of mesh and webbing (Figure 17-4). It is designed to encompass rescue subjects who are disabled or unconscious to prevent them from falling out. The fabric wraps around a per-

son's torso like a larger diaper. Because the hoisting vest requires no knowledge of it by the rescue subject, or any previous experience with it, it is appropriate for civilian rescues.

It is also very simple to use by the rescuer and is attached via a single large locking carabiner.

Horse Collar. The *horse collar* is one traditional method used by the military for extricating personnel (Figure 17-5). During the past several years there have been many incidents in which persons have slipped out of the horse collar, resulting in severe injury or death. As a result, some military search and rescue units do not use the horse collar with unrestrained civilian personnel.

> ⚠ **Warning**
>
> - The horse collar can only be used on a fully conscious individual.
> - Even an alert, well-trained individual may fall from a horse collar. The collar may impinge on nerves and result in the individual's loss of sensation in the arms. The individual may then lose his or her grip and fall from the harness.

> ⚠ **Warning**
>
> When attaching a person to a helicopter lift system, whether it be hoist or static line, use only hardware designed and rated for life support. *Never* use hardware, such as cargo hooks, designed and rated only for lifting material.

> ⚠ **Warning**
>
> Helicopters build up large charges of static electricity due to the action of the rotors against the air. This static electricity will be discharged to the ground through the helicopter or metal components, such as cable. Therefore whenever a component, such as sling or stretcher, is being lowered by a helicopter, always allow it to touch ground before reaching for it.

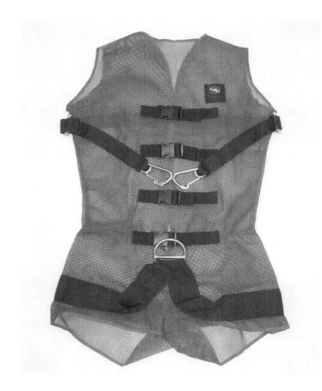

FIGURE 17-4
Screamer suit.

Many helicopter operations have replaced the horse collar with improved equipment. One example is the quick strop (Figure 7-6), which can be used for hoisting uninjured persons. The strop fits around the back or over the head of the subject. Stored in a zipper pocket on the rear of the strop is an adjustable crotch safety strap.

Jungle Penetrator. The *jungle penetrator* is a metal device with a tapered end. It has arms that swing down on which one or two persons can ride and a webbing loop to hold the user onto the device.

Because of its weight, the jungle penetrator is found on more powerful helicopters. In most cases, it will only be on military aircraft. The rescue seat (Figure 17-7) is an updated version of the jungle penetrator. The rescue seat, which is lighter weight and more compact than the jungle penetrator, is designed for hoisting persons from water or land. It will usually only be found on helicopters with hoists, normally military aircraft.

Litter Hoists. The hoisting of a litter to a helicopter has been commonly used in the military services and now is found on some civilian helicopters. There are some primary considerations for such litter hoists.

> **⚠ Warning**
>
> Due to down draft and pendulum effect, litters in a hoist may spin uncontrollably. This can complicate existing injuries and create injuries on its own.
>
> Litters that catch the downdraft, such as solid plastic litters, tend to spin more than wire basket litters. Also, litters rigged horizontal may spin more. Litters rigged slightly foot down may not spin as much.
>
> Consult local helicopter providers for specific information on rigging litters for hoists.

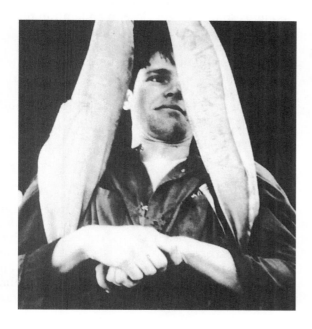

FIGURE 17-5
Horse collar.

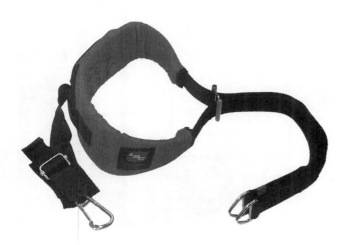

FIGURE 17-6
Quick strop.

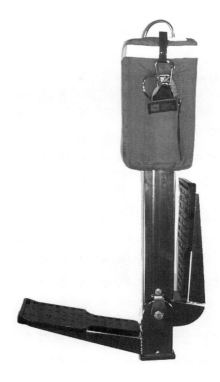

FIGURE 17-7
Rescue seat.

The spider. The litter spider must have a low enough profile so that when hoisted to the helicopter, the litter does not hang so low that the air crew is unable to bring it inside. Figure 17-8 illustrates the maximum height for a litter spider to be hoisted to a Huey model helicopter.

Tag lines. One problem with hoisting a litter is that it tends to spin and pendulum. One way to reduce these problems is to have a tag line tied to the foot of the litter and steadied by the ground crew as the litter is being hoisted. The tag line should have a simple attachment to the foot of the litter, such as a carabiner. This is so when the litter reaches the aircraft, a crewmember can quickly detach the tag line and drop it to the ground so it does not get sucked into the tail rotor.

Litter movement. Complete all necessary litter movement before attaching it to the cable. If the litter has been lowered, remove it from the cable before moving it. These actions will free the helicopter for any maneuvers it needs to make, and should a wind gust come or the wind change direction, they will prevent the helicopter from dragging the litter along the ground.

Patient protection. The patient must be protected against chill and wetness. His or her face and eyes must be protected from blowing debris.

Patient packaging. The patient, as in vertical evacuation, must be securely packaged in the litter so he or she will not slide out whatever the position of the litter. Additionally, patients packaged for helicopter hoisting must be secured so they will not slide out the end, in case of litter spin.

Rescue Nets and Baskets. Another form of helicopter rescue is the rescue net or basket. A well-designed net or basket has the advantages of being able to quickly evacuate personnel, to lift out disabled people, and to lift off several people at once. Rescue nets and baskets come in a variety of sizes from a capacity for one person to a capacity for several persons. Some nets and baskets can carry a litter containing a rescue subject. Nets and baskets are found in two basic types: collapsible and rigid (Figure 17-9).

There are safety considerations for helicopter rescue nets and baskets:

◆ The net or basket should have some rigid components so it does not close in and entrap the subject or create a feeling of claustrophobia.

◆ If used in the water, should have proper flotation so that the net or basket does not drag the subject under the water.

◆ The net or basket should create a user-friendly atmosphere so that the subject desires to climb in and does not try to hang onto the outside.

◆ The net or basket must be able to securely contain the rescue subjects so that they do not fall out.

Short Hauls

A *short haul* is a helicopter extrication technique in which a person, or persons, are connected to a rope attached to a helicopter, and the aircraft lifts off with a person or persons carried below it. The exact length of the line depends on the specific needs of the operation. In many areas, short haul has replaced helicopter rappel techniques. This is due in part to the fact that short haul techniques usually require less hover time

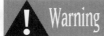

! Warning

Any litter used in the water must have a flotation kit. This kit, which includes a ballast bar on the foot end of the litter, supports the patient and litter in the water, keeps the patient's face out of the water, and prevents the litter from floating face down.

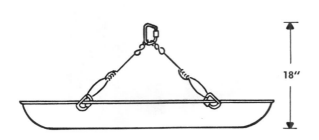

18″

FIGURE 17-8
Maximum height for litter spider.

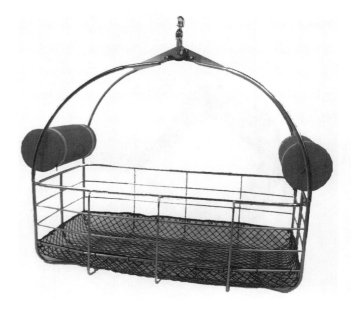

FIGURE 17-9
Example of net basket.

for helicopters. Hovering creates a strain on pilots and also on the helicopter engine and other components.

There are several specific procedures and variations that can be used with the short haul technique.

Attached Person Short Hauls

One of the simplest forms of short hauls is the attached person. This is often used in tactical operations where personnel have to be removed hurriedly. One technique for rescue is for the rescuer to be attached to a fixed line under the aircraft and to come in and pick off a rescue subject. This technique is essentially the same as a one-person rescue technique (see Chapter 13, Pickoff Rescue Techniques). As with one-person rescue techniques, the subject *should not be attached to the rescuer's seat harness but directly to the vertical system, such as the attachment to the main line rope.*

Litter Short Hauls

In a litter short haul, the crew usually flies with the litter to a landing zone near the incident site. At the landing zone, the helicopter sets down, where the crew rigs the litter. The helicopter then flies with the litter and, often, a litter tender to the incident site. There, the crew may detach the litter for the time it takes to package the patient and then return to reattach the litter and fly back to the landing zone. There, the litter with the patient, along with the crew, is placed aboard the helicopter to fly to a hospital or to meet with an ambulance.

From the patient's point of view, it is best to have a litter tender attached to the litter system to fly along with the patient. The main reason for this relates to medical considerations for the patient, primarily to ensure an open and clear airway.

There may, however, be circumstances in which the use of a litter tender on a flyaway is not practical. These often relate to altitude where the aircraft's performance is so limited that the additional weight of the tender cannot be tolerated. In these cases, the actual time of the flyaway must be kept as short as possible. In some areas, the patient is packaged on the side to help maintain an open airway.

Tied Emergency Seat Harnesses

Tied seat harnesses may be useful in an emergency when a manufactured harness is not available. How-

ever, they cannot be used for hanging in for long periods, should not be used for lead climbing, and should not be used in performing intricate or difficult high angle operations.

The Diaper Harness. The diaper harness is one of the simplest tied seat harnesses. It consists of a continuous loop of webbing (2-inch webbing is more comfortable than 1-inch webbing). The web is sewn to a very substantial buckle or connected with a ring bend (water knot) backed up. The loop is brought together in front by equalizing three portions, one between the legs, and two from either side, and attached by a large locking carabiner (Figure 17-10).

The Homemade Harness. The homemade seat harness is one harness type that is found in a number of versions throughout North America. One of the earli-

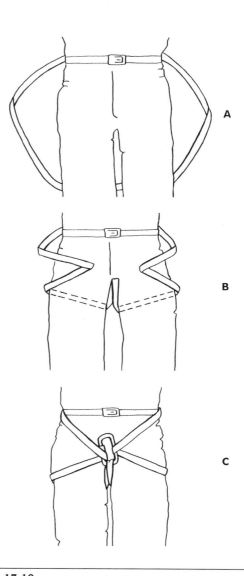

FIGURE 17-10
Diaper harness.

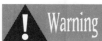

Helicopter short haul operations are complex and potentially dangerous. For short haul operations, only associate with those units whose aircraft, pilots, and crew have been certified for short haul by an appropriate agency. This could be a military service or a civilian agency such as the U.S. Office of Aircraft Services.

est descriptions was in the book, *Mountaineering, the freedom of the hills*, Seattle, 1998, The Mountaineers Press.

Procedure for tying the homemade harness (Figure 17-11)

1. Take a piece of tubular webbing 22 feet long.
2. Leaving about 4 feet of tail, tie a loop near one end using a figure **8** on a bight knot. This loop should be slightly larger than your left thigh.
3. Move over approximately 8 inches on the webbing and tie a second loop using a figure **8** on a bight. This loop should be slightly larger than your right thigh (Figure 17-11, *A*).
4. Now step into each loop and bring it up around a thigh, with the 18-inch tail on the left, the 10-inch piece at the front, and the long remaining portion on the right (Figure 17-11, *B*).
5. Take the long end and run it around the back and over the buttocks to the front.
6. Run this end under and through the 10-inch section at the front and pull everything snug (Figure 17-11, *C*).
7. Repeat step 5 (Figure 17-11, *D*).
8. Bring the end around the back again, to the side and tie it together with the 4-foot tail, using a square knot. Back the square knot up by bringing the two ends together and tying them together with a ring bend (water knot). (If enough webbing is left over, then repeat steps 5 and 6 again before tying off.)
9. Clip the tie-in carabiner across the portion where the ends have crossed the 10-inch section (Figure 7-11, *E*).
10. Now check the proportions of the harness to see if it fits the proportions of your body. You can do this by hanging in the harness just off the ground.

Alternative Approach: The Quick-Don Harness ("Swiss Seat"). One commonly used harness that can be tied quickly in emergency situations is the

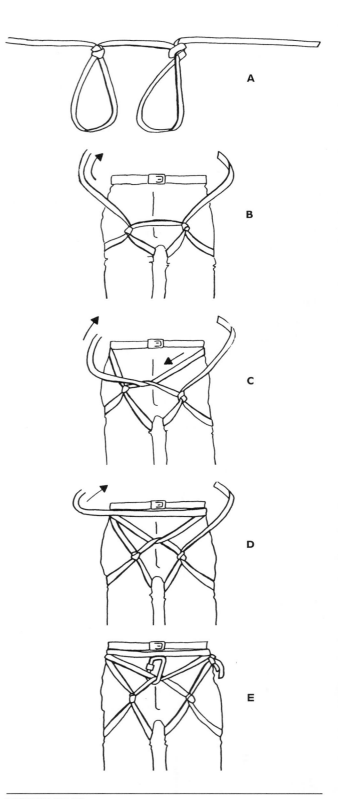

FIGURE 17-11
Homemade harness.

> ⚠ **Warning**
>
> 1. One danger posed by the quick-don harness is tying it incorrectly under stress. This could cause it to fail. For this reason, if you anticipate ever using this harness, you must consistently practice tying it so you can tie it correctly in an emergency.
> 2. If at any point the webbing is severed, the entire harness will fail.
> 3. This harness does not provide full support in some areas of the anatomy. Consequently, the webbing in this harness may constrict circulation and, possibly, impair nerve function if the wearer hangs in the harness for more than a few minutes.

quick-don harness (also known as the *Swiss seat*). This harness can usually be tied quicker than the homemade harness but it does not offer the same support or security.

Procedure for tying the quick-don harness ("Swiss seat") (*Figure* 17-12)

1. Take a length of webbing at least 13 feet long (longer if you have large buttocks or thighs).
2. Find the center.
3. Place the center in the small of the back.
4. Pull the two ends to the front and tie an overhand knot.
5. Drop the ends in front. Reach through your legs from behind and pull both ends through to the rear.
6. Now, run each end under a buttock and around the outside of the thigh.
7. Run the webbing under itself in front.
8. Pull each end in the opposite direction, around the waist, and bring them together on one side.
9. Tie off with a square knot.
10. Back up the square knot by bringing the two ends together and tying them with a water knot.

Medical Considerations

Even when they are in their best physical and mental condition, people may find helicopters intimidating. When a person is seriously injured and in a state of anxiety, a helicopter may be very frightening and could increase the medical problems. Before transporting a patient by helicopter you must:

1. Thoroughly evaluate his or her medical condition and state of mind.
2. Explain to the subject the nature of the steps that are to take place.
3. Reassure.

Some services require a litter spider to meet certain specifications before they will hoist it. One service, for example, requires that the spider be made of cable. When it is feasible, many services will have a crewman leave the helicopter to inspect the spider before they attempt to hoist it.

Critical time often can be saved when you know if the service requires specifications for the litter spider.

When an injured patient is transported without a litter tender, one of the primary dangers is blockage of the airway, which will quickly result in death. Airway blockage is often associated with the following conditions:

- ◆ Unconscious patient. When a person is lying supine (on the back) the tongue can fall back and block the airway.
- ◆ Material that is the result of the injury (such as blood or vomitus) can be aspirated into the lungs.

If a patient cannot be attended during transport, then he or she should be transported in as short a time as possible and transported in the "coma position" (on the side).

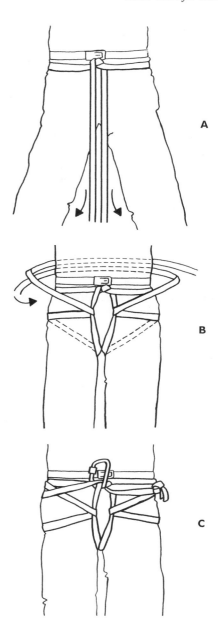

FIGURE 17-12
Quick-don harness.

Evaluation Exercises

◆ COGNITIVE AND AFFECTIVE EXERCISES ◆

1. **Describe the role of each of the following in the flight characteristics of helicopters:**
   a) Collective
   b) Cyclic
   c) Antitorque

2. How does ground effect relate to helicopter hover?

3. Describe how density altitude affects the flying of a helicopter, and what factors are used to determine it.

4. Describe how to visualize a helicopter's center of gravity.

5. List four decisions about helicopter operations that are the responsibility of the pilot.

6. When the helicopter is on sloping ground, from which direction should you approach the aircraft?

7. Name two reasons the helicopter tail rotor poses a danger.

8. Name precautions to prevent the main rotor from hitting objects that are:
   a) Small and light.
   b) Large and heavy.

9. Name four criteria to consider when selecting a helicopter-landing zone.

10. Name three reasons why hovering is often the least desirable maneuver for the helicopter pilot.

11. Name four devices that can be used on lines from helicopters to rescue individuals.

12. Name four design criteria for nets or baskets used in helicopter rescue.

13. List three actions to take before transporting a patient by helicopter.

14. Name the primary danger for a patient in a litter being short hauled without an attendant.

▼ PSYCHOMOTOR EXERCISES ▼

15. Using webbing, tie the following on yourself and then on another person:
    a) Diaper harness.
    b) Homemade harness.
    c) Quick-don harness ("Swiss seat").

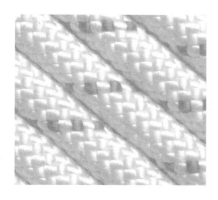

Appendix A: Standards Setting Organizations and Further Reading

STANDARDS SETTING ORGANIZATIONS

ANSI

American National Standards Institute, Inc.
11 West 42nd Street
New York, NY 10036

ANSI is concerned with standards for safety belts, harnesses, lanyards, lifelines and drop lines in areas such as construction, industry, window cleaning, and arboriculture.

ASTM

100 Barr Harbor Drive
West Conshohocken, PA 19428

ASTM is the facilitator for standards created through the full consensus method. Standards for equipment and techniques used in search and rescue are currently being developed through the ASTM process.

CE (European Committee for Standardization)

(Contact through ANSI)

CE is concerned with standards for a wide variety of products traded in the European Union, including personal protective equipment. Rescue equipment falls into this category.

NFPA

National Fire Protection Association
1 Batterymarch Park
P.O. Box 9101
Quincy, MA 02269

NFPA is concerned with standards specific to fire service applications. This includes rope and related equipment, along with performance standards for rescuers in the fire service.

UIAA

C/O American Alpine Club
710-10th Street, Suite 100
Golden, CO 80401

The UIAA sets standards for rope, helmets, hardware, and other equipment used in recreational climbing.

OSHA

U.S. Occupational Health and Safety Administration
Department of Labor
200 Constitution Avenue
Washington, DC 20210
www.osha.gov

OSHA is concerned with workplace safety.

FURTHER READING

Frank JA: *CMC rope rescue manual,* ed 3, Santa Barbara, 1998, California Mountain Company, p 208.

Graydon D: *Mountaineering: The freedom of the hills,* ed 6, Seattle, 1998, The Mountaineers, p 445.

Hudson S: *Manual of U.S. cave rescue techniques,* ed 2, Huntsville, Ala., 1992, National Speleological Society, p 260.

Leonard R, Wexler A: *Belaying the leader: An omnibus on climbing safety,* San Francisco, 1956, Sierra Club, p 85.

MacInnes H: *International mountain rescue handbook,* New York, 1972, Charles Scribner's Sons, p 218.

Ray S: *Swiftwater rescue, a manual for the rescue professional,* Ashville, N.C., 1997, CPS Press, p 243.

Robbins R: *Basic rockcraft,* Glendale, Calif., 1971, La Siesta Press, p 70.

Setnicka TJ: *Wilderness search and rescue,* Boston, 1980, Appalachian Mountain Club, p 640.

Smith B, Padgett A: *On rope: Notrh American vertical rope techniques,* new revised ed, Huntsville, Ala., 1996, National Speleological Society, p 382.

Wheelock W: *Ropes, knots, and slings for climbers,* Glendale, Calif., 1967, La Siesta Press, p 36.

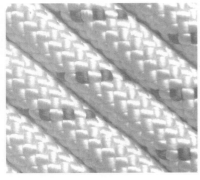

Appendix B: High Angle Skills Checklists

High Angle Skills Checklist

KNOTS

INSTRUCTIONS
As each student completes a skill check, the evaluator notes the date in the evaluator column. If the sudent demonstrates the prescribed level of competence for the skill, the instructor signs his or her initials. If the student fails, the instructor places a "U" (Unsatisfactory). If successful, the student signs his or her initials in the adjacent column to the right.

STUDENT _____

EVALUATOR(S) _____

_____

_____

	First try		Second try	
	EVALUATOR	STUDENT	EVALUATOR	STUDENT
Tie a simple overhand knot.				
Tie a simple figure 8 knot.				
Tie a figure 8 on a bight knot.				
Tie a figure 8 follow through knot.				
Tie a figure 8 bend.				
Tie a ring bend ("water knot") in webbing.				
Tie a double overhand ("barrel knot").				
Tie a double fisherman's (grapevine) knot.				

High Angle Skills Checklist

ANCHORING

INSTRUCTIONS
As each student completes a skill check, the evaluator notes the date in the evaluator column. If the sudent demonstrates the prescribed level of competence for the skill, the instructor signs his or her initials. If the student fails, the instructor places a "U" (Unsatisfactory). If successful, the student signs his or her initials in the adjacent column to the right.

STUDENT _____

EVALUATOR(S) _____

_____

_____

	First try		Second try	
	EVALUATOR	STUDENT	EVALUATOR	STUDENT
Tie and rig a tensionless hitch on anchor point.				
Tie and rig figure 8 on a bight on anchor point.				
Tie and rig figure 8 follow through on anchor point.				
Tie and rig a ring bend ("water knot") in webbing on anchor point.				
Tie and rig load sharing anchor on two anchor points.				
Rig a load distributing anchor on two anchor points.				
Rig a load distributing anchor on three or more anchor points.				

High Angle Skills Checklist

BELAYING OF ONE-PERSON LOADS

INSTRUCTIONS

As each student completes a skill check, the evaluator notes the date in the evaluator column. If the sudent demonstrates the prescribed level of competence for the skill, the instructor signs his or her initials. If the student fails, the instructor places a "U" (Unsatisfactory). If successful, the student signs his or her initials in the adjacent column to the right.

STUDENT _____

EVALUATOR(S) _____

_____

_____

	First try		Second try	
	EVALUATOR	STUDENT	EVALUATOR	STUDENT
Repeat from memory and in correct sequence the belay voice communications.				
On level ground, use a Munter hitch to belay a person moving away from the belayer.				
On level ground, use a Munter hitch to belay a person moving toward the belayer.				
Using a belay practice system, use a Munter hitch to catch a dropped weight as it is being lowered.				
On level ground, use a one-person belay device to belay a person moving away from the belayer.				
On level ground, use a one-person belay device to belay a person moving toward the belayer.				
Using a belay practice system, use a one-person belay device to catch a dropped weight as it is being raised.				
Using a belay practice system, use a one-person belay device to catch a dropped weight as it is being lowered.				

High Angle Skills Checklist

RAPPELLING

INSTRUCTIONS

As each student completes a skill check, the evaluator notes the date in the evaluator column. If the sudent demonstrates the prescribed level of competence for the skill, the instructor signs his or her initials. If the student fails, the instructor places a "U" (Unsatisfactory). If successful, the student signs his or her initials in the adjacent column to the right.

STUDENT _____

EVALUATOR(S) _____

_____

_____

	First try		Second try	
	EVALUATOR	STUDENT	EVALUATOR	STUDENT
Rappel Using a Figure 8 with Ears, and:				
1. Attach it to harness and rope correctly.				
2. Maintain control during the entire rappel.				
3. Part way down, come to a complete stop.				
4. Lock off the figure 8 descender securely.				
5. Unlock the descender and complete the rappel.				
Rappel Using a Brake Bar Rack, and:				
1. Attach it to harness and rope correctly.				
2. Maintain control during the entire rappel.				
3. Part way down, come to a complete stop.				
4. Lock off the brake bar rack securely.				
5. Unlock the descender and complete the rappel.				

High Angle Skills Checklist

ASCENDING

INSTRUCTIONS

As each student completes a skill check, the evaluator notes the date in the evaluator column. If the sudent demonstrates the prescribed level of competence for the skill, the instructor signs his or her initials. If the student fails, the instructor places a "U" (Unsatisfactory). If successful, the student signs his or her initials in the adjacent column to the right.

STUDENT _____

EVALUATOR(S) _____

_____

_____

	First try		Second try	
	E V A L U A T O R	S T U D E N T	E V A L U A T O R	S T U D E N T
Correctly tie a Prusik hitch onto a fixed rope.				
Ascend a rope safely and efficiently with an ascending system using three ascenders.				
Tie off short while ascending a fixed rope.				
Safely and efficiently change over from ascending to rappelling.				
Safely and efficiently change over from rappelling to ascending.				
Extricate oneself from a simulated jammed rappel device using ascenders.				

High Angle Skills Checklist

RESCUE BELAYING

INSTRUCTIONS

As each student completes a skill check, the evaluator notes the date in the evaluator column. If the sudent demonstrates the prescribed level of competence for the skill, the instructor signs his or her initials. If the student fails, the instructor places a "U" (Unsatisfactory). If successful, the student signs his or her initials in the adjacent column to the right.

STUDENT _____

EVALUATOR(S) _____

_____

_____

	First try		Second try	
	EVALUATOR	STUDENT	EVALUATOR	STUDENT
Correctly tie a load releasing hitch.				
Correctly release a load releasing hitch with a simulated load.				
Correctly rig a tandem Prusik belay system.				
Correctly operate a tandem Prusik belay system.				
Correctly rig a Prusik minding pulley.				
Correctly operate a Prusik minding pulley.				

High Angle Skills Checklist

PICKOFF RESCUE

INSTRUCTIONS

As each student completes a skill check, the evaluator notes the date in the evaluator column. If the sudent demonstrates the prescribed level of competence for the skill, the instructor signs his or her initials. If the student fails, the instructor places a "U" (Unsatisfactory). If successful, the student signs his or her initials in the adjacent column to the right.

STUDENT _____

EVALUATOR(S) _____

_____

_____

	First try		Second try	
	EVALUATOR	STUDENT	EVALUATOR	STUDENT
Safely and efficiently perform a pickoff rescue of a person wearing a seat harness.				
Tie onto a subject either a hasty seat harness, a hasty seat harness with a chest harness, or a hasty body harness.				
Safely and efficiently perform a pickoff rescue of a person wearing a seat harness.				

High Angle Skills Checklist

SLOPE EVACUATION

INSTRUCTIONS
As each student completes a skill check, the evaluator notes the date in the evaluator column. If the sudent demonstrates the prescribed level of competence for the skill, the instructor signs his or her initials. If the student fails, the instructor places a "U" (Unsatisfactory). If successful, the student signs his or her initials in the adjacent column to the right.

STUDENT _____

EVALUATOR(S) _____

_____

	First try		Second try	
	EVALUATOR	STUDENT	EVALUATOR	STUDENT
Repeat from memory the voice communications used in slope evacuation.				
Correctly rig a litter for slope evacuation.				
Package a rescue subject for slope evacuation.				
Correctly rig and anchor a brake system for slope evacuation using a figure 8 with ears.				
Correctly rig and anchor a brake system for slope evacuation using a brake bar rack.				
Correctly rig a tree wrap brake system.				
Correctly rig and anchor a belay system for slope evacuation.				
Correctly rig and anchor a 1:1 (counterbalance) hauling system for slope evacuation.				

High Angle Skills Checklist

HIGH ANGLE LOWERING

INSTRUCTIONS

As each student completes a skill check, the evaluator notes the date in the evaluator column. If the sudent demonstrates the prescribed level of competence for the skill, the instructor signs his or her initials. If the student fails, the instructor places a "U" (Unsatisfactory). If successful, the student signs his or her initials in the adjacent column to the right.

STUDENT _____

EVALUATOR(S) _____

_____

_____

	First try		Second try	
	EVALUATOR	STUDENT	EVALUATOR	STUDENT
Repeat from memory the voice communications used in high angle lowering.				
Correctly rig a litter for high angle lowering.				
Package a rescue subject for high angle lowering.				
Using a Litter Rigged and with a Simulated Rescue Load:				
1. Correctly anchor a brake bar rack for lowering.				
2. Correctly attach the litter to lowering rope.				
3. Correctly rig and anchor a belay for litter.				
4. Correctly lace lowering rope to brake bar rack.				
5. Correctly lower litter with simulated load, stop lowering, bring rack to full stop, tie off rack, then unlock rack to continue lower.				
6. Correctly belay a simulated rescue load during a lowering.				
7. Perform a knot pass during a simulated lowering.				

High Angle Skills Checklist

HAULING

INSTRUCTIONS

As each student completes a skill check, the evaluator notes the date in the evaluator column. If the sudent demonstrates the prescribed level of competence for the skill, the instructor signs his or her initials. If the student fails, the instructor places a "U" (Unsatisfactory). If successful, the student signs his or her initials in the adjacent column to the right.

STUDENT _____

EVALUATOR(S) _____

_____

_____

	First try		Second try	
	EVALUATOR	STUDENT	EVALUATOR	STUDENT
Repeat from memory the voice communications used in rescue hauling.				
Using a Simulated Rescue Load, Rig the Following with Appropriate Anchors, Pulley Placement, Haul Cams, and Progress Capture Device:				
1. A 1:1 haul system.				
2. A 2:1 haul system.				
3. A 3:1 haul system ("Z-Rig").				
4. A 4:1 haul "piggy-back" system.				

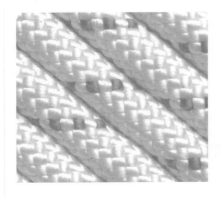

Appendix C: Assembling Your Brake Bar Rack*

COLE-STYLE RACKS

The following information is for assembling bars on the Cole-style rack (see Chapter 9, Rappelling). Be certain you also read and follow the manufacturer's instructions.

If possible, inspect the rack frame before purchase. Check it closely for any dents or cuts. Visualize frame alignment by holding it at eye level and sighting it both down the long axis and across the short axis. Check that both sides of the frame are parallel and in the same plane. A frame that is seriously out of alignment will interfere with smooth operation of the bars. If the frame is seriously misaligned, return it to the dealer for exchange.

After inspecting the rack, you are ready to assemble the bars on the rack. Now take the locking nut off the short leg of the rack.

You should make some basic decisions before finishing assembly of your rack.

The Position of the Rack on Your Seat Harness

The best position for rappelling is to attach the rack to your harness so the frame is in a vertical plane with the shorter leg on the bottom (Figure C-1). This is the best position for adding or subtracting bars or switching the rope to a different position.

With the short leg at the bottom, the open end of the frame will also be at the bottom. This means that you can keep your control hand close in front of you and easily move the rope from one side to the other. If the short end were at the top, you would have to move the rope over your head each time you add or subtract bars. This is not only annoying but also makes it more difficult to maintain control of the rope.

As mentioned before, for the rack to lie in the proper plane, it must match your seat harness front

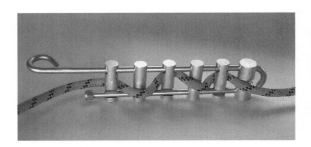

FIGURE C-1
The best position for rappelling with the rack is with the frame in a vertical plane and the shorter leg on the bottom.

attachment and carabiner. If the seat harness attachment is in a horizontal plane, such as the **D** ring on many rescue harnesses, then the seat harness carabiner will be in a vertical plane. This means that the rack should have a 90-degree offset eye. If the seat harness attachment is in a vertical plane, such as the tie-in loop on many climbing harnesses, the seat harness carabiner will be in a horizontal plane. This means the rack should have a straight eye.

Placement of the Bars on the Rack

You can thread the eyes of the brake bars either on the long or short leg of the rack frame (Figure C-2), but most users prefer them on the long side. On the longer side, you can better get disengaged bars out of your way by sliding them down the frame toward the eye.

Number of Bars to Place on Rack

For most people, it is best to install six bars on the frame. Even if you normally use less than six bars, you may encounter a situation that requires all six. You might, for example, be rappelling with extra equipment, need more control on a slicker rope, or do a pickoff rescue.

*The following Appendix is excerpted from Vines T, Hudson S: *A guide to the brake bar rack,* 1998. Portions of this paper have appeared in other publications.

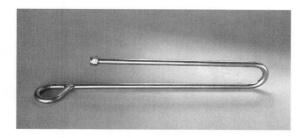

FIGURE C-2
Most users prefer to thread on the long leg of the rack frame.

Don't assume that short rappels mean fewer bars. You actually need just as many bars on a short drop as on the bottom part of a longer drop. It is only at the top of long drops that you use fewer bars. But then as you reach the bottom of the rope, you will probably need to engage all six bars.

Control Hand

Whether you use your right or left hand for control will decide how you place the bottom bar on the rack. Set up bars on the rack so that the control end of the rope exits the rack on the front of the bottom bar with all of the bars engaged. This means that you can use maximum friction advantage from all six bars.

ASSEMBLING THE BARS ON THE RACK

If, as most prefer, you plan to use the rack with the brake bar eyes attached to the long side, slide the lowest bar (the closest to the eye) on first see (Figure C-3).

Place the hole of this bar on the short leg and slide it around the top bend, down the long leg, and into position. Clip this bottom bar into the short leg to make certain you have threaded it correctly. With your harness on, and carabiner attached, clip the rack eye into the carabiner. Now visualize the rope coming across the bar to your control hand.

If it follows Figure C-1, then you have correctly threaded the bottom bar on the rack. If it does not conform to the figure, take the bar off, reverse it and thread it back on again. Thread the remaining bars on the rack.

Each of the remaining bars must be placed to face alternating directions. If you are using a large 1-inch aluminum top bar, place it on last by threading it on the short leg (Figure C-4). It has a smaller die hole, so it will not pass around the bend at the top of the rack like smaller bars.

After placing all bars on the rack, make sure they slide freely on the frame and that each bar clips in correctly. Replace the locking nut by screwing it on until it is finger tight. Finally, with a wrench, tighten it further one full turn.

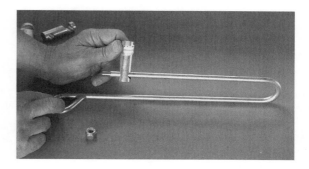

FIGURE C-3
Slide the lowest bar on the frame first.

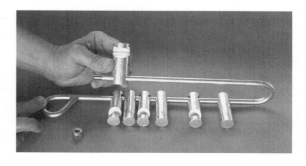

FIGURE C-4
Place the large top bar on last and on the short leg.

BRAKE BAR CONFIGURATIONS

There are some basic brake bar combinations and configurations you can use on your brake bar rack:

A. All Aluminum Set (Figure C-5)
   1-Top bar: Extra large aluminum bar with center groove.
   1-Second bar: ¾ in angled slot bar with center groove.
   4-Third through sixth bars: Angle slot bar.

B. Stainless Set #1 (Figure C-6)
   1-Top bar: ⅞ inch solid stainless steel top bar.
   2-Second through third bars: U-shaped slot bars from sheet steel with training groove.
   3-Fourth through sixth bars: U-shaped slot brake bars from sheet steel without training groove.

C. Stainless Set #2
   1-Top bar: U-shaped slot brake bars of stainless steel without training groove.
   2-Second and third bars: U-shaped slot brake bars from sheet steel with training groove.
   3-Fourth through sixth bars: U-shaped slot brake bars from sheet steel without training groove.

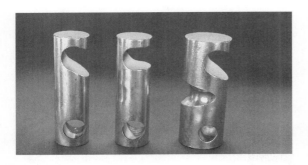

FIGURE C-5
Types of aluminum brake bars.

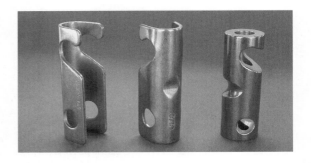

FIGURE C-6
Types of stainless steel brake bars.

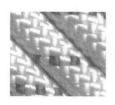

Glossary

A

Abrasion The damaging wear on rope and other software caused by their rubbing against a rough surface. *(Chapter 3)*

Anchor (1) A secure tie-in point for attaching a line (n) and (2) The act of attaching a line to an anchor (v). *(Chapter 7)*

Anchor Point A single secure connection for an anchor. An anchor point is used either alone or in combination with other anchor points to create an anchor system capable of sustaining the load on a rope rescue system. *(Chapter 7)*

Anchor System One or more anchor points rigged to provide a structurally significant connection for elements of a rope rescue system. *(Chapter 7)*

ANSI The American National Standards Institute, an organization that develops standards for equipment. *(Appendix A)*

Antitorque The use of a helicopter tail rotor to prevent the aircraft from spinning out of control. *(Chapter 17)*

Arm Rappel (Guide's Rappel) A type of rappel in which the rope wraps around both outstretched arms and across the person's back. The technique is better suited for sloping terrain than for vertical situations. *(Chapter 9)*

Artificial Anchors The use of specifically designed hardware to create anchors where insufficient natural anchors exist. *(Chapter 7)*

Ascenders Rope grab devices used by individuals to ascend a fixed rope or, with specific types of ascenders, used in the creation of hauling systems. There are basically two categories of ascenders: (1) *personal ascenders,* which are normally used for no more than one person's body weight and (2) *general-use ascenders,* which are used both as personal ascenders and in hauling systems for progress capture devices and as rope grabs. Ascenders are also called *ascent devices.* *(Chapters 5, 10)*

Ascending A means of traveling up a fixed rope with the use of either mechanical devices or friction hitches attached with slings to the user's body. *(Chapter 10)*

Ascender Sling Attachments of webbing or rope that connect a person to his or her ascenders. *(Chapter 10)*

ASTM An international organization that uses the full consensus method for setting standards. *(Chapter 2)*

Auxiliary Tender A person who rappels alongside the litter as it is being lowered in order to assist in the rescue. Duties may include medical assessment and/or primary treatment of the rescue subject, assistance in getting the litter over the edge, assistance in handling the litter on the vertical face, and assistance in loading the subject into the litter. *(Chapter 15)*

B

Backing Up A secondary or redundant system designed to provide added security. The creation of an additional independent anchor, or anchors, to sustain the high angle system should initial anchors fail. Backing up may be to the same anchor system if it is very solid or to additional anchor points. *(Chapter 15)*

Back Tie Connector from a primary anchor to a second anchor that backs up the primary anchor. *(Chapter 7)*

Back-Up Knot A second knot tied to make the first knot more secure. Also known as a *safety* or *keeper knot. (Chapter 6)*

Belay To protect against a fall by managing an unloaded rope (the belay rope) in a way that secures a person or persons from falling in case their main line rope or support fails. *(Chapters 5, 8)*

Belayer The person who performs the belay. *(Chapters 1, 8)*

Belay Device A braking mechanism through which the belay rope is run. The belayer controls the device so that should the main line or support fail, the device holds the rope and secures person or persons on belay from falling. *(Chapter 8)*

Belay Line The line attached to person or persons, which provides protection against a fall or system failure. *(Chapter 8)*

Belay Plate A simple metal plate containing one or more slots for rope and used to create rope friction with a carabiner. It is commonly used in belaying. *(Chapters 5, 8)*

Bend A class of knot that joins two rope or webbing pieces together. *(Chapter 6)*

Bight The open loop in a rope formed when it is doubled back on itself. *(Chapter 6)*

Body Rappel (Dulfersitz Rappel) A type of rappel that uses the body as friction by running the rope between the legs, across one hip, over the opposite shoulder, and to a braking hand. Because of the discomfort involved, and potential damage to body parts, the technique has largely been supplanted by other techniques. *(Chapter 9)*

Bolts Metal devices used to create permanent anchors on a rock surface by drilling a hole in the rock and setting the device in the hole. Most bolts have a mechanical means for expanding to jam themselves in the drilled hole. A *hanger* is usually attached to the bolt so that the bolt can be used as an anchor point. *(Chapter 5)*

Bombproof Jargon for an anchor or anchor system believed to be very secure. *(Chapter 7)*

Brake Bar Rack A descending device consisting of a U-shaped metal bar to which are attached several metal bars that create friction on the rope. Some "racks" are restricted to use for personal rappelling, while others may also be used for rescue lowering. Also commonly known as a *rappel rack. (Chapters 5, 9)*

Brake Hand The hand, usually the dominant one, that grasps the rope to help control the speed of descent during a rappel. *(Chapter 9)*

Brakeman Person who operates the braking device that controls the rate of descent of the load in a rescue lowering. *(Chapters 14, 15)*

Bridle See *Spider. (Chapter 15)*

C

Cams Devices used in climbing for protection or in anchoring, which lodge in a rock crack. There are "active" cams with springs to help adjust to the width of the crack and there are also "passive" cams (nuts, stoppers, and chocks) that wedge to fit the crack. *(Chapter 5)*

Carabiner A metal connector with a gate that swings open to allow rope, webbing, or climbing hardware to be inserted. The gate may be locking or nonlocking. Carabiners are used to link elements of a high angle system. It is sometimes spelled *karabiner* (outside of the United States) and is also known as *'biners* or *crabs. (Chapters 1, 5)*

Carabiner Wrap A braking technique that uses several rope wraps around a carabiner to create friction and control the descent. It is generally not considered a safe and secure technique for rappelling. *(Chapter 9)*

CE The European Union standards setting authority (European Committee for Standardization). Standards cover a wide range of products including ones for recreational climbing, industrial fall production, and rope access. *(Chapter 2)*

Center of Gravity (COG) The point where a helicopter is in balance. The center of gravity can be visualized by drawing an imaginary line from the center of the main rotor to the bottom of the aircraft. *(Chapter 17)*

Changeover To transfer from an ascending mode to a rappelling mode or from a rappelling mode to an ascending mode. *(Chapter 10)*

Chest Harness A type of harness worn around the chest for upper body support. In the high angle environment, it should never be used as the only source of support but should always be used in combination with a seat harness. *(Chapter 2)*

Chicken Loop A safety loop that fits around the ankle to secure the ascender sling and prevent the foot from slipping out of the sling should an upper connection fail and the person ascending falls over backwards. *(Chapter 10)*

Collective The mutual effect of changing pitch on helicopter rotor blades to create more or less lift. The collective is managed from a control to the pilot's left. *(Chapter 17)*

Counter Balance Hauling System A procedure for hauling that uses a 1:1 ratio and a haul team that moves in a direction opposite to the load. *(Chapter 14)*

Cyclic The control of helicopter direction of flight by changing the tilt of the main rotor. *(Chapter 17)*

D

Danger Zone The area around a helicopter where there are physical hazards or the pilot's view is restricted. *(Chapter 17)*

Density Altitude Pressure (barometric) altitude corrected for temperature and humidity. Density altitude has a profound effect on the helicopter lift and performance. *(Chapter 17)*

Descenders Metal devices that, when attached to a rappeller, create friction with the rope for a controlled rappel. Some descenders can be attached to an anchor for a controlled lowering. *(Chapters 5, 9)*

Directional A technique for repositioning a rope at a more favorable angle that would exist using only its anchor. *(Chapter 7)*

Double Line Lowering The use of two ropes attached to the litter in a lowering rigged so that they may be operated independently to change the angle of the litter. Also called *scaffold lowering. (Chapter 15)*

Dulfersitz See *Body Rappel. (Chapter 9)*

Dynamic Rope A type of rope designed for high stretch to reduce the shock on the climber and anchor system. Usually employed in systems where a high fall factor is likely. *(Chapter 3)*

E

Edge Rollers In-line, free-turning rollers that are anchored at an edge of a cliff or building to reduce rope friction. *(Chapter 5)*

Edge Tender A person connected to a safety attachment who works at the edge of a drop in a high angle lowering. Duties include assisting in getting the litter over the edge, reducing edge abrasion to the rope, and, when necessary, relaying communications between the litter tender and the brakeman. *(Chapter 15)*

Emergency Seat Harness A temporary, tied harness to be used when a manufactured, sewn seat harness is not available. *(Chapter 2)*

F

Fall Factor A calculation used to estimate the impact force on a rope when it is subjected to stopping a falling mass. It is expressed as a number to indicate the relation between rope length able to absorb energy and the distance the person falls. *(Chapter 3)*

Figure 8 Descender A device used for rappelling and, in some cases, for lowering. It is in the general shape of an 8, with a large ring to create friction on the rope and a smaller ring for attaching to a seat harness. *(Chapters 5, 9)*

Foundation Knot A simple knot that is tied as the first step in tying a more complicated knot. Examples of foundation knots include the overhand and the simple figure **8**. *(Chapter 6)*

Full Body Harness A type of harness that offers both pelvic and upper body support as one unit. *(Chapter 2)*

G

General-Use Ascenders Mechanical rope grab devices without handles that operate primarily by the force of a cam action wedging the rope against the inside of their shell. They are designed to slide in one direction on a rope and are used for both personal ascenders and for progress capture devices. *(Chapters 5, 10)*

Ground Effect The condition that occurs when a helicopter hovers close enough to the ground to compress air below itself. The result is increased lift and decreased power requirements for the helicopter, and often means the aircraft can hover in a more stable manner. When a helicopter achieves this effect, it is said to be *hovering in ground effect* (HIGE). *(Chapter 17)*

Guide Hand The hand, usually not the dominant one, that cradles the rope to help in balancing the rappeller. *(Chapter 9)*

H

Handled Ascenders Ascenders with frames large enough to accommodate built-in handles that can be comfortably gripped with the hands. Most handled ascenders have toothed cams that grip the rope. *(Chapters 5, 10)*

Haul Cam A cam ascender (or Prusik knot) that grips the rope to provide the "bite" in hauling. *(Chapter 16)*

Haul Team The group of persons who provide the power to raise the load. *(Chapter 14)*

Helmet Head covering that protects against head injury both from falling objects and from head impact. "Helmet," when used in this book, indicates head protection specifically designed for high angle work. *(Chapter 2)*

High Angle The environment in which one must be secured with rope and other equipment to keep from falling. *(Chapter 1)*

Highline A system using a rope suspended from between two points to move persons or equipment over an area that is a barrier to the rescue operation. *(Chapter 10)*

Hitch A knot that attaches to or wraps around an object or rope in such a way that when the object or rope the hitch is attached to is removed, the knot will fall apart. *(Chapter 10)*

Hoisting Vest ("Screamer Suit") A one-person rescue device made of fabric that wraps around a person's torso like a large diaper. It is connected to a line that hauls a person in operations such as helicopter rescue. *(Chapter 17)*

Hot Loading and Unloading A condition where the pilot keeps the rotor turning during loading or unloading of the aircraft. *(Chapter 17)*

Horse Collar A one-person rescue device usually used in helicopter rescue. It is connected to a line that hauls a person in operations such as helicopter rescue. *(Chapter 17)*

Hover A condition in which an airborne helicopter is maintained in a near motionless position. *(Chapter 17)*

I

Incident Command System (ICS) A standardized emergency management system developed to organize and manage all functions needed to deal with an emergency rescue. *(Chapter 11)*

J

Jungle Penetrator A metal device with a tapered end and arms that swing down on which one or two persons can ride. It is connected to a line that is hauled in operations such as helicopter rescue. *(Chapter 17)*

K

Kernmantle A rope design consisting of two elements: (1) an interior core (kern) that supports the major portion of the load on the rope and (2) an outer sheath (mantle) that serves primarily to protect the core and also supports a minor portion of the load. *(Chapter 3)*

Kevlar Trade name for a type of Aramid fiber manufactured by the Dupont Corporation and which has high tensile strength, low elongation, and high resistance to heat. *(Chapter 3)*

Knot A fastening made by tying together rope or webbing in a prescribed way. Knots include bights, bends, and hitches. *(Chapter 6)*

L

Laid Rope A rope design that consists of fiber bundles twisted around one another. *(Chapter 3)*

Litter Captain The person in slope evacuation who manages the litter team and coordinates the litter movement with other members of the rescue team. *(Chapter 13)*

Litter Attendant An individual who helps control the litter or attends to a patient's medical needs during a slope evacuation rescue. Also known as *litter tender*. *(Chapter 14)*

Litter Tender See *Litter Attendant*. *(Chapter 14)*

Load The total combined objects and persons being lowered or raised by a rope in a high angle system. Some examples include a rescue subject, a rescuer, and a subject in a litter with one or two attached litter tenders. *(Chapter 15)*

Load Releasing Hitch (LR Hitch) Any hitch that can sustain major forces without tightening and which, with the tension still on it, can be untied and released under control. Among these are the mariner's hitch, which uses webbing, and the LR hitch that uses accessory cord. *(Chapter 12)*

Load Distributing Anchor System (LDA) An anchor system established from two or more anchor points that: (1) maintains near equal loading on the anchor points despite direction changes on the main line rope and (2) reestablishes near equal loading on remaining anchor points should one or more of them fail. Sometimes referred to as *self-equalizing anchor. (Chapter 7)*

Load Sharing Anchor An anchor system established from two or more anchor points that distributes the load among the anchor points but does not adjust to direction changes on the main line. *(Chapter 7)*

Locking Carabiner A carabiner with a locking sleeve on its gate side that secures the gate shut. *(Chapter 5)*

Locking Off The technique of jamming a rope into a descender or tying off securely so that the rappeller can stop the descent or lowering and operate hands free of the rope. *(Chapter 9)*

Lowering The controlled descent of persons and equipment using rope through a lowering device. A lowering rope goes one way: down. A lowering rope has weight on it throughout the lowering operation. *(Chapter 8)*

Low Stretch Rope A type of rope designed to be used in applications such as rescue, rappelling, and ascending where high stretch would be a disadvantage and where no falls, or very short falls, are expected before being caught by the rope. The term *low stretch rope* can refer to ropes with slightly more elongation than the traditional *static ropes* or to both types of ropes. *(Chapters 3, 4)*

M

Manner of Function The method in which a particular piece of equipment was designed to be used. *(Chapter 5)*

Master Attachment Point The point at which rigging comes together for maximum strength. *(Chapters 7, 15)*

Mechanical Advantage The relationship of how much load can be moved to the amount of force it takes to move it. *(Chapter 16)*

Mechanical Ascenders Rope grab devices used by individuals to ascend a fixed rope or, with specific types of ascenders, used in the creation of hauling systems. There are two categories of ascenders: (1) personal ascenders, which are normally used for no more than one person's body weight and (2) general-use ascenders, which are used both as personal ascenders and for progress capture devices. *(Chapters 5, 10)*

Mountaineering The use of skills such as climbing, snow and ice travel, and camping to ascend a mountain. *(Chapter 1)*

Multipitch More than one rope length (normally measured in climbing rope lengths). *(Chapter 7)*

Multipoint Anchor Anchors involving two or more anchor points. *(Chapter 7)*

Munter Hitch A type of running knot that slips around a carabiner to create friction against itself. It is commonly used in belaying. *(Chapter 8)*

Munter Hitch Rappel A limited-use rappel technique using a Munter hitch attached to the seat harness carabiner. *(Chapter 9)*

N

NFPA National Fire Protection Association. A national organization that sets standards for rope and related equipment, along with performance standards for rope rescuers in the fire service. *(Chapter 2)*

Nonlocking Carabiners A carabiner without a means of securing its gate shut. *(Chapter 5)*

Nylon 6 A type of nylon used in rope manufacturing. One trade name for this type is *Perlon.* Type 6 nylon is commonly found in climbing ropes. *(Chapter 3)*

Nylon 6, 6 A type of nylon used in rope manufacturing. In North America it is manufactured by Dupont and Monsanto. Type 6, 6 nylon is commonly found in static kernmantle ropes. *(Chapter 3)*

O

One-Skid Landing A condition where a helicopter touches the portion of one skid to the ground to load or unload personnel. It is done where the terrain is unsuitable for a full landing. Also known as a *toe-in. (Chapter 17)*

1:1 Hauling System A procedure for hauling where the force needed to haul is roughly the same as the load being hauled (that is, without mechanical advantage). *(Chapter 14)*

P

Packaging The placing of a rescue subject in a litter so that the primary medical considerations are cared for and the subject is physically stabilized in the litter. *(Chapter 14)*

Pendulum To swing on a rope. *(Chapter 7)*

Perlon A trade name for one type of nylon, type 6. *(Chapter 3)*

Personal Ascenders Mechanical rope grab devices used to travel up ("ascend") a fixed rope. They are normally used for no more than one person's body weight. *(Chapters 5, 10)*

Pickoff Rescue A rescue in the high angle environment involving an uninjured or slightly injured subject in which a single rescuer usually has direct physical contact, and in which a litter is not initially used in the rescue operation. (One person rescuing another person from a perilous high angle situation.) *(Chapter 13)*

Pigtail A short piece of rope with which the litter tender is attached to the litter system. *(Chapter 15)*

Piggyback System ("Pig-Rig") A pulley system in which one hauling system pulls (or "piggybacks") on another hauling system. The term is often used for a specific type of 4:1 hauling system in which one 2:1 system is attached to ("piggybacked onto") another 2:1 system to create a 4:1 system. *(Chapter 16)*

Pitch One rope length. *(Chapter 7)*

Piton A slender metal wedge, with an eye for attachment, that is driven into a rock crack for climbing protection or for anchoring. *(Chapter 5)*

Polyester A type of fiber used in some rope manufacturing. Also known by the trade name *Dacron*. *(Chapter 3)*

Polyolefins A group of fiber types used in manufacturing ropes that are often used in water applications. In this group are polypropylene and polyethylene. *(Chapter 3)*

Progress Capture Device (PCD) A rope grab device, general-use ascender, or hitch placed on the rope in a hauling system to prevent the rope (and load) from unintentionally slipping back down as the haul system is reset. The PCD is also commonly referred to as the *ratchet. (Chapter 14)*

Prusik A type of friction hitch used in ascending and belaying. It has also come to be used by some individuals as a term synonymous with *ascending*, even when mechanical devices are used (that is, "to Prusik"). *(Chapters 5, 10)*

Prusik Loop A continuous loop of rope from which a Prusik hitch is tied. *(Chapter 10)*

Prusik Minding Pulley A pulley with specially shaped sideplates that helps manage Prusiks during a haul or belay. *(Chapter 12)*

Pulley A device with a free-turning, grooved metal wheel (sheave) used to reduce rope friction, and which has side plates to which a carabiner may be attached. *(Chapter 5)*

R

Rappel Rack See *Brake Bar Rack. (Chapters 5, 9)*

Rappelling The controlled descent on a rope using the friction of the rope against one's body or through a descender. *(Chapters 1, 9)*

Rock Climbing Ascending while making direct contact with the rock and commonly using rope and other equipment for safety should one fall. *(Chapter 1)*

Rope Grab Devices that grip the rope. There are two types: (1) mechanical rope grabs, usually made of metal, which grip the rope with a camming action and (2) rope or webbing rope grabs that use a hitch to grip the rope. *(Chapter 5)*

Rope Handler The person in a litter lowering operation who assists the brakeman with rope management. *(Chapter 14)*

Rope Rescue The performing of rescue in a high angle environment where the use of rope and related equipment is necessary. *(Chapter 1)*

Rope Rescue Technician One trained and competent in the necessary skills for rope rescue. *(Chapter 11)*

S

Safety Belt A belt-like harness worn around the waist to prevent falls from elevated positions. It should never be used as a sole means of suspension. *(Chapter 2)*

Safety Factor The ratio between the maximum load expected on a rope, equipment or system and the rope, equipment or system's breaking strength. The larger the ratio, the greater the safety factor. *(Chapter 3)*

Safety Knot See *Back-Up Knot. (Chapter 6)*

Safety Officer The individual responsible for monitoring hazardous conditions for rescuers and others. *(Chapter 11)*

Seat Harness A system of nylon or polyester webbing that wraps and supports the pelvic region to attach the wearer to the rope or other protection in the high angle environment. *(Chapter 2)*

Self-Equalizing Anchor See *Load Distributing Anchor. (Chapter 7)*

Short Haul A helicopter extrication technique in which a person, or persons, are connected to a rope attached to a helicopter and the aircraft lifts off with a person or persons carried below it. *(Chapter 17)*

Single-Line Lowering The use of one main lowering rope with a belay in litter lowering. *(Chapter 15)*

Single Rope Techniques (SRT) Ascending and descending directly on the rope without direct aid by contact with the rock. *(Chapter 3)*

Single Strand Lowering The use of one main lowering rope in litter lowering. *(Chapter 5)*

Slope Evacuation The movement of a rescue subject over terrain so rugged or angled that it requires the litter to be attached to a rope for safety and control. In slope evacuation, most of the weight is taken by the litter tenders. Slope evacuation is also known as *low angle evacuation. (Chapter 14)*

Software A category of high angle equipment that is not hardware. In this category are rope and webbing. *(Chapter 3)*

Span of Control The optimum number of rescuers that can be effectively supervised by the person in charge during a rescue operation. *(Chapter 11)*

Spectra Trade name for a high modulus polyethylene fiber with high tensile strength. *(Chapter 3)*

Spider The system of attaching a lowering rope to a litter. A spider usually has four or more legs that connect to various points of a litter to equalize loading. *(Chapter 15)*

Static Rope A type of rope designed to be used in applications such as rescue, rappelling, and ascending where high stretch would be a disadvantage and where no falls, or very short falls, are expected before being caught by the rope. Static ropes have slightly less elongation than low stretch ropes built to the same standard. Less elongation prevents loss of system efficiency due to rope stretch. *(Chapter 3)*

Stopper Knot A knot that helps provide security in rope work. Examples would be a simple figure **8** tied in the bottom end of a rope to prevent a person from rappelling off the end or tied in an end of the rope to prevent it from accidentally slipping through equipment. *(Chapter 6)*

Subject The person who is being rescued. Also called the *victim. (Chapter 11)*

System The combination of various components used in the high angle environment to construct a functioning unit. For example, lowering or anchor system. *(Chapter 1)*

T

Tag Line (1) The line that is attached to a load on a highline and is used to control the load from the far-side point. *(Chapter 16)*

Tag Line (2) A line attached to a load that can be used to maneuver the load and prevent it from snagging and to hold it away from a vertical face. *(Chapter 16)*

Tandem Prusik Belay Two triple wrap Prusik hitches, of differing lengths, set a few inches apart in series on a belay rope in order to grab the rope in case of main line failure or to hold the load while adjusting the lowering and raising system. *(Chapter 12)*

Technical Rescue The use of special knowledge, skills, and equipment to safely perform a rescue. Rope rescue is sometimes called *technical rescue. (Chapter 11)*

Tensile Strength A measurement of the greatest lengthwise stress that a rope or piece of equipment can resist without failure. *(Chapter 3)*

Theoretical Mechanical Advantage (TMA) Mechanical advantage without allowance for friction and other losses of advantage. *(Chapter 16)*

Traveling Pulley A moving pulley that is attached to a load or to a haul cam and which adds to the mechanical advantage. *(Chapter 16)*

Tree Wrap A technique of running a rope around a tree trunk to create friction for a braking effect in a litter lowering. *(Chapter 14)*

Tying Off Short A safety technique that creates an extra point of attachment during ascending by tying the person directly into the main line rope. *(Chapter 10)*

Tyrolean Another name for a highline. *(Chapter 10)*

U

UIAA The Union of International Alpine Associations. Among its activities, the organization sets performance standards for ropes, harnesses, ice axes, helmets, and carabiners to be used by climbers and mountaineers. *(Chapter 2)*

V

Vertical Caving The travel through caves that have vertical, or near vertical, sections that require the use of rope and ascending and descending equipment. *(Chapter 1)*

Z

Z-Rig Common name given to a specific type of 3:1 hauling system. The name is taken from the general shape that the rope makes as it runs through the system. *(Chapter 16)*

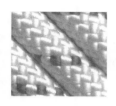

Answer Key

Chapter 1

1. A
2. B
3. D
4. C
5. A
6. A

Chapter 2

1. C
2. D
3. B
4. D
5. C
6. D
7. A
8. C
9. B
10. A
11. C
12. A
13. D

Chapter 3

1. B
2. A
3. C
4. D
5. A
6. C
7. B
8. A
9. D
10. A
11. B
12. C
13. B
14. D
15. D

Chapter 4

1. D
2. D
3. A
4. D
5. B
6. C
7. A

8. A
9. D
10. B

Chapter 5

1. C
2. B
3. A
4. D
5. B
6. D
7. A
8. C
9. C
10. B
11. A
12. D
13. A
14. B
15. C
16. D

Chapter 6

1. D
2. C
3. a) Overhand knot. Either of the following: (1) as a "foundation knot" for beginning other knots or (2) as a backup to secure other knots.
   b) Simple figure 8. Either of the following: (1) as a stopper knot for certain types of security, such as tied in the bottom end of a rope to prevent rappelling off the end, or tied in the top of rope to prevent it from accidentally slipping through equipment or (2) as a foundation knot for beginning the figure 8 follow through or the figure 8 bend.
   c) Figure 8 on a bight. To create a secure loop in a rope for connecting to any of the following: (1) safety lines, (2) persons being lowered, (3) rescue equipment such as a litter, or (4) anchor line.
   d) Figure 8 follow through. To create a loop at the end of a rope where a figure 8 on a bight cannot be tied, such as anchoring to an object you cannot get a loop over.
   e) Figure 8 bend. For joining two rope ends, such as: (1) connecting two pieces of rope or (2) creating a loop of rope by joining both ends of one rope.

f) Ring bend ("water knot"). For joining two ends of webbing, such as: (1) joining two pieces of webbing to form a longer piece or (2) tying the two ends of one piece of webbing to form a loop.

g) Double overhand backup knot. For backing up other knots.

h) Grapevine ("double fisherman's") knot. For joining two rope ends, such as: (1) connecting two pieces of rope or (2) creating a loop of rope by joining both ends of one rope.

Chapter 7

1. (1) Condition of anchor. (2) Structural nature of the anchor point. (3) Location of force on anchor point.

2. (1) Conditions where rocks or other dangerous objects might fall on the rescue subject or on the rescuers. (2) Where there are conditions between the anchor point and the rescue subject that could endanger rescuers or damage equipment such as rope. (3) Where there are no suitable anchors directly above.

3. To bring a rope into a more favorable position or angle.

4. It reduces your flexibility and limits your ability to make modifications in the anchor system.

5. (1) It is simple. (2) It reduces stress on rope and equipment. (3) It gives the flexibility to deal with changing conditions.

6. Root system.

7. (1) You may not know who tied the knot and what *kind* of knot it is. (2) Knots in webbing may eventually work their way out. (3) In webbing that has been shock loaded, the knots may have been spot-welded.

8. Tie an interior loop in the webbing using a "wrap 2, pull 1" or a "wrap 3, pull 2" technique.

9. Any of the following: Corroded metals, weathered stonework, deteriorated mortar in brickwork, vents constructed of sheet metal, flashing, gutters and downspouts, and brickwork without bulk, such as small chimneys or fire hydrants.

10. Any of the following: Structural columns, projections of structural beams, supports for large machinery, stairwell support beams, or brickwork with large bulk, such as corner walls.

11. a) Bumpers and tow hooks.
    b) Axles and cross members.

12. (1) When one anchor point is insufficient to withstand the anticipated forces or (2) when one anchor point is inconveniently placed.

13. 90 degrees.
    120 degrees.

14. Two of the following: (1) Try to keep anchor points close to one another. (2) Keep outside angle to less than 90 degrees, even better, limit angles to 60 degrees. (3) Rig load-distributing anchors with a minimum of slack in the system.

Chapter 8

1. (1) A person at risk of falling, (2) the rope attached to the person, (3) a harness worn by the person and attached to the rope, (4) a belay device, (5) the belayer, and (6) an anchor the belay device is attached to.

2. Any six of the following: (1) When a person is rock climbing or mountaineering. (2) In a rescue situation where there is danger of falling. (3) When a person is crossing an area not generally dangerous, but there is a small area of exposure. (4) When persons are unsure of themselves in attempting a new skill, such as rappelling for the first time. (5) When a person's physical or mental capabilities are diminished. (6) When environmental factors, such as potential rock falls or areas slick with ice, increase the danger of falling. (7) When one or more persons are being lowered by rope, such as in a rescue. (8) When one or more persons are being raised by rope, such as in a rescue.

3. (a) A belay is a safety to catch persons should they fall. A lowering is the controlled lowering of persons and equipment using rope through a lowering device/hardware.

   (b) A belay rope can be run either way (up or down) and does not have weight on it unless there is a fall on it. A lowering rope goes one way: down, and has weight on it throughout the lowering operation.

   (c) A one-person belay uses specialized equipment such as a personal belay device or special knots such as the Munter hitch. A lowering uses a friction device such as the large ring of a Figure 8 descender or a brake bar rack.

4.

Climber	Belayer
(1) "On belay?"	
(2)	"Belay on."
(3) "Climbing." (or: "Rappelling.")	
(4)	"Climb." (or "Rappel.")

Once placed where the climber no longer needs the belay, then the climber initiates an exchange to end the belay:

(5) "Off belay."	
(6)	"Belay off."

5. (1) The slot in the figure 8 may not be the correct size for the rope you are using. (2) Some figure 8s have slots that are not well designed for use as a belay plate. (3) A figure 8 is not as well balanced as some devices and may not be as easy to use.

6. When a top belay is not available.

Chapter 9

1. Any five of the following: (1) Being able to control the descent with minimum physical effort. (2) The rope is not damaged by heat buildup in the rappel device. (3) Anchors are not damaged by shock loading. (4) Being able to stop the rappel any time. (5) Being able to tie off securely and operate hands free of the rope and rappel device. (6) Being able to operate in any body position including upside down.
2. They both use friction of the rope on the body to slow the descent.
3. Brake.
4. Guide.
5. Short, low-angle slopes.
6. (1) The rope could become unwrapped from the leg possibly resulting in free fall to the ground. (2) Rope abrasion and pressure can injure body parts, particularly the crotch and shoulder.
7. Any two of the following: (1) You cannot use the smaller version with larger diameter rope. (2) You may find it difficult to use the smaller figure 8 descender "double wrapped." (3) It is possible for the rope wraps to slip up and around the larger ring to form a girth hitch.
8. Set an ascender or Prusik loop on the rope above the figure 8 and step into an attached sling.
9. Use a figure 8 with ears.
10. Keep the rope on the side of the descender away from the edge.
11. To prevent tangling and prevent damage to the rope from heat fusion as a result of rope cross.
12. If the main line rappel anchor failed, but the belay caught, there would be a possibility of a pendulum fall.
13. (1) Keep your body generally perpendicular to the slope. (2) Keep your feet apart, about the width of your shoulders. (3) Keep your knees relaxed and slightly flexed. (4) Take slow and deliberate steps backwards. (5) Keep your body slightly turned in the direction of the brake hand, looking down slope to select a path of travel. (6) Use your guide hand for balance. Do not support your weight with the guide hand. (7) Never take the brake hand off the rope unless the belay device is securely locked off.
14. Double wrapping the device.
15. The rope may run across seat harness webbing and damage it.
16. The preferred stance is on both feet (or alternatively, on both knees).
17. Generally, the most difficult is a horizontal angle (the anchor on the same level or lower than the rappeller), while the easiest is a vertical angle (the anchor above the rappeller).
18. The descender may become jammed and you will be stranded in a precarious position.
19. *Advantages:*
    (1) It offers greater friction; therefore greater control than most descenders. (2) It provides the ability to change friction once you have begun to rappel. (3) Its variable friction provides the ability to more comfortably rappel longer drops than most descenders.
    Disadvantages:
    (1) The brake bar rack is somewhat more complex than descenders such as the figure 8. (2) It takes a bit longer to put it on the rope. (3) It is somewhat bulkier and heavier.
20. Should not.
21. Instead of being on the rope above the device, as with other descenders, the guide hand should be resting on the bars of the rack.
22. Never less than four bars.
23. (1) If the rope wraps are not correctly put onto the carabiner, they can spiral out of the carabiner gate, resulting in a free fall. (2) The wraps can bear on the carabiner gate and break it.
24. The device could lock itself out of reach and you could be stranded on the rope.
25. In the bottom end of the rappel line tie a "stopper knot," such as a figure 8 knot.

Chapter 10

1. (1) Friction hitches. (2) Mechanical ascenders.
2. General-use ascenders grip the rope primarily by squeezing it against the inside of the ascender shell. Personal ascenders grip the rope with teeth on a cam and also press the rope inside the shell of the device.
3. Slings, webbing, rope.
4. At least two.
5. Friction hitches.
6. Smaller.
7. (1) Frame breakage. (2) Rope damage. (3) Rope slipping out of an ascender.
8. Safety lever.
9. Any three of the following: (1) The system should enable you to use your legs and feet more than your arms and hands. (2) The system should hold you upright on the rope with your body weight over the legs. (3) The system should enable you to sit and rest while on rope. (4) The system should have attachments to the seat harness, not only to the feet.
10. (1) Using three ascenders. (2) Using two ascenders and tying off short.
11. Tying off short.
12. Chicken loop.
13. The legs.
14. Go over an edge.
15. Change over to ascending.

Chapter 11

1. Any seven of the following: (1) Proper use and care of rope. (2) Proper use and care of related equipment. (3) Ability to tie appropriate knots and hitches. (4) Ability to rig safe and secure anchors. (5) Safely and confidently belay another person. (6) Rappel safely, confidently, and under control. (7) Ability to ascend safely. (8) Ability to change over from rappelling to ascending and from ascending to rappelling while on rope.
2. The rescue subject.
3. Any six of the following: (1) Always evaluate for possible hazards. (2) Don't rush. (3) Choose the least dangerous route. (4) Choose the simplest way of doing the job. (5) If there are hazards from falling objects, do not set up directly above the subject. (6) Appoint a safety officer. (7) Wear personal protective gear. (8) Set up safety lines.
4. (1) Awareness. (2) Operational. (3) Technician.
5. Three to five.
6. Incident command system or incident management system.
7. Incident commander.
8. Any three of the following: (1) Hazards. (2) Personal protective equipment. (3) Rescue rigging. (4) Personal rigging.
9. Any seven of the following: (1) Local rescue needs. (2) Jurisdictional and operational responsibility. (3) How a rescue group fits in who they report to. (4) How call out is initiated. (5) Command structure on scene. (6) Communications. (7) How the group relates to other organizations. (8) Medical control and protocols. (9) Standardized rescue procedures. (10) Regulations and standards.
10. (1) Training. (2) Medical equipment and supplies. (3) Familiarity with rescue and medical skills.

Chapter 12

1. (1) The operators must be extremely alert and prepared for failure. (2) It is very difficult to change the direction of rope travel.
2. Two triple wrapped Prusiks anchored securely and placed in line on the belay rope.
3. Any three of the following: (1) Icy rope. (2) Muddy rope. (3) High impacts. (4) Inappropriate Prusik material.
4. To shift the load off the Prusiks should they jam.
5. (1) The Prusiks are tied correctly. (2) They are neat and dressed. (3) They are the appropriate distance apart. (4) They are gripping the rope with the correct tightness.

Chapter 13

1. The subject is uninjured or only slightly injured.

2. Evaluate and stabilize the subject in terms of injury.
3. Any three of the following: (1) It is appropriate for only one person to perform the rescue. (2) There is a shortage of personnel and/or resources. (3) The urgency of the situation means there is no time to await additional personnel. (4) The benefits of a pickoff rescue outweigh the risks involved.
4. (1) The rope could hit the subject and knock him or her off. (2) If the rope is close to a panicky subject, he or she could grab your rope, stopping your rappel or causing injury or death to you and/or the rescue subject.
5. Have the rope in a bag, which is attached to you.
6. Assessment.
7. One main line rope with adequate safety factor for a two-person load, one sewn, manufactured seat harness with thigh/leg supports for rescuer, one rappel device with enough friction to handle the weight of two persons and, preferably, with variable friction, two large, locking carabiners (in addition to a locking carabiner already in the rescuer's seat harness tie-in point), one short (approximately 2 feet) sling with a loop in both ends, or an adjustable rescue pickoff strap that will support one person's weight with an adequate safety factor.
8. Directly into your rappel device tie-in point, not into your seat harness.
9. A safety check.
10. Always above.
11. (1) Continued attention to keeping airway clear. (2) If unconsciousness caused by injury, spinal precautions.
12. Any three of the following: (1) It must hold the subject upright. (2) It must prevent the subject from sliding out. (3) It must be simple to put on. (4) It must be usable in adverse conditions, such as cold, dark, and wind.

Chapter 14

1. *Slope evacuation*:
   (1) Litter tenders have most of their weight on the ground. (2) Weight of litter is supported both by tenders and rope. (3) There may be three or more litter tenders. (4) Rope is attached to one end of the litter.
   High angle evacuation:
   (1) Litter tenders have their weight supported by litter and rope. (2) Weight of litter is supported by rope. (3) At most, there are two litter attendants. (4) Litter hangs from vertical ropes.

2. Breakage of a butt weld and failure of the litter rail.
3. D
4. B

5. B
6. D
7. (1) The length of the main line lowering rope.
   (2) The availability of anchor points.
8. The rope handler assists by feeding the brakeman the rope and removing kinks and tangles before they reach the brakes.
9. Any three of the following: (1) How steep is the slope? (2) Is the footing particularly loose and treacherous? (3) Is the slope icy or muddy? (4) What would be the consequences of a fall by the litter team? (5) Are the main line brake anchors questionable? (6) Are there plenty of anchors? (7) Is there thick underbrush or large boulders?

10.
"On belay."	*(Litter captain to belayer.)*
"Belay on."	*(Belayer to litter captain.)*
"Down slow."	*(Litter captain to brakeman.)*
or	
"Down fast."	*(Should be repeated by the brakeman back to the litter captain so the captain knows that the brakeman understands.)*
"Stop!"	*(Usually the litter captain to the brakeman, but may be given by anyone who sees danger or potential problem developing.)*
"Stop! Stop! Why stop?"	*(The litter captain to brakeman. It is given when, for an unexpected reason and without command from the litter captain, the rope has stopped moving.)*
"Two - oh."	*(Given by the brakeman to the litter captain. It means there is only about 20 feet of rope left.)*
"Off belay."	*(Litter captain to belayer.)*
"Belay off."	*(Belayer to litter captain.)*

11. Such use of a personal ascender can result in failure in two potential ways: (1) The frame or other portion of the ascender may fail. (2) The sharp teeth on the cam can tear the rope sheath.
12. D
13. Any three of the following: (1) Knots on moving rope that jam in cracks. (2) Broken gear that causes system failure. (3) Systems reaching their limit. (4) Pinned arms and legs.
14. D

Chapter 15

1. Any four of the following: (1) Cliffs. (2) Buildings. (3) Industrial sites. (4) Construction sites such as tower cranes. (5) Other structures such as stacks, silos, or towers. (6) Vertical caves.
2. B
3.
"On belay."	*(Litter tender to belayer.)*
"Belay on."	*(Belayer to litter tender.)*
"Down slow"	
or	*(Litter tender to brakeman)*
"Down fast."	

"Stop!"	*(Generally the litter tender to the brakeman, but may be given by anyone who sees danger or potential problems developing.)*
"Stop! Stop! Why stop?"	*(Litter tender to brakeman. This is given when, for an unexplained reason and without command from the litter tender, the rope has stopped moving.)*
"Off belay."	*(Litter tender to belayer. The litter, rescue subject, and litter tender(s) are on the ground, or in a secure position, and in no danger of falling.)*
"Belay off."	*(Belayer to litter tender.)*

4. C
5. Take the rope in the brake hand and pull it forward hard in the direction of the load.
6. There will be greater weight on the system and greater friction will be needed.
7. (a) Single line lowering with belay.
   Advantages:
   Simpler rope work and brake management.
   Disadvantages:
   May not have adequate safety factor for weight of two litter tenders. More difficult to tilt litter from horizontal to vertical position (requires the loading of the belay line to tilt the litter).
   (b) Double line lowering.
   Advantages:
   Can be used where two litter tenders are needed, such as (1) complicated medical management of subject or (2) vertical face is too difficult for one tender to manage litter. Useful where it is necessary to shift orientation of litter.
   Disadvantages:
   Greater stress in brake systems and anchors (if both lines run through the same brake). More complex rope management. May be more difficult to keep litter horizontal if lines come to two different points on the litter.
8. D
9. A, C, and D
10. D
11. (1) The main attachment to the litter system is a "pigtail." It is attached with a figure 8 on a bight knot to the carabiners at master attachment point at the end of the main line lowering rope. (2) The litter tender is attached to the pigtail with two ascenders. To prevent the ascenders from accidentally slipping off the end of the pigtail, the lower end is brought back up and clipped into the tender's seat harness.
12. (1) Attend to the medical needs of the patient in the litter. (2) Help provide a smooth ride for the patient. (3) Communicate with and reassure the patient. (4) Prevent the litter from hanging up. (5) Shield the patient from environmental factors.

13. (1) Responding first before the litter lowering to assess the medical condition of the subject and begin primary treatment. (2) Assisting the litter tender in getting the litter over the edge. (3) Assisting in loading the subject part way down the wall. (4) Helping to maneuver the litter around obstructions.

14. (1) Where it is necessary to change the position of the litter from horizontal to vertical and back again to get it through obstacles on a vertical space or to get through a confined space. (2) On an uneven, broken up, vertical face, where two tenders need to work the litter. (3) Where medical considerations or other concerns relating to the rescue subject are too overwhelming for a single litter tender.

Chapter 16

1. Any of the following: (1) Silos. (2) River gorges. (3) Canyons. (4) Escarpments. (5) Grain elevators. (6) Sewers. (7) Tank cars. (8) Basins. (9) Utility vaults. (10) Industrial storage bins. (11) Fuel tanks. (12) Air vents. (13) Mine shafts. (14) Caves. (15) Tunnels.

2. (1) To make the raising more convenient and safer. (2) To make the raising easier.

3. Mechanical advantage: The relationship of how much load can be moved to the amount of force it takes to move it.

4. Theoretical mechanical advantage does not consider loss of force through factors such as friction, abrasion, and rope stretch. Actual mechanical advantage is the MA after loss of force through facts such as friction, abrasion, and rope stretch.

5. 1:1 - 400 lb.
2:1 - 200 lb.
3:1 - 133.33.
4:1 - 100 lb.

6. B

7. (1) 2:1 + 2:1 = 4:1. (2) 2:1 + 3:1 = 6:1.

8. They are *not* designed for the high stresses resulting from the multiplication of forces that takes place in hauling systems. The use of personal ascenders in hauling systems can result in tearing of the rope or in the structural failure of the ascender.

9. It should be positioned as far forward of the hauling system (toward the load) as possible, while still being safely in reach of the rescuers.

10. There will be too much slack in the PCD's anchor sling. This will result in two problems: (1) It can result in dangerous shock loading of the PCD, its sling, and its anchor and (2) the hauling team will lose some of the purchase it has gained when it sets the PCD to reposition for another bite.

11. (1) The friction can get very high and can result in a tremendous increase in load for the haul team. (2) It can result in severe damage to the rope and other equipment.

12. Two of the following: (1) Edge rollers. (2) Directionals. (3) Change the position of the haul rope. (4) Pad the rope. (5) Reduce the load.

13. Tag lines.

14. (1) 1:1; one main line rope, one anchor sling, two locking carabiners, one rope grab (progress capture device), plus separate belay system appropriate for the load being hauled. (2) 2:1; one main line rope, one haul rope, two anchor slings, three locking carabiners, two rope grabs (one progress capture device plus one haul cam), one pulley, plus separate belay system appropriate for the load being hauled. (3) 3:1 (Z-Rig); one main line rope, three locking carabiners, two pulleys, two rope grabs (one for hauling, one PCD), plus separate belay system appropriate for load being hauled. (4) 4:1 ("piggyback"); one main line rope, one hauling rope, three locking carabiners, two pulleys, two rope grabs (one for PCD, one for hauling), plus separate belay system appropriate for load being hauled.

15. It creates a "diminishing V," which tends to get easily snagged on brush, rock, building projections, and other objects as it advances. Also, that there are two strands of rope going over an edge to create additional friction.

Chapter 17

1. (a) Collective: varies the pitch of the rotor blades and their rate, or rpms, to create more or less lift. (b) Cyclic: tilts the main rotor to change direction of flight. (c) Antitorque: controls the tail rotor to prevent the aircraft from spinning uncontrollably.

2. Ground effect results in a cushion of air under the helicopter. This greatly assists the ability of the helicopter to hover in a safe and stable manner.

3. (1) The ability of a helicopter to lift itself is affected by the density of the air. The denser the air, the greater the lift on the rotor blades. (2) Pressure (barometric) altitude, temperature, and humidity.

4. Draw an imaginary line from the center of the main rotor to the bottom of the aircraft.

5. (1) If and when conditions are right for take off. (2) Who approaches and boards the aircraft and when. (3) Whether gear will be taken aboard and how it will be stowed on the aircraft. (4) If the mission is to be completed or aborted.

6. From downhill.

7. (1) A person may not be aware of it and walk into it. (2) The helicopter may suddenly move striking a person with the moving rotor.

8. (a) Secure small and light objects to keep them from blowing into the rotor. (b) Carry large and heavy objects low and parallel to the ground.

9. (1) Terrain. (2) Space. (3) Obstructions. (4) Nature of landing surface.

10. (1) In a hover, the helicopter is being kept in the air only by the collective (angle of the rotor blades) and engine rpm. (2) The aircraft lacks the forward momentum that could add to its lift and carry it away from danger. (3) The helicopter may be endangered by its own rotor wash that circulates to create an unstable air mass.

11. (1) Horse collar. (2) Hoisting vest. (3) Net or basket. (4) Jungle penetrator.

12. (1) The net or basket should have some rigid components so it does not close in and entrap the subject or create a feeling of claustrophobia. (2) If used in the water, it should have proper flotation so that the net or basket does not drag the subject under the water. (3) The net or basket should create a user-friendly atmosphere so that the subject desires to climb in and does not try to hang onto the outside. (4) The net or basket must be able to securely contain the rescue subjects so they do not fall out.

13. (1) Thoroughly evaluate medical condition and state of mind. (2) Explain to the patient the nature of the steps that are to take place. (3) Reassure.

14. Blockage of the airway.

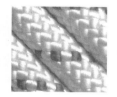

Index

Page references in *italics* indicate pages with figures.

NOTES

NOTES

NOTES

NOTES

NOTES

NOTES

NOTES

NOTES